CHILDHOOD COMMUNICATION DISORDERS: ORGANIC BASES

CHILDHOOD COMMUNICATION DISORDERS: ORGANIC BASES

Lisa Schoenbrodt, Ed.D., CCC-SLP
Chair
Associate Professor
Department of Speech Pathology and Audiology
Loyola College
Maryland

THOMSON
™
DELMAR LEARNING   Australia   Canada   Mexico   Singapore   Spain   United Kingdom   United States

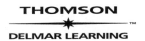

Childhood Communication Disorders: Organic Bases
Lisa Schoenbrodt, Ed.D., CCC-SLP

Vice President,
Health Care Business Unit:
William Brottmiller

Editorial Director:
Cathy L. Esperti

Developmental Editor:
Juliet Byington

Editorial Assistant:
Chris Manion

Marketing Director:
Jennifer McAvey

Art/Design Coordinator:
Robert Plante

Project Editor:
David Buddle

Production Coordinator:
Jessica Peterson

Library of Congress Cataloging-in-Publication Data

Childhood communication disorders : organic bases / [edited by] Lisa Schoenbrodt.
   p. ; cm.
Includes bibliographical references and index.
  ISBN 0-7693-0244-0
  1. Communicative disorders in children.
  [DNLM: 1. Language Disorders—physiopathology—Child. 2. Brain Diseases—complications—Child.
3. Mental Disorders—complications—Child WL 340.2
C5362 2003] I. Schoenbrodt, Lisa, 1961–
  RJ496.C67C468 2003
  618.92'855—dc21

                 2002156749

Contents

Contributors

Tracie Bullock Dickson, Ph.D., CCC-SLP
Assistant Professor, Speech-Language Pathology/Audiology
Loyola College in Maryland

Marie Kerins, Ed.D., CCC-SLP
Assistant Professor, Speech-Language Pathology/Audiology
Loyola College in Maryland

Libby Kumin, Ph.D., CCC-SLP
Professor, Speech-Language Pathology/Audiology
Loyola College in Maryland

Janet Preis, Ed.D., CCC-SLP
Assistant Professor, Speech-Language Pathology/Audiology
Loyola College in Maryland

Kathleen Siren, Ph.D., CCC-SLP
Assistant Professor, Speech-Language Pathology/Audiology
Loyola College in Maryland

Angela Strauch, M.S., CCC-SLP
Speech-Language Pathologist
United Cerebral Palsy No Boundaries Assistive Technology Center

For many years, we as faculty of the Department of Speech Pathology and Audiology at Loyola College in Maryland have offered a course based on the organic nature of childhood communication disorders. During this time, as researchers and instructors, we searched for books that addressed specific disorders in the pediatric population. While much information abounds about various organic disorders in children, the literature usually provided a brief overview and included adults as well as children. We were unable to locate a text containing information that focused specifically on pediatrics. To fill this significant gap, each chapter author of this text diligently prepared her chapter based on current research on issues surrounding the disorder. The contributing authors for this text all have extensive experience in both teaching and research in the content area presented. While the characteristics of some of the disorders may be somewhat similar in children and adults, the issues surrounding assessment and intervention clearly are not. The current text is a collaborative effort of many to address the organic bases of childhood communication disorders. While we developed this text specifically to fit the nature of such a course, it is useful not only for undergraduate upperclassmen, but for graduate clinicians and practicing professionals who need to remain current in the field.

With the current changes in standards by the American Speech-Language-Hearing Association, we are experiencing exciting times for opportunities to restructure the curriculum in undergraduate and graduate programs in speech-language pathology and audiology. We are now moving to more problem-based learning approaches, with students learning the content from clinical models. For this reason, it is important that texts, such as this one, present not only in-depth information about the disorders and the resulting communication deficits, but also a current view of assessment and intervention. While we have identified the current views and trends related to these high- and low-incidence disorders, this book is not meant to provide comprehensive coverage of all aspects related to assessment and intervention. We also assume that students have covered course content related to basic anatomy and physiology as well as "normal" language development in children in order to lay the foundation for this text.

ORGANIZATION OF THE TEXT

While some of the disabilities and the resulting communication disorders detailed in this book are high-incidence and others are considered to be low-incidence disorders, all may appear in a clinician's caseload at some point in time. Each chapter provides the same basic format. Each begins with a list of chapter objectives followed by an introduction and definition of the disorder(s). Some definitions are recognized legally, others by the underlying psychological involvement, and yet others by advocacy and support groups. The organic nature of some disorders is obvious, such as in traumatic brain injury, whereas in others, such as attention deficit disorder and learning disabilities, much controversy abounds, with research continually being conducted to further define organic dysfunction. Each chapter contains a section that details the characteristics and resulting deficits of the disorder so that clear ideas and concepts are understood as a precursor to assessment and intervention.

The sections on assessment and intervention present an overview of possibilities and related current trends in the field. The assessment and intervention sections are not meant to be an exhaustive review of every assessment tool and intervention strategy available in the market, but are geared to upperclass majors in communication disorders who are building their underlying knowledge in this area. However, the information on assessment and intervention is written broadly enough to be used by graduate students with additional input from instructors. Following these sections are two case studies that contain real-life scenarios for students to problem-solve possible educational and communication outcomes for the children presented. Review questions are available at the end of each chapter to provide thoughtful reflection on information presented in each chapter, followed by a comprehensive list of references. Appendices include a guide to assessing cognitive communication skills and a listing of web sites that may be helpful to students and clinicians who may be seeking additional information, and a glossary of terms used throughout the text is provided.

The text is organized into five parts. Part I: Neurogenic Disorders focuses on neurogenic communication disorders in traumatic brain injury (Chapter 1) and cerebral palsy (Chapter 2). Part II: Developmental Brain Differences presents information related to communication disorders in children with developmental brain differences, including attention deficit disorder (Chapter 3), learning and language learning disabilities (Chapter 4), pervasive developmental disorder (Chapter 5), and mental retardation (Chapter 6). Part III: Craniofacial Anomalies includes information on cleft lip and palate (Chapter 7). In addition to the common elements in the other chapters, this chapter presents information regarding the classification systems used and surgical management and alternative treatments for the anomalies presented. Part IV: Disorders Secondary to Environmental Factors contains information on substance abuse (Chapter 8). This chapter is structured slightly differently from the other chapters in this text in the assessment and intervention sections. The reason for this difference is that while communication disorders are present, the assessments and interventions either overlap with other disorders presented in this text or they are unique to these populations. Part V: Communication Disorders Secondary to Psychiatric Disorders concludes the text with a presentation of communication deficits in children with psychiatric disorders (Chapter 9). This chapter presents a number of psychiatric disorders that overlap with communication deficits.

The chapter authors are all experts in their content area. Each one has years of clinical experience and research with the population that translates into sound theories and practice. In addition to the above, each author teaches in that content area to both undergraduate and graduate students and has professional experience providing user-friendly information that is appropriate for students and clinicians. The format of the chapters, the expertise of the chapter authors, the objectives, review questions, and case studies are all provided to help students in training and clinicians in practice to understand the underlying organic bases of communication disorders in children.

Acknowledgments

As the editor and author of several chapters in this text, I am indebted to the many people who helped in the preparation during the various phases of this book. I would first like to thank the chapter authors for their time, effort, and undying patience in the writing and revisions of each chapter. Without them, the completion of this product would not have been possible. In addition to the chapter authors, there were several important people who helped with the tedious work of editing and collecting information, including Kelly Free, Melissa Kasper, Sunshyne Darcy, Margaret Elizabeth Sheer, Gerardine Simon, and Bernardine Kremer. Their tireless efforts are appreciated beyond what words can state. I also want to thank Juliet Byington from Delmar Learning for her continued support and encouragement as well as the reviewers and production team from Delmar Learning who provided constructive feedback throughout the process. Finally, I want to thank my family including my husband, Scott Myers, and my children, David Karl, Matthew Scott, and Amy Elizabeth, for their patience, never-ending support, and encouragement. Thank you again.

I would like to dedicate this book in loving memory of my parents,
Frederick Karl Schoenbrodt and Margaret Meyer Schoenbrodt,
who always provided support, encouragement, and love—I miss you.

PART I

Neurogenic Disorders

Chapter 1

Traumatic Brain Injury

Lisa Schoenbrodt, Ed.D., CCC-SLP

CHAPTER OBJECTIVES

Upon completing this chapter, the reader should be able to:

1. Identify and define terms relative to brain injury
2. List primary and secondary injuries resulting from traumatic brain injury
3. Identify factors affecting the outcome of traumatic brain injury
4. Describe characteristics associated with traumatic brain injury
5. Describe appropriate assessments and modifications to be used during evaluation
6. Provide intervention strategies that are important for communication

INTRODUCTION

Traumatic brain injury (TBI) is a neurogenic disorder that is considered to be of low incidence in the pediatric population. However, with recent changes in medical delivery and patients leaving acute care centers more quickly, children with TBI are returning to their schools and communities faster than in the past decade. Children with TBI present with a unique variety of speech and language as well as cognitive and motoric issues. For this reason, speech-language pathologists (SLPs) and others working with communication disorders need to be aware of all aspects of the injury in order to provide effective assessment and treatment. This chapter discusses the organic etiologies of the disorder, definitions, and characteristics, as well as effective assessment and intervention techniques.

Traumatic brain injury is the primary cause of death and disability in children today. While accidental dropping and physical abuse are the primary causes of TBI in infants, the major causes for toddlers are serious falls, vehicular accidents, pedestrian accidents, and physical abuse. In elementary school-age children, bicycle accidents are the main cause of TBI. Finally, adolescents are the most prevalent age group to suffer a TBI, most commonly due to vehicular accidents, sports-related injuries, and assault (Centers for Disease Control and Prevention, 2002).

According to the Centers for Disease Prevention and Control (2002), approximately 1.5 million cases of TBI are reported in the United States annually. Of that group, 50,000 people die and 80,000 more leave the hospital with a disability secondary to a TBI. Today an estimated 5.3 million people live with disabilities caused by a TBI. The most recent statistics indicate that people over age 75 have the highest rate of TBI, followed closely by adolescents, and finally toddlers (Centers for Disease Control and Prevention, 2002).

Epidemiological studies show that age and gender play an important role in predicting at-risk groups for TBI (Centers for Disease Control and Prevention, 2002). Boys are more likely than girls to sustain a TBI, and adolescents are at the highest risk for brain injury in the pediatric population followed by preschoolers. In addition, children who have sustained a previous head injury are more likely to sustain another one.

Terminology Related to Brain Injury

It is important to understand the terms and definitions used to describe brain injuries, and this section defines these terms as they relate to brain injury in children.

When the head is struck by an object or is abruptly stopped, the acceleration and deceleration can cause significant injury to the brain. **Head injury** typically refers to traumatic damage to the head that may fracture the bones of the skull or face and may or may not include injury to the brain. Traumatic brain injury is defined by the Brain Injury Association and is included in the 1990 reauthorization of PL 94-142, now PL 101-476, the Individuals with Disabilities Education Act (**IDEA**). According to the Individuals with Disabilities Act (1991), TBI is defined as an acquired brain injury caused by an external physical force, resulting in total or partial functional disability, or psychosocial impairment, or both, which adversely affects a child's educational performance. The term applies to open or closed head injuries resulting in impairments in one or more areas, including cognition; language; memory; attention; reasoning; abstract thinking; problem solving; sensory, perceptual, and motor abilities; psychosocial behavior; physical functions; information processing; and speech. The term does not apply to congenital or degenerative brain injuries induced by birth trauma.

A **closed head injury** (CHI) is one where there is no penetration or opening from the outside through the dura mater. In a closed head injury, the damage is more diffuse or generalized. Damage can occur anywhere in the brain and may cause variable behavior and learning problems. In an **open head injury** (OHI), the skull is penetrated (e.g., a gunshot wound), and the damage is localized to the site of penetration.

The term *traumatic brain injury* indicates that there is evidence of brain involvement that is demonstrated by (a) an altered level of consciousness (lethargy, confusion, and coma) or (b) neurological signs, for example, localized weakness that indicates that the brain was injured (Christensen, 2001).

What Happens to the Brain When It Is Injured?

Injuries that are caused by trauma are classified as primary (or immediate) and secondary (or delayed).

Primary or Immediate Injuries

Primary injuries occur at the time of the trauma, and are due to the direct movement of the brain inside the skull. The movement results in the slamming and rubbing of the brain, which may cause contusions, or bruises. The location of the contusions depends upon the site and the circumstances of the injury. For example, if the skull is hit with a blunt object, the contusion will be in the cortex at the point of contact. In addition, there may be another bruise on the opposite side of the brain, approximately 180 degrees from the initial bruise. These contusions are frequently referred to as coup (the French word for hit) and contre-coup (opposite the hit) contusions (see Figure 1-1).

A severe CHI involves greater speed and energy, and the head is often moving at the time of the injury. CHI contusions occur when the head is suddenly stopped but the brain keeps moving forward until it stops on impact, hitting the inside of the skull. The brain then smashes into the bony protrusions around the frontal and possibly the temporal lobes, resulting in a more severe injury (Christensen, 2001).

Primary injury can also result from shearing and rotation of the axons, known as **diffuse axonal injury** (DAI), which occurs diffusely throughout the brain rather than in one localized area. DAI is often referred to as a shearing injury. The axons in the brain are particularly susceptible to the rotation of the brain at the time of injury. As the head and brain accelerate, these structures spin violently and then come to a quick stop. As a result, the brain twists on itself, stretching the axons so far as to physically pull them apart (see Figure 1-2). The separation creates an immediate loss of neuron function followed by the death of that neuron (Blosser & DePompei, 2003; Kaufman & Dacey, 1994).

Secondary or Delayed Injuries

Primary injuries cannot be modified, as they are the direct result of a traumatic incident. Secondary injuries, however, can be prevented or minimized during the acute treatment stage. Several types of secondary injuries may occur, including (a) bleeding (hemorrhage), (b) herniation syndrome, and (c) edema or swelling.

Bleeding

Bleeding can occur over and within the brain tissue as a result of torn or disrupted vessels. Bleeding within the brain is referred to as an intracerebral hemorrhage; a bleed into the ventricles is known as an **intraventricular hemorrhage** (IVH); and bleeding into the spaces of the brain is referred to as (a) an epidural hematoma (between the skull and the dura), (b) a subdural hematoma (under the dura), or

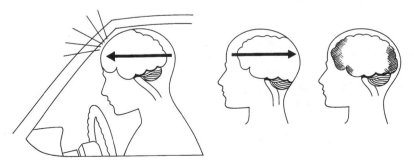

Figure 1-1
Coup/Contre-Coup Contusions
(From C. Jones and J. Lorman, *Traumatic Brain Injury: A Guide for the Patient and Family* [rev. ed. 2001]. Stow, OH: Interactive Therapeutics. Reprinted with permission)

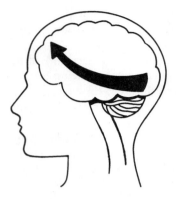

Figure 1-2
Results of Brain Acceleration: Axonal Stretching
(From C. Jones and J. Lorman, *Traumatic Brain Injury: A Guide for the Patient and Family* [rev. ed. 2001]. Stow, OH: Interactive Therapeutics. Reprinted with permission)

(c) a subarachnoid hemorrhage (under the arachnoid layer of the meninges and into the cerebrospinal fluid) (Bruce et al., 1979; Christensen, 2001; Kaufman & Dacey, 1994). The outcome of a bleed varies with respect to the amount of blood lost, how fast the blood accumulates, and the location of the bleeding. Because there is little "extra" space available in the skull, any additional blood that occupies space means that intracranial pressure may increase within that area or that more room may have to be made for excess blood. If the accumulation of blood or the hemorrhage occurs slowly, then the brain has time to adjust by either eliminating some of the cerebrospinal fluid or decreasing the amount of blood in the blood vessels. If the blood loss or hemorrhage is rapid, the pressure on the brain increases; this is known as increased intracranial pressure (ICP). ICP can result in insufficient circulation of blood flow to the brain, causing further injury due to the lack of oxygen to the brain, otherwise known as hypoxic ischemic injury.

Herniation Syndrome

A second type of delayed injury is **herniation syndrome,** which occurs if a localized mass or area of swelling pushes on and deforms the shape of the brain. When the brain attempts to squeeze itself into another area within the intracranial space, high pressure on that area of the brain and the surrounding blood vessels occurs. Herniation may result in further localized brain injury and stroke.

Edema

Edema, or swelling of the brain, is due to fluid leakage. Edema can cause increased ICP and can either be localized to the area of impact or diffuse. Swelling of the brain is more common in children than adults and may cause deficits similar to those caused by bleeding in the brain.

Severe cases of edema can be monitored through an intracranial pressure monitor that is surgically implanted inside the head. This monitor effectively records information about internal pressures, which allows the early detection of potential problems. Both primary and secondary injuries are indicators of the degree of an injury's severity and of the variables related to the outcome of a TBI.

Severity of Injury

The severity of a brain injury is categorized as mild, moderate, or severe. The outcome of a TBI is predicted by several factors, including (a) degree and length of coma, (b) duration of post-traumatic amnesia, (c) evaluation of the child's premorbid level of health, and (d) preexisting learning or educational problems.

Degree and Length of Coma

The Glasgow Coma Scale (GCS) (Jennett & Teasdale, 1981) is commonly used in assessing degree and length of coma. The GCS measures eye opening, as well as motor and verbal responses, on a scale from 0 to 15 (see Table 1-1). This scale is typically used in the hospital as a means of evaluating the degree and severity of the TBI. A mild head injury is defined as a GCS of 13 or better with either no loss of consciousness or loss of consciousness for less than 20 minutes. A moderate head injury is defined as a GCS of 8 to 12 with loss of consciousness for more than 20 minutes and an accompanying fracture with contusions. A severe head injury is defined as a GCS of 7 or less accompanied by intracranial hematoma, fracture with neurological deficit, bruising, or contusion of brain tissue. The relationship between the GCS score and outcome was not studied extensively in children with TBI, causing the instrument's predictive validity to be questioned (Lehr, 1990).

Coma is defined as a period of unresponsiveness or unconsciousness, though the medical community disagrees as to the indicators that coma has ended. In a rehabilitation setting, coma is considered to have ended when the child begins to follow simple commands, which indicates that the child is able to have some interaction with the environment and correlates to long-term outcome (Christensen, 2001). Another classification system similar to GCS is the International Classification of Diseases, which categorizes TBI as (a) mild (less than 1 hour of coma with momentary or no loss of consciousness), (b) moderate (1–24 hours of coma), or (c) severe (24 or more hours of coma).

Table 1-1 Glasgow Coma Scale

Eye Opening	
spontaneous	E4
to speech	3
to pain	2
nil	1
Best Motor Response	
obeys	M6
localizes	5
withdraws	4
abnormal flexion	3
extensor response	2
nil	1
Verbal Response	
orientated	V5
confused conversation	4
inappropriate words	3
incomprehensible sounds	2
nil	1
Coma score (E + M + V) = 3 to 15	

Source: From Jennett, B., & Teasdale, G. (1981). *Management of head injuries.* P. 78. Philadelphia: F. A. Davis Company. Reprinted with permission.

Post-Traumatic Amnesia

A second indicator for outcome is **post-traumatic amnesia** (PTA). PTA is defined as a period of amnesia or memory disturbance occurring after the trauma and is characterized by confusion, disorientation, and agitation. Children can recall many old memories that were in long-term storage prior to the accident; however, memory of new information is impaired, causing disorientation and confusion with regard to daily events.

PTA provides a good indication of how severely memory and cognition will be affected over the long term. This fact is particularly true for children who experienced no coma or one of very short duration. PTA severity is classified as (a) mild—less than 1 hour, (b) moderate—1 to 24 hours of PTA, (c) severe—1 to 7 days of PTA, or (d) very severe—more than 7 days of PTA. PTA ends when the child can continuously lay down new memories.

Premorbid Level of Health

The child's premorbid level of health is also an indicator of outcome. This indicator references the status of the child's physical and mental health prior to the accident. Studies (Ylvisaker & DeBonis, 2000) suggest that children who have had a previous TBI are more likely to sustain a second. In addition, children diagnosed with other health concerns such as attention deficit disorder or seizure disorder may have a less optimal outcome than children who have no history of health problems (Arroyos-Jurado, Paulsen, Merrell, Lindgren, & Max, 2000; Massagli & Jaffe, 1994).

Preexisting Learning or Behavioral Problems

Just as premorbid health can help predict the outcome of a TBI, so can any previously existing learning or educational deficits. Studies showed that children diagnosed with attention deficit disorder have a greater likelihood of incurring a TBI than their peers without attention deficit disorder. In addition, preexisting learning disabilities need to be considered when the child is formally assessed for educational placement following a TBI.

Age

One additional factor in evaluating outcome of TBI that is well worth mentioning is the age at the time of injury. One common myth about TBI holds that the younger the child at the time of injury, the better the outcome. In fact, the opposite is true. Children who sustain a TBI before age 9 display greater cognitive deficits overall, including a reduction in intelligence scores and increased difficulties in reading. The reason for this outcome is again related to the brain: the immature skull is thinner and thus more easily damaged by trauma. The immature brain also has limited protective covering, and there is incomplete myelination of the neurons of the brain. Young children have a greater risk of increased intracranial pressure, diffuse swelling, and secondary brain injuries (Arroyos-Jurado et al., 2000; Chapman & McKinnon, 2000).

Another factor related to age is that the younger the child, the greater the likelihood of long-term cognitive impairment due to the lack of formal learning that has occurred. Preschool children have not experienced as much formal school learning as elementary school children; therefore, they do not have as much stored information simply because of their younger age. The pediatric TBI population is also unique in that there is the potential for delayed onset of deficits. Evidence suggests that children who sustained a TBI before age 2 could be at increased risk for the later onset of seizures.

Neurological Deficits Secondary to TBI

Additional medical difficulties that occur after TBI include various types of neurological problems, such as postconcussion syndrome, headaches, seizures, and motor impairments.

Postconcussion Syndrome

A **concussion** is a mild head injury, which may or may not include a brief loss of consciousness, and may be followed by a short period of change in mental status without any focal neurological signs, known as **postconcussion syndrome** (P-CS). Symptoms of this syndrome include (a) headache, (b) fatigue, (c) memory loss (for new information), (d) depression, (e) impaired concentration, (f) increased sensitivity to sound, (g) emotional lability (frequently changing emotions), and (h) disinhibition (acting on inappropriate thoughts or actions) (Christensen, 2001). These symptoms may resolve spontaneously after weeks or months, though in a small percentage of children, some persist. It is extremely important that educators recognize these symptoms as indicators of P-CS syndrome and not as signs of laziness or a lack of motivation.

Headaches

Headaches occur more frequently following a mild TBI than after more severe injuries. There are many types of headaches that can occur following a TBI, including (a) those related directly to the head trauma, (b) those related to tension, (c) head and neck pain resulting from whiplash, and (d) migraines that result from TBI. Tension headaches are frequently triggered by the stress and/or pressure related to the social and academic challenges faced upon return to the home and school community. While not as intense as migraines, tension headaches still produce a dull ache and may interfere with day-to-day functioning. Migraines occur frequently in children and may be triggered or worsened by trauma. If such headaches cause significant impairment in functioning, appropriate medical intervention may be necessary.

Seizures

Seizures occur when there is excessive or disorderly firing of the neurons, which leads to changes in neurological functioning and disruption in the normal functioning of the brain. The level of alertness, abnormal sensations, and unusual movements are indicators of this abrupt change in functioning. Early post-traumatic seizures are not uncommon and usually occur in the first 7 days following the trauma; they are not positively correlated with the severity of injury or the likelihood that seizure activity will continue. Late seizures (those occurring more than 1 week after the TBI) are more positively correlated with the chance of developing post-traumatic epilepsy—which is between 5 and 7 percent, particularly if the child has incurred a mild head injury. The chance of developing epilepsy increases to 11 percent, however, if the TBI is severe. Risk factors reported to coincide with developing post-traumatic seizures include focal injuries, such as hematoma (bleeding or the development of blood clots), wounds that involve the penetration of the dura, and factors such as prolonged coma or PTA (Chapman & McKinnon, 2000; Christensen, 2001).

Motor Impairment

As with seizures, a small percentage of children who sustain a TBI may develop long-term motor problems. Types of potential motor impairments that may occur include weakness; lack of ability to plan and control movements; abnormal muscle tone; inability to sit or stand or to maintain posture and balance; tremors; and lack of overall coordination.

A particularly important category of motor impairment includes any that affect the child's ability to swallow, which can impact nutrition. Swallowing difficulties are more common in severe TBI and may occur during both the oral and pharyngeal stages of swallowing. The oral phase involves moving food around in the mouth, chewing, preparing the food for swallowing, and gathering the food into a **bolus.** During the pharyngeal phase, muscles move the bolus from the mouth through the pharynx, past the larynx, and into the esophagus. The entire process requires fine motor coordination.

If the child exhibits difficulty with either of these phases, she or he may eat inefficiently or be unable to prepare the food properly for swallowing. Eating or drinking may become a slow, laborious, and sometimes life-threatening process. Choking may occur, and the possibility of **aspiration** pneumonia (infection or wheezing caused by passing too much food into the lungs) exists.

CHARACTERISTICS OF CHILDREN WITH TRAUMATIC BRAIN INJURY

All of the primary, secondary, and neurological complications discussed previously are the result of the diffuse damage caused by the traumatic incident. A TBI, even in its mildest form, can result in alterations in thinking and behavior. Cognitive changes produce the most disruption to the child and the family in their attempt to return to a "normal" life and are often more debilitating than disruptions in motor behavior. The following section offers greater detail regarding the characteristics or deficits of children following TBI, specifically in the areas of cognition, perceptual or sensory (visual) deficits, behavior, and communication.

Cognition

Problems in cognition can take a variety of forms. Overall general intellectual ability is assessed through the use of intelligence testing. A common assessment tool that is used for children is the Wechsler Intelligence Scale for Children-Third Edition (WISC-III). Through a series of subtests, the assessment provides summative data resulting in a Verbal IQ (VIQ), a Performance IQ (PIQ), and a Full Scale IQ (FSIQ). While intelligence testing may give some "hard" data as to the level at which the child is functioning, one should employ caution in interpreting these data following a TBI.

The results from IQ testing only describe how the child is functioning at the time of testing. Change or variability in performance is one of the hallmarks of TBI, and can occur within the first year after the injury and beyond. In addition, IQ tests are standardized on children of the same age who have *not* sustained a TBI. Therefore, the information cannot be used as a predictor as to how children who have sustained a TBI will perform in the real world. In addition to deficits in overall general intelligence, TBIs can also result in problems in memory and new learning. Difficulties in these two areas, along with previously discussed variability of performance, are critical to understanding children with TBI (Arroyos-Jurado et al., 2000; Trudeau, Poulin-Dubois, & Joanette, 2000).

One recovery scale that measures cognitive functioning that may be used in conjunction with IQ testing is the Ranchos Los Amigos Scale of Cognitive Functioning (Hagan & Malkmus, 1979). This scale gives a general description of cognitive behaviors to be expected at each stage of recovery. It is important to note that patients in recovery may remain in one stage for a long period of time, be in more than one stage at a time, or move rapidly through all stages (Blosser & DePompei, 2003). Malkmus revised the scale in 1982 to include cognitive-communicative descriptions for recovery levels (see Table 1-2). This scale is more widely used for persons age 14 and over than for younger patients.

Table 1-2   Rancho Scale of Cognition and Language, Levels of Cognitive Functioning and Associated Linguistic Behaviors.

Level I. No Response

General Behaviors

Patient appears to be in a deep sleep and is completely unresponsive to any stimuli presented.

Linguistic Behaviors

Receptive: No evidence of processing of linguistic input.

Expressive: Absence of verbal and gestural expression.

Level II. Generalized Response

General Behaviors

Patient reacts inconsistently and nonpurposefully to stimuli in a nonspecific manner. Responses are limited in nature and are often the same regardless of stimulus presented. Responses may be physiological changes, gross body movements and vocalization. Responses are likely to be delayed. The earlier response is to deep pain.

Level III. Localized Response

General Behaviors

Patient reacts specifically but inconsistently to stimuli. Responses are directly related to the type of stimulus presented, as in turning head toward a sound or focusing on an object presented. The patient may withdraw an extremity and vocalize when presented with a painful stimulus. He or she may follow simple commands in an inconsistent, delayed manner, such as closing eyes, squeezing or extending an extremity. Once external stimuli are removed, the patient may lie quietly. He or she may also show a vague awareness of self and body by responding to discomfort such as pulling at the nasogastric tube or catheter or resisting restraints. He or she may show a bias toward responding to some persons, especially family and friends, but not to others.

Linguistic Behaviors

As the patient progresses through this phase, linguistic behaviors emerge.

Receptive: Progresses from localizing to processing, retaining and following simple commands which elicit automatic responses: inconsistent and delayed. May demonstrate limited graphic processing.

Expressive: Emergence of automatic verbal and gestural responses. Negative head nods, requiring less head control, before positive. Single-word expressions or several words used as "holophrastic" responses. Expression is dependent upon elicitation by an external stimulus.

Level IV. Confused-Agitated

General Behaviors

Patient is in a heightened state of activity with severely decreased ability to process information. He or she is detached from the present and responds primarily to his or her own internal confusion. Behavior is frequently bizarre and nonpurposeful relative to the immediate environment. He or she may cry out or scream out of proportion to stimuli even after removal, may show aggressive behavior, attempt to remove restraints or tube or crawl out of bed in a purposeful manner. He or she does not discriminate

Linguistic Behaviors

Severe disruption of frontal-temporal lobes, and resultant confusion, becomes apparent.

Receptive: Marked disruption of integrity of auditory mechanism, with severe decreases in ability to maintain temporal order of phonemic events rate of processing and ability to attend to, retain, categorize and associate information. Graphic processing is equally affected. Compounded by disinhibition and inability to inhibit response to internal stimuli.

continued

Table 1-2   *(continued)*

among persons nor objects and is unable to cooperate directly with treatment efforts. Verbalization is frequently incoherent or inappropriate to the environment. Confabulation may be present; pateitn may be hostile. Gross attention to environment is very brief and selective attention often nonexistent. Being unaware for present events, patient lacks short-term recall and may be reacting to past events. He or she is unable to perform self-care activities without maximum assistance. If not disabled physically, he or she may perform automatic motor activities such as sitting, reaching, and ambulating as part of the agitated state but not as a purposeful act nor on request, necessarily.

Expressive: Marked disruption of phonological, semantic, syntactic and suprasegmental features. Characterized by disinhibition, incoherence; bizarre and unrelated to environment. Frequently, literal, verbal and neologistic paraphasias are present, with disturbance of logico-sequential features and incompleteness of expression. Prosodic features are disturbed secondary to inability to cognitively monitor and adjust rate, pitch, vocal intensity, etc.

Level V. Confused-Inappropriate

General Behaviors

Patient appears alert and is able to respond to simple commands fairly consistently. However, with increased complexity of commands or lack of any external structure, responses are nonpurposeful, random or, at best, fragmented toward any desired goal. He or she may show agitated behavior but not on an internal basis, as in Level IV; rather as a result of external stimuli and usually out of proportion to the stimulus. The patient has gross attention to the environment, is highly distractible and lacks ability to focus attention to a specific task without frequent redirection. With structure he or she may be able to converse on a social-automatic level for short periods of time. Verbalization is often inappropriate; confabulation may be triggered by present events. Memory is severely impaired, with confusion of past and present in reaction to ongoing activity. Patient lacks initiation of functional tasks and often shows inappropriate use of objects without external direction. He or she may be able to perform previously learned tasks when structured, but is unable to learn new information. He or she responds best to self, body, comfort and, often, family members. The patient usually can perform self-care activities with assistance and may accomplish feeding with supervision. Management on the unit is often a problem if the patient is physically mobile as he or she may wander off, either randomly or with vague intention of "going home."

Linguistic Behaviors

Marked by presence of linguistic fluctuations according to degree of external structure present and familiarity-predictability of linguistic events.

Receptive: Processing improved, with increased ability to retain temporal order of phonemic events, but persistence of semantic and syntactic confusions. Length of retained input is limited to phrases or short sentences. Rate, accuracy and quality remain significantly reduced, with auditory processing better than graphic.

Expressive: Disruption of phonological, semantic, syntactic and prosodic features persists. Characterized by disturbance of logico-sequential features: irrelevancies, incompleteness, tangential, circumlocutious and confabulatory expression. Decrease in literal paraphrasias; neologisms and/or verbal paraphasias persists. Length of utterance may be decreased or increased, depending on inhibition-disinhibition factors. Expressive responses are stimulus-bound. Word retrieval deficits become apparent, as characterized by delay, generalization, description, semantic association and/or circumlocution. Disruption of syntactic features evidence beyond concrete level of expression or with increase in length of output. Graphic expression is severely limited; gestural expression is limited and incomplete.

Level VI: Confused-Appropriate

General Behaviors

Patient shows goal directed behavior, but is dependent on external input for direction. Response to discomfort is

Linguistic Behaviors

Receptive: Processing remains delayed, with difficulty retaining, analyzing-synthesizing input: Processing of audi-

continued

Table 1-2   *(continued)*

appropriate and he or she is able to tolerate unpleasant stimuli, e.g., NG tube, when need is explained. He or she follows simple directions consistently and shows carryover for tasks learned; e.g., self-care. He or she is at least supervised with old learning, unable to maximally assissted for new learning with little or no carry-over. Responses may be incorrect due to memory problems but are appropriate to the situation. They may be delayed to immediate and he or she shows decreased ability to process information with little or no anticipation or prediction of events. Past memories show more depth and detail than recent memory. The patient may show beginning awareness of the situation by realizing he or she doesn't know an answer. He or she no longer wanders and is inconsistently oriented to time and place. Selective attention to tasks may be impaired, especially with difficult tasks and in unstructured settings, but is now functional for common daily activities. The patient may show vague recognition of some staff and has increased awareness of self, family and basic needs.

tory input improves to compound sentence level; graphic stimuli processed at short sentence level. Self-monitoring capacity emerges.

Expressive: Expression reflects internal confusion-disorganization, but is appropriate to situation or idea. Information retrieval and expression reflects significantly reduced new learning and displacement of temporal and situational contexts. Social automatic expression is essentially intact; expression remains stimulus-bound. Tangential, irrelevant responses are diminished in familiar, predictable situations; re-emerge in open-ended communicative situations requiring referential language. Confabulatory responses and neologisms extinguish. Literal paraphasia persists only if specific apraxia is present. Word retrieval errors occur in referential language but seldom in confrontation naming. Length of utterance remains reduced unless marked disinhibition is present, resulting in inability to channel flow of ideas-expression. Limited graphic expression emerges. Gestural expression increases. Prosodic features reflect "voice of confusion": equal stress, monopitch and monoloudness.

Level VII. Automatic-Appropriate

General Behaviors

Patient appears appropriate and oriented within hospital and home settings, goes through daily routine automatically but robot-like, with minimal to absent confusion and has shallow recall for what he or she has been doing. He or she shows increased awareness of self, body, family, bood, people and interaction in the environment. The patient has superficial awareness of but lacks insight into his condition decreased judgment and problem solving and lacks realistic planning for the future. he or she shows carryover for new learning at a decreased rate. The patient requires at least minimal supervision for learning and safety purposes. He or she is independent in self-care activities and supervised in home and community skills for safety. With structure, he or she is able to initiate tasks or social and recreational activities in which there is now interest. His or her judgment remains impaired. Prevocational evaluation and counseling may be indicated.

Linguistic Behaviors

Majority of linguistic behaviors appear "normal" within familiar, predictable, structured environments, but persistent deficits are apparent in open-ended communication and less structured settings.

Receptive: Reductions persist in rate and quality of auditory and graphic processing regrading length, complexity and competitive stimuli. Retention improves to short paragraph level, but difficulty discerning salient features, organizing/integrating input and absence of detail persists.

Expressive: Automatic level of language is apparent in referential communication, verbal reasoning; primarily self-oriented and concrete. Tangential expression and irrelevancies evidenced in abstract linguistic attempts. Word retrieval errors persist, with reduced frequency. Length of utterance and gestural expression approximate normal. Graphic expression increases to short paragraphs; syntactic disorganization, simplistic, with irrelevancies. Prosodic features remain aberrant.

continued

Table 1-2   *(continued)*

Level VIII. Purposeful-Appropriate

General Behaviors	Linguistic Behaviors
Patient is alert and oriented, and is able to recall and integrate past and recent events and is aware of and responsive to his culture. He or she shows carryover for new learning if acceptable to him or her and his other life role and needs no supervision once activities are learned. Within his or her physical capabilities, the patient is independent in home and community, skills. Vocational rehabilitation, to determine ability to return as a contributor to society, perhaps in a new capacity, is indicated. He or she may continue to show decreases, relative to premorbid abilities in quality and rate of processing, abstract reasoning, tolerance for stress and judgment in emergencies or unusual circumstances. His social, emotional and intellectual capacities may continue to be at a decreased level for him, but functional within society.	Language capacities may fall within normal limits. Otherwise, problems persist in competitive situations and in response to fatigue, stress and emotionality reducing effectiveness, efficiency and quality of performance. Receptive: Rate of processing of auditory and graphic input remains reduced but unremarkable upon testing. Retention span remains limited at paragraph level, but improved with use of retrieval-organization strategies. Analysis, organization, integration are reduced in rate and quality. Expressive: Syntactic and semantic features fall within normal limits; verbal reasoning, abstraction remain reduced. Graphic expression usually falls below premorbid level. Prosodic features fall within normal limits unless dysarthria is present.

Source: Adapted from Malkmus, D. (1981). Cognition and language, models and techniques of cognitive rehabilitation. Second Annual International Symposium, Indianapolis, Indiana.

Memory

Memory is critical to the "sense of continuity of self, to an appreciation of cause-effect relationships, and to the acquisition of new knowledge" (Brady, 2001, p. 142). Learning of any kind, particularly academic learning, involves memory, which is thus an important indicator of learning ability. While TBI often disrupts memory of new information, memory of old information (information that is well learned) is preserved even following a severe TBI. This preservation of old information can be misleading when testing prior to the child's return to school. Academic, speech and language, and intelligence testing may show scores that indicate that the child has lost few academic skills following the TBI. For the "novice" in TBI, one might assume that the child can go back to the same classroom and return to "normal." In fact, the assessments have tapped into the child's old memory of overlearned material. These assessments do not always evaluate new learning, which needs to be assessed before a child returns to the classroom setting.

New learning is the result of information stored in short-term memory, which is not permanent. Short-term memory lasts for a few seconds at a time but can be extended with continuous rehearsal of information. Short-term memory can be disrupted if any distraction occurs before the information is transferred into long-term memory for permanent storage. Short-term memory can be very unstable following TBI. In the school setting, memory deficits can be manifest as difficulty with recalling events from earlier in the day or previous days. The child may not complete assignments simply because he or she did not remember, not because he or she is showing noncompliant behavior. Difficulty retrieving information in an organized manner may also be symptomatic of a memory deficit. In this situation, the child may need information repeated again and again in order to store it in short-term memory. Further complicating the problem, a child with TBI has difficulty using strategies such as chunking and rehearsal on her or his own. Even when taught these strategies, distractions may still impede this child's ability to utilize them (Brady, 2001; Savage & Wolcott, 1999).

Attention

Attention problems are the most persistent symptom following TBI. Attention is a prerequisite to all other cognitive activity. In order for someone to perceive, remember, or manipulate information, one must attend to it on some level. Location and different types of brain injury may result in different attention problems. The most basic of these dysfunctions is coma, which results from injury to the brain stem. Injury to the sensory input unit (the temporal, parietal, and/or occipital lobes) may manifest as omissions and/or errors in processing and integrating incoming signals. Difficulty managing, allocating, and directing attention in a purposeful, productive manner results from an injury to the frontal lobe (Brady, 2001). Specific types of attention include sustained, selective, alternating, and divided attention.

Sustained Attention. Sustained attention, often referred to as attention span or concentration, involves the ability to respond consistently for the amount of time needed to complete a task. The length of time of response and consistency of response to be maintained over time are important aspects of sustained attention. Problems with sustained attention appear more often in the early stages of recovery. Children have difficulties with previously nondemanding tasks, such as watching a television program (Brady, 2001).

Selective Attention. Selective attention involves the ability to focus on "relevant stimuli in the presence of a distraction—and is often referred to as freedom from distractibility" (Brady, 2001, p. 153). Deficits can result in difficulty focusing attention and filtering out distractions. After sustaining a TBI, the child may not follow instructions in class or pay attention to the lesson because he or she is unable to filter out distractions, whether in the surrounding environment or internal feelings or thoughts. Problems in selective attention can cause numerous difficulties for a child in a "normal" environment with many competing noises.

Alternating Attention. A difficulty with alternating attention means the child encounters problems when shifting focus from one task to another. Children with TBI may have difficulty transitioning from one activity or task to the next, for example, moving from topic to topic in a conversation or even going from class to class. If teachers give advance warning of a change in events or specific directions for beginning a new task, the child may have better success in alternating attention. Problems in alternating attention may not always be apparent in younger children with TBI since alternating attention involves cognitive processes that are more complex and may not be evident until children begin school.

Divided Attention. Children with divided attention deficits exhibit difficulties in attending to many tasks or multiple components of a task. Examples of behavior requiring divided attention include the ability to talk on the phone while typing on the computer, or more typically, doing homework while watching television. This type of attention is not generally seen in younger children with TBI and may appear later as a residual effect of the TBI (Brady, 2001; Savage & Wolcott, 1999).

Executive Functioning

Executive function involves a cluster of cognitive processes necessary for organized, goal-directed behavior. Executive functioning involves the ability to think about and plan responses. Executive function deficits are very common following TBI and can involve any of the following (Ylvisaker & DeBonis, 2000):

- Difficulty setting goals
- Difficulty planning tasks
- Difficulty in self-monitoring
- Difficulty in self-evaluation
- Inability to evaluate individual strengths and needs realistically
- Problems in initiation
- Difficulty controlling and suppressing behavior

The responses of the executive system are related to deficits in the area of the frontal lobes. Since a TBI almost always affects the frontal lobes, many deficits in executive functioning are guaranteed. One executive function that is controlled by the frontal lobes is inhibition, which involves the ability to control or suppress impulsive, automatic responses to a stimulus, whether external, such as a comment or gesture from a person, or internal, such as feelings of fear or aggression. For example, a child who is teased has the ability to inhibit the initial response of reacting to the teasing, which may be hitting, by thinking of the various consequences of his or her actions before reacting. The child with TBI may have deficits in executive functioning, and may not be able to inhibit the initial response, thus facing far greater consequences of his or her actions.

Impaired planning ability, another deficit, also has an impact on post-TBI functioning. Symptoms of impaired planning vary and range from solving problems in an unrealistic manner to difficulty with organization of steps in order to perform a task to perservation on a thought or activity. The child may encounter difficulty in self-evaluation of a task. It is also possible that the child may have difficulty performing the task because she or he cannot interpret abstract language and may be too literal in comprehension. Problems in handling abstraction and poor judgment are also implicated in the executive system following TBI.

Impaired abstraction means the child is unable to generalize thinking to other situations, a behavior often referred to as "stimulus-bound," since the brain recognizes and reacts to the actual objects in that particular environment. More subtle difficulties may include the inability to differentiate between variations in facial expression. The child may misinterpret a facial expression of someone who is showing concern, reading the expression as anger or disappointment instead. These abstraction difficulties also affect the ability to comprehend and interpret literal language. The child with TBI has difficulty interpreting abstract language such as idioms and metaphors, therefore making it more difficult for the child to continue to "fit in" and not look awkward with peers. Poor judgment is another characteristic that is frequently evident following TBI. The child may be unaware of his or her problems, or deny having difficulties. Decision making is impaired and may cause safety issues at both home and school. For example, a child who was typically capable of preparing an afternoon snack, like popcorn in the microwave, may forget to put the popcorn in the microwave and turn it on anyway, thus causing danger to himself or herself and damaging the appliance as well.

The final aspect of the executive system to be discussed is initiation, lack of which is underscore. Many times, following TBI, children appear unmotivated or dull and teachers may categorize them as lazy or as exhibiting behavior problems. Such children require continual prompting in order to get up and get dressed, start assignments in school, and engage in or initiate conversation. It is important to emphasize to teachers and caregivers that the behaviors that result from a lack of initiation are organically and not behaviorally based.

Perceptual and/or Sensory Deficits

Sight, sound, touch, taste, and smell can be lost or damaged following a TBI. The child may become more sensitive to touch or be unable to see objects in a different part of the visual field. The child may encounter difficulty perceiving spatial orientation of objects, or difficulty with depth perception. The post-TBI child also may have problems scanning and visually searching information in an organized way, which can affect reading comprehension. Loss of smell and taste is also possible.

Visual processing is particularly critical to self-care, work, play, and school academics. The visual system is widely distributed throughout the brain; therefore, disruptions of the visual system are likely following a TBI, although they may not be immediately apparent. When damage to the visual system involves cranial nerve dysfunction (from swelling and bleeding, or other sources of pressure), numerous problems can occur, including:

- Ptosis: the drooping of the eyelid
- Dilation of the pupil: the inability of the pupil to get smaller in response to light
- **Strabismus**: a condition in which both eyes cannot focus on the same point due to the fact that one eye deviates upward, outward, and/or inward, resulting in double vision
- Inability of both eyes to focus on the side opposite the injury, resulting in a fixed gaze to one side or the other

Most of these problems will resolve on their own as the swelling subsides. Other less transitory deficits include visual-perceptual problems.

Visual-Perceptual Problems

If damage occurs to the right side of the brain, unilateral visual neglect, which refers to inattention to or failure to respond to anything that is in the opposite field of view occurs. Neglect is a failure of attention due to loss of spatial awareness and may occur even though the child has intact vision. Children experiencing neglect are not aware that they are not attending to that part of the environment. The problems may be subtle, in that the child may start in the middle of the page when writing, may not return to the left margin when reading, or may complete only the right half of the page of a worksheet. Most forms of neglect improve over time; however, some of the more subtle signs may persist but can be compensated for through various techniques, such as placing items in a vertical rather than horizontal array.

Another type of visual-perceptual problem involves deficits in interpreting spatial information. Many activities, particularly in the classroom, rely on the interpretation of spatial information. Following directions, for example, involves the interpretation of words with visual-spatial meanings. Words such as *over, under, behind, inside,* and the like may become confusing, particularly to a child who is hearing instructions from the teacher in the classroom. In this case, the child, who is overwhelmed by too many pictures and displays on the walls and is overly stimulated by the amount of noise in the classroom, will experience difficulty following through on a spoken direction like, "Take out your book, put it on top of your desk, put your paper inside your book, and put your pencil beside the book." By the time the child processes this information, the class has already moved on to another activity. The child with TBI may also experience difficulty manipulating graphs, charts, and other visual displays in the classroom. Processing problems may make it difficult for the child to locate the classroom or her or his house. Reading a map and telling time are also difficult, as these tasks require the comprehension and manipulation of space. Problems interpreting spatial information also have an effect on visual-motor integration, or the ability to convert information received through the eyes mentally into a plan for motor output.

Visual-motor integration is important in moving the body through visual space, such as walking, but is also important in activities such as copying, writing, and drawing. Difficulties with visual-motor integration can certainly impair motor speed and motor planning, both important skills for functioning in school. Deficits in physical capabilities and cognition, as well as the organic nature of some neurological insult, may lead to behavior problems.

Behavior

The interpretation and control of feelings involves cognitive abilities and emotions. Many behavioral manifestations may occur following TBI, including:

- Impulsivity
- Disinhibition
- Poor judgment
- Dependency
- Aggression
- Apathy or indifference
- Lack of goal direction
- Depression
- Emotional lability
- Social withdrawal
- Denial

Behaviors such as agitation, frustration, impulsivity, depression, and disinhibition are the most common. An individual's ability to cope with these problems depends upon both the extent of neurological damage and the presence of any premorbid psychological conditions, such as moodiness or depression.

Survivors of brain injury often experience frustration during the rehabilitation process for a variety of reasons. They may be unable to perform tasks that were easy prior to the trauma, or they do not understand the words and actions of others, or they are disoriented in their surroundings and thus do not understand where they are or why. All these feelings of frustration may cause children to become verbally and physically aggressive to those around them. This agitation is not directed toward any one person, which is difficult for most family members to understand. The emotions displayed are simply their way of coping with all the difficulties and demands that they are experiencing.

When the brain is injured, the child may lose the ability to monitor behavior in a socially acceptable way. The child may be uninhibited or impulsive, and may act out of character. Adolescents may act inappropriately on sexual impulses. Others may demonstrate social immaturity by making inappropriate comments and noises. This type of behavior can be very embarrassing for family members.

Going out to dinner in a restaurant may end in extreme frustration and embarrassment when the child with TBI curses loudly at the table and makes burping noises throughout dinner. Coping with this problem not only requires a great deal of patience from teachers and family members, but also prompting and cueing in order to help the child control her or his behavior.

Following TBI, children may become self-centered and demanding. Oftentimes, friends and family members may withdraw from them, which complicates issues of self-esteem, a loss of which is common in children with brain injuries. Children may see themselves as less than persons following the injury. For example, the straight A high school athlete who was counting on a scholarship to a top-notch university must face the fact that not only may he be unable to play sports again, but he may not be able to handle his course load any longer and may not be going to the school of his dreams. This loss often seems insurmountable and these feelings can result in depression and thoughts of suicide.

Communication

Children who have sustained a TBI can face many problems with communication—the giving and receiving of information. These difficulties may be only temporary and improve over time, but can be permanent. Communication problems often persist for years, depending on the severity of the TBI.

Expressive Speech Problems

Effective speech requires coordination of structures involved in phonation and articulation. A brain injury may affect these areas. Overall, however, speech problems are less common than language problems in children with TBI (Blosser & DePompei, 2003).

Following TBI, children may experience dysarthric or dysfluent speech in the initial phases of recovery. Dysarthric speech is slow and labored, sometimes accompanied by imprecise articulation. Dysfluent speech, otherwise known as stuttering, is characterized by repetition of sounds, syllables, words, or phrases, which impairs the overall flow of speech. Both conditions make intelligibility of speech difficult. Other speech problems that can result from a brain injury include:

- Speech sound production difficulties: include dysarthria (discussed above), apraxia, or dyspraxia. In **apraxia,** a child is unable to plan and execute the movements necessary to produce sounds or words.
- Vocal problems: include problems with resonance involving the way in which the air vibrates within the oral and nasal cavities, which can result in a child's voice sounding too nasal. Problems with voice quality can result in a hoarse, breathy, or other atypical voice quality.

Language Problems

Language problems are more common than speech problems in children with TBI. These problems can range from mild to severe and may be temporary or permanent. One reason that children with TBI have language problems is that language abilities are closely linked to cognitive functions. In particular, language abilities are related to executive function of the brain, including:

- Attention
- Memory
- Conceptual organization

- Speed of processing
- Analysis and synthesis of environmental cues and conversation

When these executive functions are disrupted by brain injury, language ability may also be impaired, resulting in difficulties in (a) learning new vocabulary; (b) word retrieval; (c) following multistep directions; (d) understanding idioms, metaphors, and figurative language; and (e) solving problems (Trudeau et al., 2000; Ylvisaker & DeBonis, 2000).

Conversational skills are part of the subset of pragmatic skills, involving the social use of language. Again, depending upon the severity of the injury, children will display a variety of pragmatic problems, conversational skills and friendship-making skills being two of the more obvious problem areas. Pragmatic skill deficiencies can overlap with behavioral problems such as disinhibition. As stated earlier, post-TBI children frequently have difficulty "turning on and off" inappropriate comments and gestures due to the injury. Though the child is doing his or her best to fit in, inappropriate comments may be incorporated into language use, thereby alienating friends. This cycle can spin out of control, leading to depression and other problems. Equally as frustrating is the child who has difficulty expressing basic wants and needs, due to deficits in speech production or in the ability to use language. This child may need a communication board or a communication device in order to better express herself or himself (Schoenbrodt, 2001).

In addition, children may have many difficulties with conversational speech. Their conversations may be tangential, meaning that they talk around the topic and switch topics frequently, leaving fragments or tangents of unfinished conversation. Conversational speech may also be characterized by irrelevant information, and often is confabulatory, or made up (the information provided is not real or true). While conversational skills will improve, many of the above characteristics may continue and much cueing and prompting may be necessary for the child to become an effective communicator.

The combination of all of the characteristics of TBI—physical, emotional, cognitive, communication, and sensory—and the variability of the severity of the injury create a need for continuous evaluation and reevaluation of deficit areas. Individuals providing assessment need to be knowledgeable about the sequelae that result from the injury.

ASSESSMENT

An in-depth multidisciplinary evaluation of the child with TBI is necessary to identify cognitive strengths and weaknesses, establish baseline behavior, and provide information for litigation purposes. Every child with TBI is unique. Cognitive, psychomotor, and psychosocial profiles are unpredictable and cannot be generalized from one child to the next. Variability is one of the hallmarks of TBI and can be seen throughout all stages of recovery. This is the reason why continuous evaluation is critical. When conducting assessments, the evaluator must keep in mind the child's premorbid level of functioning as a mechanism for comparison in determining educational placement and the level of support services needed (Schoenbrodt & Smith, 1995; Schoenbrodt, 2001).

A multidisciplinary or team approach to evaluation and coordination of services is important for many reasons:

1. If each specialist and each classroom teacher evaluates and develops goals and objectives independently, a fragmented program may evolve that can cause even more confusion for the child.

2. If each evaluator operates independently, valuable crossover of goals, objectives, and ideas for intervention is lost, decreasing the chances of generalization of skills to all environments.
3. While each evaluator is responsible for his or her area of expertise (e.g., the speech-language pathologist administers speech and language testing), the team of evaluators decides on which assessments should be administered based upon the child's individual profile. If evaluators operate independently, skills testing may overlap, artificially increasing the time needed to evaluate the child fully and increasing the risk that the results will be skewed by fatigue (to be discussed later).

Speech and Language Evaluation

Two types of speech and language assessments should be used when evaluating a child with TBI: formal (or standardized) assessments and informal (or naturalistic) assessments. Standardized testing is necessary to document comparable scores and to establish eligibility for educational and support services. Because few formalized assessments have been normed on children with TBI, clinicians should combine formal assessments with careful observation of language and communication in a variety of settings and contexts (Ylvisaker, Urbanczyk, & Feeney, 1992). A comprehensive, multidisciplinary formal assessment battery should evaluate functioning in the following areas: intellectual, executive, problem-solving, attention, concentration, memory, speech, language, perceptual-motor, and academic abilities. In a speech and language battery, tests should specifically sample behaviors in:

- Language (syntax, semantics, pragmatics)
- Speech (articulation, fluency, voice quality)
- Word finding

During the evaluation, the examiner should document the occurrence of any of the following characteristics:

- Level of attention
- Tolerance of stress (time constraints, noise, frustration)
- Degree of cueing and prompting necessary
- Use of compensatory strategies
- Processing time
- Delayed response or slowed performance
- Anxiety
- Fear of failure
- Fatigue

If any of the above characteristics are noted, modifications may be necessary during the testing session. For example, fatigue is common in children with TBI, thus assessments may need to be broken down into several testing sessions. Likewise, if children evidence visual field deficits, printed material may need to be enlarged or presented to the nonaffected side. Many researchers have suggested additional modifications. Blosser and DePompei (2003, p. 103) compiled the following list of testing modifications:

1. Allowing untimed testing
2. Dividing testing into several sessions to prevent fatigue or loss of attention

3. Lengthening the test time to determine if attention to task decreases or if a child can persevere
4. Introducing auditory or visual distractions, such as testing in a classroom, cafeteria, or busy physical therapy area
5. Reducing distractions in a one-on-one quiet environment to determine maximum performance potentials
6. Enlarging printed materials or placing fewer items on each page
7. Permitting different types of response modes, such as gesturing or writing, rather than relying strictly on verbal responses
8. Restating test directions by using simpler directions or by making directions more lengthy and complex
9. Using pictures or printed cards to reinforce an understanding of test procedures
10. Repeating and cueing to determine if multiple bits of information will stimulate recall
11. Selecting various subtests of different tests according to the needs of the individual
12. Observing pragmatic language skills during testing to sense appropriate use of problem solving, questioning, turn taking, and self-monitoring

While modifications in testing may be necessary, the SLP must adhere to all instructions and time constraints outlined in the standardized assessment. Adhering to these rules is necessary to ensure that the results are reliable and valid. Failure to institute some modifications, however, may result in the loss or misinterpretation of the child's performance. For example, if a test item is supposed to be answered in 20 seconds, a potential modification may be for the SLP to mark the item as incorrect if the child does not respond within the time constraints, but then allow the child a longer period of time in which to answer. The child may need additional time to process the information to give a correct response. Without modification, the evaluator might conclude that the child does not have the knowledge to complete the test, when in reality, he or she simply needs more processing time (Carney & Schoenbrodt, 1994; Schoenbrodt & Smith, 1995; Schoenbrodt, 2001).

Interpretation of Standardized Tests

Though standardized testing is important in the evaluation process, the clinician must remember that most instruments have not been normed on the population with TBI. Therefore, interpretation of scores should provide insight into the strengths and weaknesses of the student but should not be considered definitive. Information obtained on a formal assessment can be deceiving. A student may obtain an "average" score on the administered assessment but be unable to function appropriately at home or in the school environment. Conversely, a child may function below average on many assessments, but be able to function adequately in daily life activities. In general, the results obtained from the standardized testing battery should be interpreted cautiously. For this reason naturalistic or informal assessments are an essential portion of the overall evaluation of communication of the child with TBI.

Informal Assessment

Naturalistic assessments are carried out in the child's natural environment and are not standardized. These assessments can provide important information about the child's language functioning that may not be apparent with standardized tests. Informal assessment can take many forms, including interviews, questionnaires, behavioral observations, curriculum-based language assessments, and narrative language samples.

Interviews and Questionnaires

Interviews and questionnaires can provide the SLP with more in-depth information from parents and teachers about communication problems that may be occurring at home or in the classroom (Blosser & DePompei, 2003) (see Appendix A). Possible questions include:

1. How do communication problems affect the child's ability to indicate wants and needs?
2. How well is the child able to hold appropriate conversations with family members or peers?
3. Is the child able to express the need for clarification or repetition of assignments?

Behavioral Observations

Both the SLP and the classroom teacher should observe the child in a variety of settings and contexts, such as the gymnasium, cafeteria, playground, and classroom. An observation in the cafeteria, for example, yields information regarding the child's ability to process information in a noisy environment, to communicate under time constraints (ordering food in the lunch line), to communicate effectively in conversation, to find required vocabulary, and so on. Standardized assessments cannot adequately provide such valuable information.

Curriculum-Based Language Assessment

Curriculum-based language assessment (CBLA) is another form of informal assessment. CBLA assesses:

- The types of language skills and strategies the child has for processing the language of the curriculum or classroom content areas (math, social studies, science, etc.)
- The resources the child is using to handle the class curriculum
- The skills the child has in place to process classroom information more efficiently
- Any modifications that could be made in the curriculum or its presentation to make it more accessible to the child

In CBLA, the child's schoolwork is reviewed with the understanding that it is only the end product and does not give insight into the process the child uses to complete the work. For example, a review of the child's science quiz may uncover an obvious pattern of errors, but fail to offer insight into why the child is having difficulty or how she or he solved the problem.

The child should be observed in different classroom environments at various times of the day in order to record the potentially problematic language and communication demands in the curriculum. The diagnostic information obtained from CBLA can identify the language demands of the curriculum and how well the child handles them. CBLA is the best way of gathering functional information for use in developing meaningful instructional goals for the child.

For instance, the SLP may observe that the teacher frequently gives directions to the class orally but does not write them on the board. If the child with TBI has difficulty processing language, he or she may never be able to write down the information, let alone comprehend what was said. Goals for intervention would then include working on methods to teach the child how to focus on important pieces of oral information instead of being concerned with everything that is said. The SLP may teach the child to listen for key words like "turn to page . . . " or "your assignment is . . . " In addition, the clinician may talk to the teacher and the child about modifications that may be needed in the classroom, such as tape recording directions so that the child can listen to them as many times as needed.

Narrative Language Samples

Another form of naturalistic assessment is narrative assessment—evaluating a child's ability to tell or retell a story. These types of evaluations are important because being able to produce and understand narratives is vital to both academic success (reading and writing) and to participation in conversations (Chapman, 1995; Chapman, Levin, & Lawyer, 1999; Roth, 1986).

Several methods can be used to obtain narrative samples:

1. Having the child relate a personal experience
2. Having the child create a fictional story from pictures or from a given story stem, such as, "One night in a dark and scary woods . . ."
3. Having the child retell a story after hearing the story presented orally or after viewing a videotape
4. Having the child relate a narrative about routine events in daily life (e.g., getting ready for school)

In general, it is more difficult for children to create a novel story than to retell a story or tell about an everyday event. For this reason, it is important that as many narrative samples as possible be obtained in each of the above four areas.

Once the narrative samples are obtained, they are analyzed for story grammar elements (Stein & Glenn, 1979, 1982), including introduction of the characters, a theme or plot, and a closing or resolution. The samples are also analyzed for narrative style and cohesiveness, that is, does the story make sense and flow from one thought to the next? In addition, mean length of utterance and type token ratios (the calculation of the variety of words that are used) can be obtained from the samples.

The information collected through each of these types of informal evaluation reveals a great deal about the child's communication needs at school and in less formal settings (playground, lunchroom, with peers) and should be evaluated along with the information collected through standardized tests for a complete evaluation of the post-TBI child. Continuing brain development can also make it difficult to predict success from test scores, because brain function may or may not continue to improve. Furthermore, there is no way to know how quickly improvement will occur. The combination of both informal and formal evaluations therefore yields a better descriptor of communication competence than either assessment alone and this helps to develop more effective intervention plans.

INTERVENTION

Traumatic brain injury presents a number of deficits that require intervention. As with any population, the most suitable interventions are those that are evidence-based. Currently, many of the interventions used with children with TBI are not evidence-based, but are based on clinical experience. Many states are now mandating that efficacy studies be conducted regarding intervention. Carney et al. (2000) provided a review of evidence-based rehabilitation practices for TBI. The results of their findings (with adults) showed that while many interventions based on clinical experience were effective, clinical relevance could not be established. Their findings lead to the strong suggestion that clinical practice models based on research models and studies utilizing both are needed. The following interventions presented are not all evidence-based due to the paucity of information in this area. However, some clinical interventions are presented here with advice to the reader that more information regarding evidence-based interventions will likely be appearing in this decade.

As with assessment, intervention should be interdisciplinary in order to promote carryover and generalization to all environments. Effective intervention for speech and language involves a collaboration between teachers and specialists who are working with the child. The goals of speech-language intervention will depend on a number of factors, including: (a) chronological age; (b) the developmental age or stage at which the child is functioning; (c) the extent of damage from the TBI; (d) the degree of current functioning at home, at school, and in the community; and (e) the amount of family support available. Overall, intervention should focus on helping the child function in various environments. Rather than teaching or reteaching skills through drills, it is more helpful to teach skills in a meaningful way that will encourage transfer of skills to all settings.

Motor Speech Disorders Intervention

Problems with motor speech disorders may involve phonation, respiration, articulation, and resonation. For children with motor speech disorders, oral motor therapy, phonation exercises, and articulation therapy may be implicated. In most instances, speech production problems are resolved without direct intervention (Blosser & DePompei, 2003). If motor speech problems persist and production or intelligibility is impaired, alternative forms of communication may be explored, such as electronic communication boards, sign language, picture communication boards, and other means.

Language Disorders Intervention

Language disorders are more common than speech disorders in children with TBI. For children with language disorders, therapy may focus on one or more of the following areas.

Vocabulary

The development of vocabulary is crucial for both comprehension and speaking. Children need to develop vocabulary that is meaningful in a variety of settings, including home, school, work, extracurricular activities, and social activities. The child needs to learn not only classroom vocabulary, but also common slang expressions used in conversational speech. Visualization techniques are helpful as well as the use of categorization to aid in word retrieval. Word webs are also effective in helping children to expand ideas and increase word vocabulary.

Pragmatic Skills

Pragmatic skills for language usage are often deficit areas for children with TBI. Conversational and social skills are best taught in settings with peers. In the beginning of therapy, a quiet therapy room with a small group of peers may prove the best setting in which to teach conversational skills. In order for the child to transfer these skills successfully to more natural environments, however, intervention needs to move out of the therapy room into the cafeteria, playground, restaurant, or job setting. By monitoring the child's communication in a variety of settings, the SLP can help the child evaluate where communication breakdowns occur. Therapy can then continue to incorporate problem-solving cognitive skills so the child acquires the ability to think about language and effective communication.

Cueing or prompting in conversational speech may be effective in decreasing circumlocution (talking around a topic without getting to the point). For example, the SLP might put her finger on her chin to signal to the child that he is off-topic. This cue may be enough for the child to stop and think about what he is saying and get back on topic. This cueing system should then be taught to peers, teachers, and family members to help the child communicate more effectively in conversation.

Organizational Skills

Organizational skills should also be taught to facilitate language learning. Examples of such skills include:

- Classification
- Categorization
- Association
- Sequencing

Humor

The child with TBI may also need help in understanding and using humor appropriately. If the child cannot understand humor, she or he will not "get" jokes and will have trouble fitting in with peers. He or she may also fail to recognize sarcasm. Understanding and using humor involves abstract language and is a higher-level skill. Cartoons, comic strips, and books of jokes and riddles can also be used. The list of possible interventions outlined in this section is clearly not all-inclusive. The type and degree of intervention necessary depends upon the severity of the injury and the residual outcomes.

Intervention begins in the hospital, rehabilitation, and school setting, depending upon the severity of the injury. Children who have sustained a mild TBI may never have been in the hospital, and the school may be the first to notice deficits. Most children, however, will generally return to school at some point in time. The SLP may act as a case manager, or a service coordinator, particularly in the school setting.

CASE MANAGEMENT

As part of the child's educational team, the SLP should play an active role in coordinating the child's transition from the rehabilitation center to the school. **Speech-language pathologists** have knowledge of the neurological deficits and educational needs following a TBI that provides a foundation to act in the role of case manager (Blosser & DePompei, 2003; Russell, 1993).

As the case manager, the school SLP should be in contact with the rehabilitation center before the student returns to school. Information should be obtained regarding the nature of the trauma, assessment scores, the severity of injury, and any initial impressions regarding outcome for the purpose of educational placement.

Additionally, those educators and specialists who will be involved with the student with TBI upon return to school should schedule a visit to the rehabilitation center during the student's stay. Telephone contact between both facilities should be conducted frequently, even after the child returns to school. A recent study showed that teachers reported that observations conducted in the rehabilitation center, followed by classroom training, was an effective way to enhance their understanding of the needs of the student with TBI (Feeney & Urbanczyk, 1992). The specialists and professionals from the rehabilitation center should also be invited to attend individualized education plan (IEP) meetings in order to facilitate the transition process.

As the case manager, the SLP should provide information to the child's teachers regarding the injury and the impact it can have on the student's ability to function in school. The SLP should present information regarding the child's current level of performance in comparison to premorbid performance. Educators should also be made aware of the differences between children having TBI versus children with disabilities, as children with TBI frequently exhibit characteristics similar to those of children with learning disabilities, though some basic differences are evident (see Table 1-3).

One major difference is that the child's learning and communication deficits were acquired as a result of a traumatic injury. In many cases, the child had no learning difficulties prior to the trauma. According to DePompei and Blosser (1986, p. 69), the child has:

Table 1-3   Similarities and Differences in Characteristics of Children with Traumatic Brain Injury (TBI) and Children with Learning Disabilities (LD)

Children with TBI	Children with LD
Acquired. Sudden onset.	Congenital defect. Usually early onset.
Documented history of coma in many cases.	No coma.
Cause attributed to event such as motor vehicle accident, gun shot wound, etc.	Cause not clear.
Documented post-traumatic amnesia (PTA) affecting memory.	Memory deficits not related to PTA.
Noticeable differences in premorbid skills and post-trauma abilities.	No pre/post effect.
New learning difficult, can remember old skills.	Learning may be slow with continued progress in new learning.
Range of deficits from mild to severe.	Range of deficits from mild to severe.
Poor social/pragmatic skills secondary to injury.	Poor social/pragmatic skills secondary to language impairment.
Inability to comprehend post-traumatic deficits.	Good comprehension of learning strengths and weaknesses.
Seizure medications given for traumatically induced seizures.	No antiseizure medication.
Marked impairment of progress initially indicating a need for frequent monitoring of progress. At the school level, annual review and dismissal meetings should be held monthly until progress stabilizes.	Slow, steady progress. Monitoring of progress may take place at the school level one or two times a year to document gains.
Once in school change of classroom placement may be needed if progress occurs.	Relatively stable. Classroom placement remains constant.
Needs modification in testing due to impairments (fatigue, distractibility, etc.) secondary to TBI.	Needs modification in testing due to impairments (distractibility, language deficits, etc.) of the LD.
Family may not accept child's school placement and needs due to problems coping with the deficits presented secondary to the sudden trauma.	Family generally understands strengths and weaknesses of child as well as the LD because onset was early and gradual.

1. A sense of being normal that persists from the premorbid period
2. Discrepancies in ability levels
3. A previous history of successful experiences in academic and social settings
4. Inconsistent patterns of performance
5. Variability and fluctuation in the recovery process, resulting in unpredictable and unexpected spurts of recovery
6. More extreme problems with generalizing, integrating, or structuring information
7. Poor judgment and loss of emotional control, which cause the student to appear emotionally disturbed at times
8. Cognitive deficits that, though present in other disabilities, are more uneven in extent of damage and rate of recovery
9. Combinations of disability conditions that do not fall into usual categories of disabilities
10. Inappropriate behaviors that may be more exaggerated than the behaviors of students with other disabilities
11. A learning style that requires the use of a variety of compensatory and adaptive strategies
12. Some intact high-level skills that make it difficult to understand why the student has difficulties in performing lower-level tasks
13. A previously learned base of information that facilitates rapid learning

The SLP should share this information with the child's teachers so that they will be able to develop an awareness of the child's strengths and weaknesses and be able to program for the child in the classroom. In addition, teachers should be aware that the child may require a rest period during the school day due to physical fatigue or a need for emotional release. Requirements for class assignments may also need to be modified.

As a case manager, the SLP has several important roles: (a) to provide information to the educators managing the student in the classroom; (b) to monitor frequently the progress of the student, which may be variable due to the constantly changing nature of postinjury medical, behavioral, and cognitive deficits; (c) to act in conjunction with the monitoring of the student, making updates to the IEP and enacting changes in placement due to these variables; and (d) to act as a liaison for the student when the family is under emotional stress and may lack the knowledge necessary to act as an advocate for their child (Schoenbrodt & Smith, 1995; Schoenbrodt, 2001).

FAMILY ISSUES

The family of the child with TBI plays an important role in facilitating the child's integration into the school and the community. As a result of the trauma, the family also experiences major alterations of roles, rules, and internal responsibilities in its adjustments to the affected family member. The impact on the family of the child with the TBI begins with the telephone call that informs them of the injury and continues through the rehabilitation process and a lifetime of outpatient care (DePompei & Zarski, 1989). Many studies document that TBI affects all aspects of family life and that major changes in structure and organization are inevitable (Prigitano & Klonoff, 1988; Ylvisaker, Szekeres, Henry, Sullivan, & Wheeler, 1987).

The stress resulting from the changes in routine, social status, family health, and patient behaviors has a major impact on a family's ability to adjust to the child with TBI. In addition, the family of the person with the TBI has particular difficulty with the mourning process. Unlike the death of a family member, TBI means that the individual with TBI remains with the family, often in the same physical state but in an altered cognitive state (DePompei & Zarski, 1989).

The family must mourn the characteristics of the child that were lost while learning to respond to the differences in the person, a step that is crucial to the outcome of the child with the TBI. The family often is faced with overwhelming economic burdens in providing the required long-term care. The family of a younger child with TBI is faced with the concern that they will be "parenting" forever. On the other hand, the family of an adolescent is faced with handling a child who was once independent who is now dependent again. This situation is further complicated when the adolescent is aware of prior independence and feels "babied" by parents when he or she is fully aware of prior boundaries.

The functional family eventually draws internal and external support to respond to new needs of the family member and maintains hope for the future. A dysfunctional family is unable to focus on any factor other than the trauma and tends to concentrate on the individual's weaknesses rather than strengths.

CONCLUSION

The neurological and cognitive sequelae that result from TBI vary greatly in terms of severity across the population. For this reason, a child with TBI must be considered unique and be treated on an individual basis.

Communication is essential in all aspects of life, thus communication needs should be identified and monitored continuously throughout the acute care stage as well as through the child's reentry to a school or possibly work setting. Goals for successful communication should also be monitored and frequently revised to match the child's needs in the environment. Plans for intervention should take into consideration functioning in all areas, including cognitive, motor, and behavioral. The ultimate goal should be to enable the child to function effectively at home, in school, and in the community.

Case Study 1: Nina's Case History

Nina is a 9-year, 10-month-old girl who was referred for a complete multidisciplinary assessment subsequent to a severe traumatic brain injury sustained while she was a passenger restrained in the backseat of a car. The current assessments were requested to aid in the transition from the rehabilitation center to the school.

Nina currently resides with her mother, father, and older brother. There is no reported family history of psychiatric illness or learning disabilities. According to parental reports, there were no problems with the pregnancy or labor. Nina was delivered at a weight of 8 pounds, 11 ounces. Early developmental milestones were reported within normal limits. Nina is very active in the neighborhood, and has many friends.

Nina was attending third grade in elementary school at the time of the injury. A review of her records indicated above average performance on report cards and the Comprehensive Test of Basic Skills (CTBS) given at the school. Nina's mother reported that she was diagnosed with ADHD one year ago and was taking medication prior to this injury. School records and teacher reports indicate that Nina had difficulty staying on-task, following directions, avoiding careless mistakes, sustaining attention, and controlling her emotions.

Nina was injured as a restrained backseat passenger. According to medical records, the car she was riding in was hit on the right rear passenger side. Nina lost consciousness at the scene of the accident. She was stabilized at a local hospital and was intubated and resuscitated. She was transferred to a trauma center, where a Glasgow Coma Scale score of 5 (intubated) was reported upon admission.

According to medical records, Nina had a massive injury to the right side of the face and experienced a great deal of blood loss. Her left pupil was small and reactive, while the right pupil was unable to be assessed. A head CT scan revealed two large areas of hemorrhagic contusions. Blood and air were seen within the contusions as well as in the left temporal lobe. There were also extensive temporal bone fractures with disruptions of the inner ear structures bilaterally. Coma duration was noted as 7 weeks. An end of PTA was noted two months after admission, indicating a duration of 6 to 7 weeks between the termination of coma and the termination of post-traumatic amnesia. Conductive hearing loss was identified in the left ear as well as complete hearing loss in the right ear.

Premorbid intellectual skills were judged to be within the average range. Current neuropsychological testing revealed a discrepancy between verbal and performance on the WISC-R, suggesting that nonverbal intellectual skills are currently stronger than language-based problem-solving abilities.

Formal and informal speech and language evaluation revealed receptive and expressive language skills to be in the below average to well below average level for concepts and directions, word classes, semantic relationships, paragraph comprehension, formulating sentences, recalling sentences, and assembling sentences. During the testing, it was observed that Nina required increased time to process information when responding to a question. When Nina was provided with additional time to respond, as well as with visual, auditory, and phonemic cues to elicit words, this increased her ability to answer questions. Word finding deficits, processing deficits, attention deficits, and hearing loss will significantly impact her ability to perform within academic and social environments.

An informal speech and oral motor evaluation revealed mild oral motor deficits secondary to a TBI. Nina presented with slightly decreased strength and mobility of her tongue. Despite mild weakness, oral motor skills appeared to be adequate for speech and eating. Nina tolerated a regular diet with thin liquids.

Results of the multidisciplinary evaluation team revealed that Nina requires direct speech language therapy upon reentry to school, as well as significant modifications to the classroom. As Nina's language skills are changing frequently, it is recommended that she be reevaluated weekly for the first month and then monthly for at least the next year.

Case Study 2: Ron's Case History

Ron is a 6-year, 10-month-old student who was referred for a multidisciplinary assessment following a CHI secondary to a motor vehicle accident. Ron was comatose for four days and received surgery for a subdural hematoma. He remained in a rehabilitation center for one month following the injury. At that time, he was evaluated and weaknesses were demonstrated in attending, following directions, vocabulary, word retrieval, and verbal expression skills.

The current evaluation is being conducted prior to his return to school. Behaviorally, Ron accompanied the examiner willingly and engaged in conversation easily. He was somewhat silly, and inappropriate giggling was noted. His attention to tasks was varied. As tasks became more difficult, off-task behavior was noted. Frequent redirection and breaks were needed in order to complete the testing. In addition, Ron demonstrated slow processing and frequently asked for repetition and/or clarification of oral directions and information. His expressive vocabulary was characterized by frequent restarts, word retrieval, sequencing, and organizational difficulties. Spontaneous conversation was tangential, requiring the listener to clarify and question what was said continually.

Formal and informal evaluations were conducted to evaluate speech and language functioning. The results of the evaluation showed that Ron demonstrates a speech or language impairment characterized by moderate deficits in auditory processing, language content, language structure, and language usage. Overall language skills were in the below average range, with individual scores ranging from average to significantly below average. An individual strength was noted in his ability to perceive relationships between words. Weaknesses were noted in knowledge of antonyms, knowledge of form and meaning of grammatical morphemes, knowledge of synonyms, word knowledge in linguistic context, comprehension of intended meaning, ability to initiate and maintain conversation, and knowledge of form and meaning of grammatical morphemes and comprehension of syntax in spoken narratives.

The results of the evaluation showed that Ron's speech and language impairment significantly impact his performance throughout the school day. The impairment affects his ability to comprehend oral information and lectures, follow directions, answer questions, understand, integrate, and use curriculum vocabulary, express thoughts and ideas in a clear, concise manner, and interact with peers and adults within an educational environment.

As a result of the evaluation, the multidisciplinary team recommended speech and language therapy to focus on remediation of weaknesses and modifications in his academic program, including reducing rate, length, and complexity of oral directions and input; repeating and clarifying directions; preteaching vocabulary and concepts; providing listening, memory, organization, and retrieval strategies; and providing opportunities for participating in social skills groups with peers. Ron's family is encouraged to help with these modifications in his home environment. The assessment team at his school should reevaluate his progress in 30 days to be sure recommendations and modifications are in place.

REVIEW QUESTIONS

1. What is the importance of utilizing standardized and naturalistic assessments in evaluating communication problems?
2. What are the most common communication deficits? Provide examples of each.
3. Explain the types of problems a child with TBI may experience upon returning to school.
4. As a speech-language pathologist, explain what you think your role on a transition team should be.
5. Locate an empirical research article that documents assessment and/or intervention procedures useful for children with TBI.
6. Explain the issues you think families of child survivors of trauma face throughout rehabilitation.

REFERENCES

Arroyos-Jurado, E., Paulsen, J., Merrell, K., Lindgren, S., & Max, J. (2000). Traumatic brain injury in school-age children: Academic and social outcome. *Journal of School Psychology, 38*(6), 571–587.

Blosser, J., & DePompei, R. (1989). Head injured students returning to school: Recovery and treatment. *Topics in Language Disorders, 9,* 67–77.

Blosser, J., & DePompei, R. (2003). *Pediatric traumatic brain injury* (2nd ed.). Clifton Park, NY: Delmar Learning.

Brady, K. (2001). How TBI affects learning and thinking. In L. Schoenbrodt (Ed.), *Children with traumatic brain injury: A parent's guide* (pp. 133–176). Bethesda, MD: Woodbine House.

Bruce, D., Raphaely, R., Goldberg, A., et al. (1979). Pathophysiology, treatment, and outcome following severe head injury in children. *Child's Brain, 5*, 174–191.

Carney, J., & Schoenbrodt, L. (1994). Educational implications of traumatic brain injury. *Pediatric Annals, 23*(1), 47–52.

Carney, N., Chestnut, R., Maynardt, H., Mann, N., Patterson, P., & Helfend, M. (2000). Effect of cognitive rehabilitation on outcomes for persons with traumatic brain injury: A systematic review. *Journal of Head Trauma Rehabilitation, 14*(3), 277–307.

Centers for Disease Control and Prevention. (2002). Traumatic brain injury-SafeUSA. Retrieved 10/12/02 from http//www.cdc.gov/safeusa/home/tbi.htm.

Chapman, S. (1995). Discourse as an outcome measure in pediatric head injured patients. In S. Broman & M. E. Michel (Eds.), *Consequences of traumatic head injury in children: Variability in short and long term outcomes* (pp. 95–116). New York: Oxford University Press.

Chapman, S., Levin, H., & Lawyer, S. (1999). Communication problems resulting from brain injury in children: Special issues of assessment and management. In S. McDonald, L. Togher, & C. Code (Eds.), *Communication disorders following traumatic brain injury* (pp. 235–270). East Sussex, UK: Psychology Press Ltd.

Chapman, S., & McKinnon, L. (2000). Discussion of developmental plasticity: Factors affecting cognitive outcome after pediatric traumatic brain injury. *Journal of Communication Disorders, 33*, 333–344.

Christensen, J. (2001). What is traumatic brain injury? In L. Schoenbrodt (Ed.), *Children with traumatic brain injury* (pp. 1–23). Bethesda, MD: Woodbine House.

DePompei, R., & Blosser, J. (1986). Strategies for helping head injured children find success returning to school. *Language, Speech, and Hearing Services in Schools, 18*, 292–300.

DePompei, R., & Zarski, J. (1989). Families, head injury, and cognitive-communicative impairments: Issues for family counseling. *Topics in Language Disorders, 9*(2), 78–89.

Feeney, J., & Urbanczyk, A. (1992). Educational programming following acquired brain injury. Paper presented at the Annual Conference on Cognitive Rehabilitation, Richmond, VA.

Hagan, C., & Malkmus, D. (1979, November). Intervention strategies for language disorders secondary to head injury. Short course presented at the annual convention of American Speech Language Hearing Association, Atlanta, GA.

Jennett, B., & Teasdale, G. (1981). *Management of severe head injuries.* Philadelphia: F. A. Davis.

Kaufman, B., & Dacey, R. (1994). Acute care management of closed head injury in childhood. *Pediatric Annals, 23*(1), 18–27.

Lehr, E. (1990). Psychological management of traumatic brain injuries in children and adolescents. Gaithersburg, MD: Aspen.

Malkmus, D. (1982, August). Levels of cognitive functioning and associated linguistic behaviors. Paper presented at Models and Techniques of Cognitive Rehabilitation, London, UK.

Massagli, T., & Jaffe, K. (1994). Pediatric traumatic brain injury: Prognosis and rehabilitation. *Pediatric Annals, 23*(1), 29–37.

Roth, F. (1986). Oral narrative abilities of learning-disabled students. *Topics in Language Disorders,* 7(1), 21–30.

Russell, N. (1993). Educational considerations in traumatic brain injury: The role of the speech language pathologist. *Language, Speech, and Hearing Services in the Schools, 24*(2), 67–75.

Savage, R., & Wolcott, G. (1999). *An educator's manual: What educators need to know about students with brain injury.* Washington, DC: Brain Injury Association, Inc.

Schoenbrodt, L. (2001). How TBI affects speech and language. In L. Schoenbrodt (Ed.), *Children with traumatic brain injury* (pp. 177–204). Bethesda, MD: Woodbine House.

Schoenbrodt, L., & Smith, R. (1995). *Communication disorders and interventions in low incidence pediatric populations.* Clifton Park, NY: Delmar Learning.

Stein, N., & Glenn, C. (1979). An analysis of story comprehension in elementary school children. In R.O. Freedle (Ed.), *New directions in discourse processing* (pp. 53–120). Norwood, NJ: Ablex.

Stein, N., & Glenn, C. (1982). Children's concept of time: The development of a story schema. In W. Friedman (Ed.), *The developmental psychology of time* (pp. 255–282). New York: Academic Press.

Trudeau, N., Poulin-Dubois, D., & Joanette, Y. (2000). Language development following brain injury in early childhood: A longitudinal case study. *International Journal of Language and Communication Disorders, 35*(2), 227–249.

Ylvisaker, M., & DeBonis, D. (2000). Executive function impairment in adolescence: TBI and ADHD. *Topics in Language Disorders, 20*(2), 29–57.

Ylvisaker, M., & Goebbel, E. (1987). *Community re-entry for head injured adults.* Boston: Little, Brown.

Ylvisaker, M., Szekeres, S., Henry, K., Sullivan, D., & Wheeler, P. (1987). Topics in cognitive rehabilitation. In M. Ylvisaker (Ed.), *Communication for head injured adults.* Austin, TX: ProEd.

Ylvisavaker, M., Urbanczyk, B., & Feeney, T. (1992). Social skills following traumatic brain injury. *Seminars in Speech and Language, 13*, 308–321.

Chapter 2

Cerebral Palsy

Angela Strauch, M.S., CCC-SLP

CHAPTER OBJECTIVES

Upon completing this chapter, the reader should be able to:

1. Identify cerebral palsy as a nonprogressive motor disorder that varies in severity and characteristics
2. Understand that cerebral palsy can occur before or during birth, or within the first five years of life
3. Identify dysarthria and apraxia as two expressive language disorders that frequently co-occur with cerebral palsy
4. Identify factors associated with cerebral palsy that affect gross motor and fine motor skills, including walking, speaking, and eating
5. List several impairments that frequently co-occur with cerebral palsy
6. Describe interventions, such as surgery, augmentative communication, pharmacological approaches, and behavior modification
7. Identify psychosocial issues that affect self-esteem

INTRODUCTION

Cerebral palsy (CP) is a motor disorder that presents with a variety of characteristics and secondary disorders. **Speech-language pathologists** (SLPs) and others who work with this population of people should be aware of the organic bases of this disorder in order to provide effective treatment. This chapter discusses the etiologies and types of cerebral palsy, as well as effective assessment and intervention techniques.

Cerebral palsy is caused by damage to the motor systems of the brain. This damage affects the person's ability to perform basic functions such as walking, swallowing, and speaking. In order to understand how cerebral palsy affects speech, it is necessary to review the neurology of the speech process.

NEUROLOGY OF THE SPEECH PROCESS

Speech production is a complex process involving major mechanisms throughout the nervous system. It is produced through the integration of three primary motor systems: the pyramidal system, the extrapyramidal system, and the cerebellar system.

Pyramidal System

The **pyramidal system** is responsible for voluntary movement of the speech muscles. It is comprised of three important pathways, the corticospinal, corticobulbar, and corticopontine tracts, which aid in the transmission of messages to other parts of the nervous system. Damage to these tracts can cause severe upper and lower motor neuron disorders.

Neurons are the basic nerve cells of the nervous system that are responsible for all neural behaviors, including speech, language, and hearing. They transmit neural impulses, or electrical signals, to glands, muscles, and other neurons. They contain two processes, the dendrites and the axon. **Dendrites** are projections from the neurons that receive neural stimuli. In contrast, the **axon** is a projection that conducts a nerve impulse away from the neuron and synapses, or transmits a nerve impulse to another neuron, a gland, or a muscle (Love & Webb, 1996). In order to understand the speech motor disorders of children with CP, it is necessary to discuss two neuron groups, the upper and lower motor neurons.

The neurons along the corticobulbar tract, which send axons from the cerebral cortex to the nuclei (a group of nerve cells in the central nervous system that have the same function) in the brainstem are called **upper motor neurons.** These neurons are contained within the brain, brainstem, and spinal cord. Neurons that send motor axons to the peripheral nerves (cranial and spinal nerves) are called **lower motor neurons.**

Damage to the upper and lower motor neurons can greatly affect speech production (Brookshire, 1997). When there is damage anywhere along the corticobulbar tract, upper motor neuron damage occurs. As a result, the muscles become spastic, or tight. Spastic muscles are characterized by resistance to movement, called **hypertonia.** The effects of upper motor neuron damage on speech include slow speech characterized by limited flexibility of the articulators and decreased flexibility of the speech muscles.

When a lesion occurs in the pathway of the lower motor neurons, neural impulses are not transmitted to the muscles (denervation). As a result, the muscles innervated by the cranial or spinal nerves lose muscle tone and become soft and flabby, or flaccid (Love & Webb, 1996). This loss of muscle tone is called **hypotonia.** As a result, vocal quality, pitch patterns, resonance, and articulation are affected.

Extrapyramidal System

The **extrapyramidal system** is responsible for regulating extraneous movements. It is involved with maintaining proper tone and posture and changing facial expressions. One important component of the extrapyramidal system is the **basal ganglia,** a group of subcortical nuclei that influence the initiation and maintenance of movement. Damage to the basal ganglia can result in **dyskinesias** (involuntary movement disorders), including reduction in movement (**akinesia**), excess movement (**hyperkinesia**), and too little movement (**hypokinesia**) (Love & Webb, 1996). The damage also produces uncoordinated speech that is characterized by tremors that reduce intelligibility.

Cerebellar System

The **cerebellar system** works in conjunction with the pyramidal and extrapyramidal systems to provide the coordination for motor speech. It is divided into three lobes: the anterior lobe, which is responsible for regulating posture; the posterior lobe, which regulates coordination of muscle movement; and the flocculondular lobe, which controls equilibrium. The cerebellar system provides smooth, coordinated, and precise movements required for connected speech production. Damage to this system can cause **ataxia** (general incoordination of motor acts), **adiadochokinesia** (the inability to perform rapid alternating muscle movements), hypotonia, or tremors (Love & Webb, 1996). All of these impairments negatively affect speech production.

These three systems play an integral part in the motor processes involved in speaking. When a person is asked a question, the message is received and comprehended in **Wernicke's area,** a speech and language center in the temporal lobe responsible for comprehension. In order for the person to respond, the message travels through the **arcuate fasciculus,** a long subcortical tract that connects the posterior and anterior speech and language areas in the cerebrum, to Broca's area in the frontal lobe. **Broca's area** is a speech and language center that is important for the expression of language. It is here that the verbal response is developed.

Once the response is developed, the brain sends the message to the corticobulbar tract. Through the corticobulbar tract, impulses are sent to the **cranial nerves,** which originate in the brainstem and provide sensory and motor information to the oral, pharyngeal, and laryngeal musculature. The cranial nerves are identified by their names and by a roman numeral. Those involved in speech production include (a) trigeminal—V, (b) facial—VII, (c) glossopharyngeal—IX, (d) vagus—X, (e) accessory—XI, and (f) hypoglossal—XII. Duffy (1995) discussed the individual functions of each of these nerves that combine to form the process of speech. These functions are shown in Table 2-1.

CONSEQUENCES OF CEREBRAL PALSY

The National Information Center for Children and Youth with Disabilities (1997) describes cerebral palsy as a condition caused by damage to the brain, usually occurring before, during, or shortly following birth. "Cerebral" refers to the brain and "palsy" to a disorder of movement or posture. According to the United Cerebral Palsy Association (2001), CP is a term used to describe a group of chronic conditions affecting body movement and muscle coordination. These disorders are not caused by problems in the muscles or nerves. Instead, damage to motor areas in the brain disrupts the brain's ability to control movement and posture adequately. In other words, it is not the muscles or the nerves themselves that have something wrong with them. It is the damaged parts of the brain that send the wrong messages to the muscles. CP results in poor coordination, poor balance, abnormal movement patterns, or a combination of all three (Miller & Bachrach, 1995). CP is not communicable, inherited, or the primary cause of death (Pincus, 2000).

When CP occurs before or during birth, it is called **congenital** CP. Acquired CP is the name given to the disorder when it occurs after birth. However, it can be acquired only until a person reaches age 5. It is believed that injuries to the brain that occur after age 5 result in neurological impairments similar to those observed in adults. Therefore, the damage to the brain would be considered a stroke or traumatic brain injury (Pellegrino & Dormans, 1998).

Table 2-1   Cranial Nerves Involved in Speech Production

Nerve	Motor Functions	Sensory Functions	Effects of Damage
Trigeminal Nerve V	Innervates muscles of mastication, the tensor tympani (muscle involved in hearing), and the tensor veli palatini (muscle involved in raising the velum).	Transmits pain, thermal and tactile sensation from the face and forehead, mucous membranes of the nose and mouth, and conveys deep pressure and kinesthetic information from the teeth, gums, hard palate, and temporomandibular joint.	Transmits pain, thermal and tactile sensation from the face and forehead, mucous membranes of the nose and mouth, and conveys deep pressure and kinesthetic information from the teeth, gums, hard palate, and temporomandibular joint.
Facial Nerve VII	Innervates the stapedius muscle (involved in hearing) and the muscles of facial expression.	Involves the provision of taste to the anterior two-thirds of the tongue.	Paralyzes muscles on the entire ipsilateral (same side) side of the face.
Glossopharyngeal Nerve IX	Provides motor supply to the stylopharyngeus muscle (muscle of the pharynx).	Transmits sensory information to the pharynx, tongue, eustachian tubes, soft palate, tonsils, ear canals, and tympanic cavity.	Causes reduced pharyngeal sensation and a decreased gag reflex.
Vagus Nerve X	Innervates the muscles of the soft palate, pharynx, and larynx.	Provides sensation to the palate, pharynx, and larynx.	Affects resonance, voice quality, and swallowing and causes decreased peristalsis for bolus transport.
Accessory Nerve XI	Innervates sternocleidomastoid and trapezius muscles.	None	Reduces head rotation and the ability to elevate shoulder on the affected side.
Hypoglossal Nerve XII	Innervates all intrinsic muscles and all but one extrinsic muscle of the tongue.	None	Causes atrophy, weakness, and fasciculations (uncontrollable twitching) of the tongue.

The United Cerebral Palsy Association reports that between 500,000 and 700,000 American children and adults currently have CP. One would assume that these statistics would decrease as medical improvements are made. However, medical advances have saved the lives of children who previously would have died at birth (Miller & Bachrach, 1995); thus the incidence of CP has remained constant.

CAUSES OF CEREBRAL PALSY: CONGENITAL

In most cases, the cause of congenital CP is unknown. Some factors that may play a role in its development include:

- Infections during pregnancy
- Jaundice in the infant
- Severe oxygen shortage in the brain
- Trauma caused by a difficult birth

- Rh incompatibility
- Bleeding in the brain
- Low birth weight

Children born with a very low birth weight (less than 3 pounds, 5 ounces) represent half of the reported cases of CP (Pellegrino & Dormans, 1998). In addition, the incidence of CP in multiple births is much greater than that of a singleton (single birth).

Prenatal Causes

Though there is no one cause of CP which occurs prior to birth, several risk factors involving the mother are identified. Pellegrino and Dormans (1998) identified the following factors:

- Thyroid disorder
- Previous pregnancy loss
- Mental retardation
- Bleeding in the third trimester of pregnancy
- High blood pressure
- Seizure disorder
- Alcohol or drug abuse

Other causes of the development of prenatal CP include genetic or chromosome abnormalities, radiation exposure, prenatal infections, and congenital malformations.

Perinatal Causes

When an infant is born prematurely, the blood vessels in the brain are very fragile and may bleed into the **ventricles** (inner fluid spaces) of the brain. As a result, an **intraventricular hemorrhage** (IVH) may occur. An IVH is defined as bleeding into the normal fluid spaces (ventricles) within the brain and occurs when blood vessels in the brain burst. When the IVH is severe, it frequently causes neurological damage and often results in the occurrence of CP (Pellegrino & Dormans, 1998).

The cause of CP in a full-term baby is most often related to **hypoxic-ischemic encephalopathy** (HIE), which is a brain dysfunction caused by insufficient oxygen and blood flow during the birth process. For example, meconium aspiration syndrome is a condition where aspiration of the first bowel movement occurs during labor and delivery. This condition causes respiratory compromise and frequently results in HIE. HIE commonly occurs when the umbilical cord is wrapped around the child's neck during labor and delivery. The developmental stage of the full-term baby's brain makes the child vulnerable to damage in the basal ganglia. Therefore, CP in full-term babies is typically characterized by uncoordinated and uncontrolled muscle movements (Pellegrino & Dormans, 1998).

CAUSES OF CEREBRAL PALSY: ACQUIRED

Approximately 10 to 20 percent of people with CP acquire the disorder after birth. Acquired CP can result from severe brain infections (meningitis, encephalitis), a lack of oxygen to the brain (**asphyxia**), or **traumatic brain injury,** most commonly from a motor vehicle accident, fall, or child abuse (Pincus, 2000).

CLASSIFICATION OF CEREBRAL PALSY

Since motor ability and coordination vary greatly in children with CP, it is difficult to classify the various types (Miller & Bachrach, 1995). Classification involves the site of lesion and effects on movement and the identification of affected extremities. When classifying CP by the site of the lesion, professionals use the terms *spastic, athetoid, ataxic,* and *mixed.* Figure 2-1 depicts the percentage of the population that exhibits each type of CP.

Spastic Cerebral Palsy

Spastic CP occurs when there is damage to the pyramidal system of the brain. It is the term used to describe muscle tone that is hypertonic. It is the most common form of CP, as it occurs in 70 to 80 percent of all cases (Pellegrino & Dormans, 1998). A person with spastic CP presents with impaired control of voluntary movements due to rigid muscles that are permanently contracted. Attempts to complete a motor activity result in increased tensing of the muscles. For example, when people with spastic CP attempt to drop an object from their hand, the muscles become tighter and prohibit the release of the object.

Athetoid Cerebral Palsy

Athetoid CP is the result of damage to the extrapyramidal system. It results in mixed (sometimes hypertonic and sometimes hypotonic) muscle tone and impairs the person's ability to control involun-

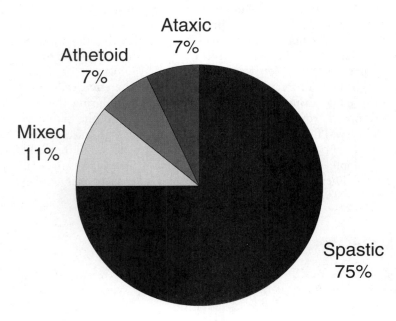

Figure 2-1
Prevalence of the types of cerebral palsy.

tary movements. It affects 5 to 10 percent of persons with CP and is the least common type. Athetoid CP is characterized by slow, writhing, involuntary movements. These uncontrolled movements make it difficult for the person to grasp objects, such as eating utensils, and to coordinate muscles for ambulation (walking). The muscles of the face and tongue can also be affected, resulting in grimaces, odd facial expressions, or drooling (Pincus, 2000).

Ataxic Cerebral Palsy

Ataxic CP is caused by damage to the cerebellum and affects coordination. It is characterized by hypotonia and affects 5 to 10 percent of the CP population. Persons with ataxia present with unsteady, shaky movements, or tremors. They typically experience balance and coordination problems, which negatively affect ambulation, writing, and dressing (Pincus, 2000).

Mixed Cerebral Palsy

People who exhibit a combination of two or more of the types of CP (spastic, athetoid, ataxic) are said to have mixed CP. This form of the impairment results in a mixture of hypertonicity (high tone or tightness of the muscles) and hypotonicity (low tone or floppiness of the muscles).

Affected Extremities

Cerebral palsy is also classified by the extremities that are affected:

- **Hemiplegia**—one arm and one leg on the same side of the body are affected
- **Diplegia**—both legs are involved, but the arms are not affected
- **Triplegia**—three limbs are affected
- **Quadriplegia**—all four extremities are affected

Following this dual-descriptive model, a doctor would be able to classify the disorder based on both site of lesion and affected extremities. For example, a person with tight muscles and involvement of only the legs is classified as having "spastic diplegia." Similarly, a person with rigidity and involvement of all four limbs has "spastic quadriplegia." CP can affect a person's motor skills mildly or severely. The location and extent of the brain injury determine the severity of the CP.

DIAGNOSIS OF CEREBRAL PALSY

The diagnosis of CP is a lengthy process requiring a great deal of observation over time. Three main factors contributing to the diagnosis of CP are the acquisition of developmental milestones, muscle tone, and muscle function (Miller & Bachrach, 1995). Developmental milestones include reaching for toys, sitting, crawling, walking, and speaking a first word. Since these milestones are based on motor function, delays may suggest CP. Parents will typically begin to notice that their child's motor skills may be different from those of other children around 6 months of age. The child may round her or his shoulders when sitting to avoid falling backward, use only one hand when reaching, or arch her or his back when rolling over (Gersh, 1991). As the infant matures, the concern of CP may arise as development of milestones becomes increasingly delayed.

Observation of muscle tone and function are two other important factors in the diagnosis of CP. Abnormal muscle tone, atypical movements, and lasting infantile reflexes are red flags for the diagnosis. Some of the these abnormalities include:

- Variable muscle tone—tone may change from floppy to stiff
- Asymmetry of movement—one side of the body moves more easily than the other
- Weak oral motor skills—poor tongue and lip control, especially during feeding
- Persistent primitive reflexes—reflexes like the asymmetric tonic neck reflex (ATNR) and Babinski reflex persist longer than 6 months and 1 year of age, respectively

Some symptoms of CP can occur during the first six months of life. These include lethargy, irritability, **bradycardia** (slow heart rate), feeding difficulties, seizures, and trembling of the arms and legs (Gersh, 1991). These symptoms alone are not sufficient for the diagnosis of CP, as they must accompany muscular issues and delayed developmental milestones. The use of magnetic resonance imaging (MRI) and computerized topography (CT) scans assists physicians in ruling out other motor impairments when the diagnosis of CP is questionable.

CHARACTERISTICS OF CHILDREN WITH CEREBRAL PALSY

The characteristics of children with CP vary based on the site and severity of the brain damage. Typically, deficits can be found in four areas of functioning: motor, sensory, cognitive/linguistic, and other co-occurring impairments.

Motor Impairments

Cerebral palsy is solely a motor disorder that affects people's abilities to control their muscles. It is not the direct cause of cognitive, visual, hearing, or attention impairments. Therefore, understanding how CP affects gross and fine motor functions is critical.

Gross Motor: Lower Extremities

The gross motor impairments of the lower extremities (legs) vary greatly. Some children with CP require the use of a wheelchair, walker, or cane (see Figure 2-2). Others walk with a distorted gait or without any noticeable impairment. The rigidity of the muscles frequently causes the feet to turn inward or the legs to "scissor," or cross, when the child attempts to walk. In contrast, CP may also cause the child to take uncontrolled and uncoordinated large steps when walking. A prosthetic device called an **ankle foot orthosis** (AFO) or brace is used to maintain the proper positioning of the ankle and calf.

Commonly, children with CP develop dislocated hips and tight hamstring, calf, and ankle muscles. Medical or surgical interventions are required to decrease the tone. Botox, or botulism, is used to paralyze a muscle group and allow for increased range of motion. Surgical interventions include clipping a muscle, such as the hamstring, to facilitate stretching and improve mobility.

Fine Motor: Upper Extremities

In most cases, CP affects both the lower and upper (arms) extremities. Weakness or tightness of the muscles makes even the simplest tasks difficult. Fine motor deficits of the upper extremities affect the

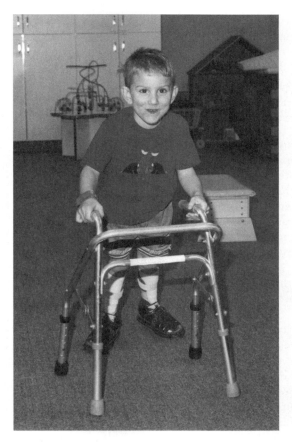

Figure 2-2
Young boy with cerebral palsy using a walker to assist with mobility.

children's abilities to dress themselves, toilet themselves, write, feed themselves, and use simple tools such as scissors. It is not uncommon for the wrists to be "stuck" in a pronated, or downward, position. This prohibits the rotation of the wrist and makes daily tasks, such as self-feeding, difficult. Hand and wrist splints are often utilized to ensure the proper positioning of the fingers and wrist.

Fine Motor: Speech

The speech characteristics of people with CP are as varied as those of the CP itself. For many people with the disorder, speech is affected mildly or not at all. Mild articulation errors caused by hypertonicity or hypotonicity may be present. For others, their speech is severely impaired by one of two speech motor disorders called dysarthria and apraxia.

Dysarthria is defined as a group of motor disorders characterized by disturbed muscle control resulting from damage to the central or peripheral nervous system or to the speech musculature. This disorder affects respiration, phonation, articulation, resonance, or prosody and can result in paralysis, decreased range, force, intelligibility, timing, and regulation of speech muscles (Carter, Yorkston, Strand, & Hammen, 1996). The types of dysarthria vary depending on the site of the brain damage.

Love and Webb (1996) discussed the varieties of dysarthria that are most common in children with CP. These include spastic, dyskinetic, and ataxic dysarthrias.

- Spastic dysarthria—caused by damage along the corticobulbar tract of the pyramidal system (upper motor neuron lesions). Characteristics include decreased muscle tone and range, dysphagia, articulation errors, hypernasality, decreased rate of speech, a perceptually harsh and strained vocal quality, and decreased variation in loudness. Spastic dysarthria is most commonly seen in children with spastic CP.
- Dyskinetic or flaccid dysarthria—caused by damage to the extrapyramidal system (lower motor neuron lesion). Characteristics include hypotonic muscle tone, dysphagia, articulation disorders, involuntary movements, hypernasality, breathiness, stridor, prevocalizations, and monotone pitch and loudness. Dyskinetic dysarthria is most commonly seen in children with athetoid CP.
- Ataxic dysarthria—caused by damage to the cerebellar system. Characteristics include articulation and prosody errors, tremors, increased rate of speech, impaired production of repetitive sounds, unequal stress, and loudness and pitch variability. Speech appears to be explosive. Ataxic dysarthria is most commonly seen in children with ataxic CP.

Given the similarities among all three types of dysarthria, differential diagnosis cannot be determined by articulatory errors alone. Vocal and prosodic features play a vital part in the perceptual judgment of the dysarthrias (Love & Webb, 1996).

Apraxia is defined as an impaired ability to execute voluntarily the appropriate movement of speech in the absence of paralysis, weakness, and the incoordination of the speech muscles (Love & Webb, 1996). In other words, it is a disorder of motor planning rather than that of muscle weakness. It is caused by a lesion in the motor areas of the brain. Though there are several different types of apraxia, the most common type seen in children with CP is developmental apraxia of speech.

Developmental apraxia of speech is a condition where the impaired movements of the articulators cause issues with sound production. It is characterized by atypical sounds, voicing, and repetition errors, as well as errors of **metathesis** (transposition of phonemes in words) (Hall, Jordan, & Robin, 1993). Consequences of this disorder can include delayed development of speech and language, and delayed achievement of developmental milestones of language (production of one- and two-word utterances) (Love & Webb, 1996). It is identified only by irregular **prosody** (intonation of speech) and atypical sound errors that cannot be attributed to dysarthria.

It is often difficult to differentiate apraxia of speech from dysarthria. Observations of subtle differences must be made to determine the correct diagnosis. Apraxia is characterized by inconsistent speech errors and articulatory movements, while the speech errors of dysarthria are more consistent and involve distorted sounds. In addition, people with dysarthria demonstrate some impairment of the nonspeech musculature (weakness, paralysis, or involuntary movement). These impairments are not observed in people with apraxia (Love & Webb, 1996). The site of the lesion plays a role in the differential diagnosis. Dysarthria is typically associated with several lesions at different sites in the brain. Apraxia, however, is caused by a unilateral left hemisphere lesion (Yorkston, Beukelman, & Bell, 1988).

Fine Motor: Respiration

The respiratory system is made up of the upper airway (nose, mouth, pharynx, and larynx) and the lower airway (tracheal tree and lungs). Normal respiration involves three phases of breathing: quiet, forced, and speech breathing. During quiet breathing, there is active inspiration and passive expiration. Forced breathing consists of active inspiration and exhalation. Finally, speech breathing uses active inspiration and expiration against the resistance of the vocal folds (Dikeman & Kazandjian, 2003). For children with CP, the processes of respiration are not as clearly defined. Respiration is often compromised by immature lungs and respiratory distress, asthma, aspiration pneumonia, **sleep apnea** (intermittent interruptions of breathing during sleep), and **chronic obstructive pulmonary disease** (COPD), an irreversible lung disorder. It is important to note that not all respiratory issues are caused by lung inefficiency. The lungs may be healthy, but the access to them or to the contributing systems may be impaired (Driver, 2000). Some respiratory issues are outgrown, while others persist and compromise respiration severely enough to require intervention. Two types of respiratory management are tracheostomy and ventilation.

A **tracheotomy** is the surgical placement of a plastic or metal tube through the outer surface of the neck and into the trachea to create an airway (Dikeman & Kazandjian, 2003). The **stoma** (hole), which remains after the procedure, is called a tracheostomy. Placement of a tracheostomy tube provides a secure airway, long-term access to the airway, and an interface if ventilation becomes necessary (Driver, 2000). Following the surgery, airflow is diverted through the tracheostomy tube and out of the neck, rather than through the upper airway. If a tracheostomy tube is placed and the child is unable to maintain adequate respiratory functioning, mechanical ventilation may be required.

Mechanical ventilation is the process by which negative or positive pressure is provided to assist or substitute for the inspiratory muscle function needed for breathing (Bach & Ishikawa, 2000). This support is necessary when the normal exchange of air in and out of the lungs is compromised and **hypoventilation** (inadequate ventilation) occurs. The process of mechanical ventilation begins when a ventilator machine is attached to the tracheostomy by a plastic coil tube. A preset volume of oxygen is delivered into the lungs to inflate them. The lungs then begin to deflate passively and air leaves the lungs. The ventilator then repeats the cycle (Dikeman & Kazandjian, 2003). Mechanical ventilation assists in maintaining the respiratory process when the child is unable to control it himself or herself. Both the tracheostomy tube and mechanical ventilation alter the process by which air enters and leaves the body. Therefore, use of these interventions affects speech and feeding and swallowing.

Effects on Speech. In order for speech to occur, a sound source for phonation and the ability to articulate to produce intelligible speech must be present (Driver, 2000). The presence of a tracheostomy tube with a cuff, an internal balloon that surrounds the outer portion of the tracheostomy tube, and ventilator prohibits or reduces airflow to the upper airway. Therefore, the vocal folds do not vibrate and sound production does not occur. To allow for the production of speech, one-way speaking valves can be attached to the tracheostomy tube (when mechanical ventilation is not required). One example of a speaking valve is the Passy-Muir Tracheostomy Speaking Valve. This valve consists of a thin silicone membrane that opens on inhalation and allows air to enter the lungs through the tube. The membrane closes on exhalation, resulting in the diversion of air upward through the larynx and out the nose and mouth. This process provides the airflow necessary for speech production. Before a speaking valve can be placed, an assessment of oral motor function and upper airway status must occur. For example, if vocal fold paralysis, dysarthric speech, or other airway dysfunctions are observed, a speaking valve is no longer a viable option (Driver, 2000). In addition, a trial of finger occlusion should occur when the cuff is deflated to determine if the person can independently produce sound. This process involves the manual occlusion of the tracheostomy so the air in the person's lungs is forced into the upper airway. If this trial is successful, a speaking valve is not required.

Speech production in conjunction with mechanical ventilation requires the deflation of the cuff. The purpose of the cuff is to prevent air from escaping around the tube when the air is moving from the lower to upper airway and to reduce the risk of aspiration. The deflation of the cuff allows air to rise to the upper airway and vibrate the vocal folds (Dikeman & Kazandjian, 2003). Given the cuff's protective purpose, its deflation could cause respiratory compromise. For some children, the respiratory situation is too compromised to allow for the placement of speaking valve or cuff deflation. In those cases, alternate forms of communication must be explored.

Effects on Feeding and Swallowing. The coordination of respiration and swallowing are essential in the oral feeding process. For children who have depended on a tracheostomy tube or mechanical ventilation since birth, feeding and swallowing can be severely impaired. When food is introduced, lack of experience may cause oral defensiveness. In addition, limited experience with handling secretions may cause desensitization or decreased glottic closure and affect the swallowing process.

The placement of a tracheostomy tube can negatively impact swallowing. It is possible for the tracheostomy tube to "anchor" the larynx and cause reduced laryngeal elevation and epiglottic closure during a swallow. In addition, a lack of airflow through the pharynx and larynx can cause desensitization of those areas and increased risk of aspiration. The use of a speaking valve equalizes air pressure, increases sensation in the upper airway, and, therefore, improves the child's ability to swallow (Driver, 2000).

The process of swallowing involves several fine motor functions, including (a) forming of the **bolus** (a chewed piece of food ready to be swallowed) intraorally, (b) propelling the bolus posteriorly, (c) raising the larynx, (d) closing the velopharyngeal port, (e) inverting the larynx, and (f) closing the true vocal folds. When muscle function is affected, swallowing becomes more difficult and less effective. For children with CP, weakness of the muscles of the lips, tongue, and pharynx inhibits the production of a strong swallow, leaving residue in the mouth and throat. Swallow function and airway protection can also be compromised by delayed reflex and decreased glottic closure, which may allow food or liquid to enter the airway. In order to understand how swallow function is impaired, it necessary to review the process of a normal swallow. Dikeman and Kazandjian (2003) discussed the three phases of the swallow: oral phase, pharyngeal phase, and esophageal phase.

Oral Phase. The oral phase of the swallow begins when the bolus of food is placed in the mouth. In a normal swallow, the lips close to prohibit anterior leakage, or food spilling out of the mouth. The mandible and tongue work to move the food laterally onto the teeth for mastication. At the same time, the velum or soft palate rests against the base of the tongue to prevent food from entering the nasal cavity. Once the food is masticated and held in a ball (bolus) in the middle of the tongue, the transit to the posterior section of the mouth begins. The tongue presses the bolus of food against the hard palate and thrusts it posteriorly to the **hypopharynx,** or portion of the throat below the base of the tongue. As the bolus passes through the faucial arches, the pharyngeal phase begins.

Pharyngeal Phase. The pharyngeal phase begins as the bolus passes through the faucial arches. The larynx begins to move anteriorally and superiorally and the epiglottis inverts to protect the trachea. The arytenoids rock forward toward the epiglottis and the true vocal folds and epiglottis close. Intraoral pressure forces the bolus down while the pharyngeal constriction assists in the clearance of the bolus. At this time, the esophageal phase begins.

Esophageal Phase. During the esophageal phase, the bolus of food passes through the opening at the top of the esophagus called the **cricopharyngeal sphincter,** or upper esophageal sphincter (UES). This sphincter is typically closed and seals off the entrance to the esophagus. It is the elevation of the larynx in conjunction with the relaxation of the muscle in the cricopharyngeal sphincter that allows food to enter the esophagus (Dikeman & Kazandjian, 2003). The food is then propelled through the lower esophageal sphincter (LES) into the stomach via esophageal peristalsis.

Fine Motor: Feeding

Difficulties with jaw control and tongue, lip, and cheek mobility resulting from high or low muscle tone complicate feeding for the child with CP (Anderson, 1991). Decreased tongue strength can cause a forward thrusting of the tongue that pushes the food anteriorly toward the lips and limits the lateralization of the bolus to the teeth for mastication. Consequently, a sucking pattern is observed where the tongue mashes the bolus against the hard palate, and the food is swallowed without having been chewed. An open mouth posture is common in children with CP as low tone in the mandible and lips inhibits closure and results in drooling and anterior bolus leakage. If the muscles of the larynx and epiglottis are weak, insufficient protection of the airway occurs. Similarly, high muscle tone can constrict the pharynx and make swallowing laborious. The consequences of compromised muscle strength often result in the need for alternate feeding methods. These methods include the placement of tubes through the nose (**nasogastric tube**) or directly into the stomach (**gastrostomy tube**). Liquid nourishment is then sent through the tube into the person's body to ensure proper nutrition.

Feeding issues not related to swallowing are prevalent in the child with CP. High muscle tone or extraneous movements cause the child to burn excessive calories and develop weight issues. If sensory problems are present, the child may refuse any nourishment by mouth, which results in poor nutrition and weight loss (Anderson, 1991). Feeding programs are often developed to ensure proper nutrition. They may consist of foods high in calories to supplement weight loss or varying textures of foods (i.e., pureed foods, thickened liquids) to assist in decreasing sensitivity.

If feeding becomes compromised by weakness of the muscles involved in swallowing, alternate feeding techniques must be considered. When the coordination of swallowing is lacking, food, liquid, or saliva may be aspirated into the lungs. **Aspiration** is the entry of food, liquid, or foreign objects into the airway that can lead to chronic lung damage; it plays a major role in the illness and death of children with CP (Pellegrino & Dormans, 1998). The symptoms of aspiration include coughing, gagging, choking while eating, and difficulty breathing when eating. For children without a strong cough or gag reflex, aspiration can be "silent" or unnoticeable because no symptoms are observed. When dietary changes are unsuccessful at eliminating the aspiration, a feeding tube is considered.

Fine Motor: Visual-Motor Impairments

Approximately 40 percent of people with CP have a co-occurring visual impairment (Pellegrino & Dormans, 1998). A variety of factors predispose a person to visual difficulties, including prematurity and a lack of oxygen to the brain, which result in damage to the retina, optic nerve, or occipital lobe. In the educational system, a child is considered to have a visual impairment when it interferes with the ability to learn (Miller & Bachrach, 1995). Some visual problems seen in children with CP include:

- **Strabismus**—an eye muscle imbalance resulting in inward or outward turning of one eye. It is frequently referred to as "cross-eye" and can cause double vision.

- **Nystagmus**—an eye disorder that causes jerking movements of the eye in either a vertical or a horizontal direction.

Most visual impairments can be corrected with surgery, corrective lenses, or eye patching. Visual deficits experienced by children with CP affect not only motor function, but also perceptual skills.

Sensory Impairments

Visual-Perceptual Impairments

Visual impairments often affect the sensory organization of the child with CP. For example, nystagmus may alter balance and cause a delay in motor milestones such as crawling and walking. **Diplopia,** or double vision, distorts vision and makes it difficult to discriminate between foreground and background. Consequently, the child may frequently trip over objects. A visual field cut, or loss of vision in a section of the visual field, is common in children with hemiplegia and affects depth perception (Pellegrino & Dormans, 1998). Other sensory visual impairments include:

- Refractive errors—which include nearsightedness, farsightedness, and astigmatism or distorted vision.
- **Retinopathy of prematurity**—which is a condition that commonly occurs in children born prematurely and results from oxygen-related damage to the blood vessels of the retina. It frequently causes severe visual impairments, including blindness.
- **Optic atrophy**—which is damage to the optic nerve that prohibits the brain from receiving visual stimuli and transferring it into a visual image.
- **Cortical blindness**—which is caused by damage to the brain that prohibits the conversion of visual stimuli into a visual image. In other words, the eye and optic nerve are functioning properly, but are not receiving the visual messages from the brain.

Visual-perceptual impairments play a role in the child's ability to operate a power wheelchair, walk, complete spatial activities (i.e., puzzles), and reach for objects.

Hearing Impairments

Another disorder that frequently occurs in conjunction with CP is a hearing impairment. Approximately 15 percent of children with CP develop a hearing impairment caused by bleeding in or a lack of oxygen to the brain (Miller & Bachrach, 1995). There are two types of hearing impairments, sensorineural and conductive. A **sensorineural hearing loss** occurs when the inner ear or auditory nerve is damaged. A **conductive hearing loss** is caused by a problem in the outer or middle ear that prohibits the conduction of sound into the inner ear or auditory nerve. A **mixed hearing loss** can occur when a person with a sensorineural hearing loss develops a conductive hearing loss. The severity of hearing impairments ranges from slight to profound and can negatively affect the speech and language of the child with CP.

Auditory Processing

Auditory processing describes the process by which the brain uses information received through the sense of hearing (Foltz, DeGangi, & Lewis, 1991). For children with CP, **auditory processing disor-**

ders are often observed. These difficulties are manifested in short-term memory auditory deficits, auditory sequencing, and organizing ideas. Compensatory strategies are utilized to decrease the severity of these deficits.

Sensory Integration

Children with CP frequently suffer from sensory impairments, which affect their **proprioception,** or awareness of the position of the body in space. It is very common for children with CP to lean to one side when sitting and to be completely unaware of their postures. Tactile defensiveness is another common sensory impairment. The feeling of wet paint on their hands or feet often results in a sensory integration "overload" that causes crying, refusing to participate in the activity, or attempting to remove the paint from the body part. Continued experiences with varied textures assist the children in decreasing the defensiveness.

Cognitive/Linguistic Impairments

Cognition

Intelligence can be defined as the ability to reason, conceptualize, solve problems, think, and adapt in the environment (Blacklin, 1991). It is determined based a standard test of intelligence that measures the intelligence quotient (IQ). People who achieve a score between 70 and 130 on an IQ test are said to have normal intelligence. When the score falls below 70, the person is considered to have mental retardation. **Mental retardation** is defined as below average intellectual functioning that includes adaptive limitations. The causes of mental retardation are similar to those of CP; however, it is the location of lesion in the brain that differentiates the disorders. Due to damage to the brain, some form of mental retardation (mild, moderate, or severe) is found in two-thirds of people with CP (Miller & Bachrach, 1995). Physical limitations make it difficult to test the cognition of a person with CP. The inability to speak or complete a motor task may impede testing and produce a score that is not commensurate with true cognitive ability.

Since CP is a motor disorder, it does not necessarily manifest itself as a cognitive disorder. Many children with CP do not demonstrate any cognitive deficits. They are impaired only by their motor function and are able to succeed in the cognitive tasks of daily life.

Language and Communication Impairments

Language is a complex system of symbols manifested in speech, writing, and gesture (Solot, 1998). It can be receptive (comprehension) or expressive (output), verbal or nonverbal. Language can include gestures, words, head shakes, and reaching. The five general systems of language are:

- **Phonology**—the sound system
- **Morphology**—form
- **Syntax**—grammar
- **Semantics**—meaning
- **Pragmatics**—social aspects/language use

The development of language is influenced by several factors. First, children begin to learn language by interpreting environmental experiences and affecting events. For example, when a child cries and a caregiver responds, he learns that his communication results in attention. When children suffer from motor, sensory, cognitive, and linguistic impairments, their ability to affect the environment is altered. For example, weak cries and decreased facial expressions impair the child's ability to communicate intent. In response, the child's communicative attempts are not reinforced and a passive nature develops. A second factor in the development of language is parent-child interaction. Parents assist in stimulating the child's language by reacting to verbal and nonverbal communication. When communicating with an unresponsive child, parents often become frustrated by the lack of communication and limit their own interaction. Without reciprocity from the parent, it is difficult for normal language and communication skills to develop. A final factor affecting language development is experience. Children learn language by modeling their peers. For children with CP, motor and cognitive deficits limit their interactions with peers and the opportunities for language development (Solot, 1998).

Language deficits associated with CP have several possible etiologies, which include damage to the language-processing areas of the brain, mental retardation, hearing and vision loss, and attention disorders. The specific language impairments developed by the child with CP depend on the site of the lesion in the brain.

Learning Disabilities

When a child has normal cognitive functioning with isolated deficits in learning, he is said to have a **learning disability** (LD) (Trauner, 1988). The result is an impaired ability to read, write, organize, spell, think, and listen. The two main areas of dysfunction associated with learning disabilities are processing and discrepancies in achievement. A person with an LD processes information differently than people not affected by the disorder. Processing involves the reception, use, storage, retrieval, and expression of information. When processing is impaired, the result is compromised understanding and use of written and spoken language. The discrepancy occurs between the person's ability and achievement. Despite normal cognitive functioning, the LD impairs performance and the child appears to be lower functioning. Since the characteristics of LD are associated with higher-level functioning, the disorder is not diagnosed until preschool or the early school years (Gersh, 1991). Consequences of a learning disability can include **dyslexia** (severely impaired reading skills), **dysgraphia** (severely impaired writing skills), and difficulty with reading comprehension, written and oral expression, and auditory processing.

Other impairments can occur in conjunction with CP that are neither motor- nor sensory-based. However, like the motor and sensory disorders, these impairments affect the child's social skills, academic achievement, and daily functioning. These additional impairments include growth issues, seizures, behavioral issues, and attention deficits.

Additional Impairments

Growth Issues

Delayed growth can be caused by poor nutrition or neurological factors. Since swallowing difficulties are common, the child may not take in enough nutrition to increase height or weight. Hormone imbalances caused by damage to the brain may also stunt growth (Miller & Bachrach, 1995). Muscles that are too weak or too tight also affect the growth of the child. Meals commonly take an hour to complete, with little food having been ingested. Poor lip closure and a tongue thrust also contribute to the loss of food. Therefore, the child does not receive adequate calories and nutrition to grow at a normal rate.

Seizures

Seizures occur when there is an episode of disorganized activity in the brain that results in abnormal involuntary movements or alterations of consciousness (Pellegrino & Dormans, 1998). They may involve one or both hemispheres of the brain and range in severity from mild to severe. Grand mal seizures typically occur in children with CP. This type of seizure involves the entire body and includes a loss of consciousness, alternating rigidity and relaxation, and periods of lethargy or disorientation (Miller & Bachrach, 1995). Myoclonic seizures are less severe and include brief periods of involuntary jerking of the arms and legs. Most seizures can be controlled with medication.

Behavioral Issues

Behavioral issues are not any more common in children with CP than in children with normal development; however, they do occur. One type of behavior problem is **self-injurious behaviors** (SIB), which are chronic and repetitive behaviors that a person inflicts on self to cause physical harm. They include head banging; pinching, biting, and scratching oneself; and repeated vomiting (Miller & Bachrach, 1995). Behavior modification programs are required to decrease the behaviors.

Children with CP have limited control over their environment. Their physical impairments limit their ability to react when upset (e.g., run out of the room) or to break a rule (e.g., purposefully run the wrong way in a race). To compensate, they often develop behavioral control issues. For example, the child may not open his mouth during feeding as a way to manipulate the environment. He may drive in the wrong direction during a power wheelchair race or ignore verbal directions. The opposite behaviors may be seen in more passive children. Some children are content to sit in a room without causing disruption. Their low affect and docile nature sometimes compromise their success in school. If a child does not require a great deal of attention, he or she may be ignored by a caregiver or teacher and receive limited interaction.

Attention Deficits

Children with learning problems often have a mixture of symptoms that include inattention, distractibility, impulsivity, and hyperactivity (Vigil & van Kleeck, 1996). These difficulties affect their academic progress, social interactions, and self-control. For children with CP, attention deficits further segregate them from their nondisabled peers. These deficits impact their ability to make friends, play with others, and follow the rules of a game. Impulsivity can impact test scores when the child chooses an answer before fully processing the information. Group participation in class is difficult for children with CP as they daydream or call out an answer instead of raising their hand. Medication and compensatory strategies can be used to assist the child in decreasing attention deficits and improving academic and social skills. The varying impairments associated with CP make the input of numerous professionals essential. These professionals interact to provide comprehensive assessment and therapeutic services for the child.

MULTIDISCIPLINARY MANAGEMENT

A multidisciplinary evaluation of the child with CP is essential to determine strengths and weaknesses and identify the need for intervention. While CP itself is not progressive, there are many co-occurring impairments that affect cognition and communication. For example, most learning disabilities are not identified until the child is close to age 5. The course of CP is difficult to predict due to the variability of the co-occurring impairments. Therefore, consistent monitoring provides for early identification of changes in functioning. The input of professionals representing various areas of expertise assists in determining and maintaining the most appropriate services for the child. These professionals include:

- **Orthopod**: a doctor who specializes in medical and surgical treatment of the bones, joints, and ligaments
- **Developmental pediatrician**: a doctor who works with children with developmental disabilities
- **Physical therapist**: a therapist who provides assessment and intervention for gross motor impairments
- **Occupational therapist**: a therapist who provides assessment and intervention for fine motor impairments
- Speech-language pathologist: a therapist who provides assessment and intervention for speech, language, oral motor, and communication skills
- **Social worker**: a person who assists families in coping with their social, emotional, physical, or financial needs
- **Special educator**: a person who provides specialized education services for people with emotional, physical, or social disabilities
- **Psychologist**: a person who provides counseling and makes recommendations for issues relating to behavior

Team Approaches

When a group of professionals evaluates and treats a child, one of following three approaches is followed: multidisciplinary approach, interdisciplinary approach, or transdisciplinary approach (Pellegrino & Meyer, 1998), as discussed below.

- Multidisciplinary approach: this type of intervention involves a varied group of professionals who treat the child independently of each other, frequently in the same place. The shared location of the professionals allows for collaborative opportunities.
- Interdisciplinary approach: this type of intervention involves professionals who work together to solve issues and problems. For example, an occupational therapist and a speech-language pathologist collaborate on a child's feeding assessment to ensure that fine motor issues and swallowing are both addressed appropriately.
- Transdisciplinary approach: this type of intervention involves professionals who address similar goals and utilize similar methods. For example, a special educator and a speech-language pathologist (SLP) may use the same method to improve sequencing goals.

For the child with CP, the interdisciplinary approach is the most effective because this assessment style allows for the improved coordination of care and an agreement regarding the goals being addressed. Some of the most important people involved in the interdisciplinary management are the child's family members.

Family Involvement

Family members play an important role in the management of the child's intervention. Pincus (2000) reported that family support and personal determination are two of the most important aspects that decide which individuals with CP will most likely achieve their long-term goals. While the interdisciplinary team of professionals can make suggestions for the child, it is family who ultimately makes the decisions regarding the child's care. In addition, the family is responsible for following through on the therapy recommendations. For example, the child may need to wear braces every night to lengthen the hamstrings or drink thickened liquids to prevent aspiration. Active family participation and support assist in creating the most complete and appropriate program for the child.

SPEECH AND LANGUAGE ASSESSMENT

The continued assessment of children with CP is essential due to the variable nature of the co-occurring impairments. For children with CP, the speech and language assessment process can be a long one. Impulsivity, attention difficulties, behavioral issues, cognitive impairment, and physical limitations may play a part in complicating the assessment. The assessment process, completed by a speech-language pathologist (SLP), involves two types of testing: formal and informal. Both components are necessary to ensure that the SLP gains the whole picture of the child.

Formal Testing

Formal or standardized testing is important in identifying the child's strengths and weaknesses. Tests are chosen based on the child's age, ability, and extent of physical limitations (Gersh, 1991). However, there are no tests normed for children with CP and, therefore, the children's true skills may not be represented. For example, a child's dysarthric speech may negatively affect the outcome of expressive language testing or physical limitations may limit the manual manipulation of objects required for some testing items. A complete formal assessment by the SLP should test several areas, including:

- Receptive language
- Expressive language
- Speech
- Vocabulary
- Pragmatics
- Oral motor skills
- Memory
- Auditory comprehension
- Literacy

It is important for the evaluator to note any characteristics that may be indicative of a learning disability, as the child would benefit from early intervention. In addition, any behavioral issues, distractibility, or impulsivity should be documented during testing, as they will negatively affect school performance.

For children with CP who demonstrate physical limitations, distractibility, or increased response time, modifications within the formal assessment process may be necessary to assist them in completing the test items. These modifications may include:

- Use of a word processor for completing written work
- Use of an augmentative and alternative communication device to answer questions
- A quiet room without distractions

- Testing broken down into several sessions to avoid fatigue
- Repetition of directions for children with auditory processing difficulties
- Frequent redirection to task
- Enlargement of testing pictures for children who are visually impaired
- Use of eye gaze when physical impairments limit pointing abilities
- Untimed testing for those children with physical impairments or delayed processing

The results of standardized testing do not always coincide with the child's functional potential. A child who achieves a high score in a quiet testing area may not be able to perform in a classroom full of distractions. In addition, a child who does not test well might be stronger in the functional use of the skills. Therefore, the use of informal testing is essential to gain information about the child in her or his naturalistic setting.

Informal Testing

The use of informal testing provides the SLP with information regarding the child's performance when no testing demands are placed on him or her. While this type of testing does not provide the examiner with age equivalents or standard scores, it gives an accurate picture of the child's functional speech and language skills. Two types of informal testing are interview and behavioral observation.

Interviews

The use of interviews can provide insight into the child's function in the natural environment, and frequently identifies problems that were not evidenced in formal testing (Gerring & Carney, 1992). For children who do not perform well in a testing situation, the parent interview is essential for providing information regarding the child's true skills. It is important, however, that the clinician record that this information was by parent report and not directly observed. Though parent report of children's language skills is often a valid proxy, parents may have the tendency to exaggerate their child's skills. Therefore, the use of "by report" will qualify the information.

Interviews with teachers are also important. Like the parent, the teacher interacts with the child on a daily basis and becomes aware of her or his strengths and weaknesses. The information provided by the teacher will be helpful in determining classroom modifications and functional speech and language goals that will enhance classroom learning.

Behavioral Observations

The SLP should also observe the child in a variety of settings to determine how effectively he or she communicates and understands in each one (see Figure 2-3). Gerring and Carney (1992) named several aspects that should be taken into consideration when interpreting an observation. These are:

- Parameters of the task
- Environmental factors
- Guidelines for assessing the quality or quantity of the behavior
- Degree of cueing and compensation required to complete the task

Given the large number of variables included in observation interpretation, it is necessary to complete several observations in a variety of settings. Once the assessment process is complete, specific goals for speech and language intervention are created and implemented.

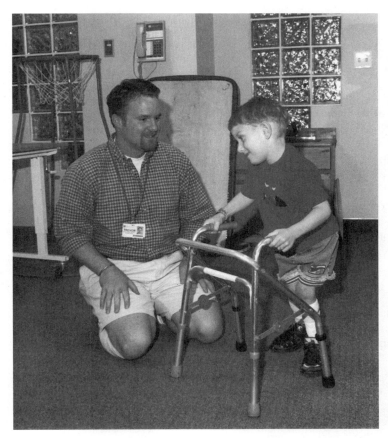

Figure 2-3
An SLP performs multiple behavioral observations of a child with cerebral palsy to assess his communication skills.

SPEECH AND LANGUAGE INTERVENTION

Though CP is not progressive, it requires intervention that will assist in maintaining or improving the child's current level of functioning. The SLP, in conjunction with other professionals, is responsible for several aspects of the child's intervention. These areas include speech, language, oral motor/feeding, and communication.

Speech Disorders

Speech disorders may include developmental articulation errors and motor speech disorders (dysarthria and apraxia). Traditional articulation therapy can be utilized when the articulation errors are developmental in nature and not associated with motor involvement. Intervention for motor speech disorders is more complicated. The therapist must focus on improving oral motor skills, respiration, vocal quality, and resonance. The underlying neuromotor impairment of motor speech disorders may make intelligible speech an unrealistic goal for the child (Yorkston et al., 1988). If the motor speech disorder is too severe and not improving with intervention, then alternate forms of communication should be considered.

Communication

Communicative impairments can occur as a result of a motor speech disorder, placement of a tracheostomy tube, cognitive delay, or other impairment. When traditional speech and language therapy techniques are unsuccessful, alternative forms of communication can be explored. **Augmentative and alternative communication** (AAC) is defined as communication methods that range from the use of gestures, sign language, and facial expressions to the use of alphabet or picture boards and sophisticated computer systems (Glennen, 1997). The purpose of AAC is to augment (supplement) or act as an alternative to speech. For example, a child with CP can use an AAC device to interact with friends, participate in the morning opening exercises, and make choices throughout the day. Communication intervention is an essential part of intervention due to the number of children with CP who have impaired speech skills. Alternative forms of communication not only provide the child with a means of expression, they also assist in improving self-concept when they are used to answer questions in class.

Language Disorders

The language impairments of children with CP vary depending on the severity of involvement. Language intervention focuses on improving skills in the areas of pragmatics, receptive and expressive language disorders, and oral motor and feeding disorders.

Pragmatics

According to Bernstein (1993), the most important area of linguistic growth during the school-age years is in language use, or pragmatics. During this time, children begin to develop conversational and presuppositional skills. They become more aware of their conversational partner's needs. For children with CP, speech impairments and a lack of social interaction may limit the use of pragmatics. The role of the SLP is to present the child with social situations to allow for increased conversational opportunities and experience. These should occur in small group or classroom settings to ensure that all of the child's pragmatic needs are being addressed. This type of intervention supports a functional approach to pragmatic improvement.

Receptive and Expressive Language

Deficits in the areas of receptive and expressive language are common in children with CP due to developmental disabilities, learning disabilities, or lack of experience. Because language is a crucial part of academics (i.e., spatial and temporal concepts in math, descriptive concepts and writing stories in English, and following complex directions in science), the SLP frequently works in conjunction with the child's teacher. The SLP can introduce strategies that the child can generalize to the classroom. In addition, the SLP can provide support in the classroom to ensure that the child keeps pace with peers.

Children with CP often demonstrate deficits in vocabulary skills. Vocabulary is developed through experiences such as social interaction and exploring new situations. For children with CP, some of these experiences may be limited due to physical impairments. The SLP works to improve the child's vocabulary by providing these experiences through thematic units (i.e., all vocabulary is associated with one topic), reading books, and firsthand experiences. When poor vocabulary skills are related more to neurological deficits than to a lack of experience, the SLP must provide the child with compensatory strategies in conjunction with the experiential intervention.

Oral Motor/Feeding

Poor **oral motor** skills affect the child's ability to speak, eat, and manage drooling. In order to manage the varied swallowing and feeding issues of the young child, individualized treatment plans must be developed (Arvedson, 1993). The SLP customizes an oral motor stimulation program consisting of deep pressure and stroking of the lips, tongue, cheeks, and gums. The deep pressure assists in improving muscle tone, while the stroking works to provide sensory input and alleviate oral defensiveness. The SLP must also determine how these weak oral motor skills affect swallowing and feeding.

The SLP works in conjunction with the occupational therapist to determine a feeding program for the child. For some children with impaired chewing and swallowing patterns, alterations to their diet are necessary. The SLP may recommend pureed foods or thickened liquids to ensure the child's safety when eating. Intervention may also include the introduction of adaptive equipment to assist the child in feeding herself or himself. This equipment may consist of dishes with "lips" for easier scooping and curved spoons for improved access to the mouth.

The SLP plays many roles in the intervention of the child with CP. However, each role is an important one. These children adapt to new situations more successfully when they receive early intervention. Through the early intervention process, the child receives the modifications needed to be mobile, to communicate, to feed self, and to gain independence. This intervention assists in creating a more positive self-image for the child, which is necessary as he or she enters school. However, children with CP often develop psychosocial issues and require professional intervention due to the physical differences caused by their impairment.

PSYCHOSOCIAL ISSUES

Young children with cerebral palsy are frequently unaware that they are different from other children their age. Their determination and ability to modify tasks lead them to the belief that they can do whatever their friends do. As they enter school, they become increasingly aware of their disability. It is not uncommon for children with CP to ask when they can stop using a walker or start writing with a pencil. Since many children with CP do not have cognitive impairments, they begin to realize that this disorder is permanent and that it makes them different from others. Therefore, building self-esteem is essential for children with CP so they feel a sense of belonging and develop relationships with their peer group.

School Age

When children with CP enter elementary school, they begin to develop an awareness of their differences. They may be unable to attend their community school with their siblings and friends because it is not accessible. Participation in gym, music, or art classes may be difficult due to motor impairments. At this age, these children should be given information about their disability so they can develop personal motivation and investment in dealing with their personal issues (Trachtenberg & Rouse, 1998).

The family's acceptance of the disorder is key in helping the child cope. The child should be included in family activities, chore lists, and decisions. When parents and siblings view the child as worthwhile, the child generally has a good self-image (Trachtenburg & Rouse, 1998). A positive self-concept will assist the child outside the home as well.

People outside of the home environment, like classmates, may not be as accepting as family members. Children may tease or exclude the child with CP from activities. Teachers can play a vital role in assisting the child in development of a sense of belonging by creating situations where she or he can succeed. However, teachers who are unfamiliar with CP may not have the knowledge of adaptations that can assist the inclusion of the child.

Adolescence

The impairments of CP make adolescence an even more difficult time for the teenager with CP, who must cope with physical differences as well as typical adolescent issues such as identity crises, varied emotions, increased independence, and peer pressure.

During adolescence, teenagers begin to develop a sense of independence by obtaining a driver's license and attending activities without their parents. Motor impairments often prohibit adolescents with CP from gaining this independence. They may be forced to rely on their parents for transportation, assistance with hygiene, or even feeding. All of these factors work to isolate these teenagers from their peer group.

Most adolescents with CP have the same sexual feelings as those of their peers. However, a history of ridicule or rejection may make them unwilling to chance dating (Miller & Bachrach, 1995). Poor self-image caused by delayed growth may also inhibit these teenagers from seeking a relationship.

It is during the adolescent years that most parents seek counseling for their children with CP. The social and emotional issues that they face may become too overwhelming for the teenagers and their families. Therefore, professional advice is invaluable in assisting the teenagers in pursuing activities in which they can be successful.

Young Adulthood

The transition to adulthood continues to be a social and emotional trial for young adults with CP. It is during this time that they may desire to move out of their parents' house and into an independent setting. However, the impairments of CP often dictate that the young adult have some supervision or assistance in his or her new home (Trachtenburg & Rouse, 1998). During this time, people determine their career path in life. Career choices may be limited more by motor impairments than by cognitive issues. Assistive devices are available to increase employment opportunities for people with CP and integrate them into a workplace. For example, voice recognition software allows a person to use the voice as a replacement for hands when creating a word processing document. In addition, joysticks, similar to those on power wheelchairs, serve as an alternate access method for persons who have difficulty controlling a computer mouse.

In their study, Magill-Evans and Restall (1991) found that adolescents with CP showed an increase in self-esteem as they entered young adulthood. This increase may be attributed to greater choice of environments in which to interact, reduced exposure to negative situations, or increased independence to choose activities in which they are successful. For adults with CP, quality of life is primarily influenced by the attitudes they have toward themselves and the attitudes of other people. The participation of all parties involved and the acceptance of professional guidance can assist the person with CP and loved ones in overcoming the physical limitations associated with CP (Miller & Bachrach, 1995).

The impairments of CP can deeply affect the social and emotional well-being of anyone diagnosed with the disorder. Familial acceptance, professional advice, and participation in activities for people with disabilities (i.e., Special Olympics) can assist in building a strong self-image. A positive self-concept will lead the person with CP to personal and professional success.

CONCLUSION

The effects of CP vary from one child to another. The severity and location of the brain damage play a major role in the manifestation of the CP. The effects of the disorder can range from complete physical and cognitive involvement to a barely noticeable limp. Each child is unique and his or her needs should be assessed and met based on specific strengths and needs.

Cerebral palsy can severely affect language and speech production, communication, and swallowing. These impairments can impact the child's socialization, academics, and vocation goals. Therefore, timely assessment and intervention play an integral part in preparing the child for the future. Due to the multiple impairments that can co-occur, assessment and intervention must be ongoing processes.

Family members play an important role in supporting the child with CP. Once family members accept and understand the child's disability, they can work to assist the child in understanding the disorder and creating a positive self-concept. Parent advocacy helps the child receive beneficial services. The most successful multidisciplinary team is one that includes the parents. The team of people who work with children with CP is an interdisciplinary group of professionals who work together to meet the child's needs. Frequent co-treatment and consultations occur to ensure that comprehensive treatment is provided.

The occurrence of CP has remained constant over the past several years due to medical advances that have decreased the morbidity rate of newborns. Since CP is not curable, continued development of assistive devices, medical and surgical interventions, knowledgeable professionals, and acceptance is essential in helping the person with CP meet personal and professional goals.

Case Study 1: The Effects of CP on a Preschool Child

Tameka is a 7-year-old female who presents with spastic quadriplegia. Therefore, her motor impairment is characterized by muscle rigidity in all four extremities and limited range of motion. Her co-occurring impairments include strabismus, developmental delay, reactive airway disease, and status post orthopedic surgery.

Tameka was born prematurely at 26 weeks' gestation and developed respiratory distress syndrome (RDS), a pulmonary disease caused by pneumonia, aspiration, or a traumatic injury that often results in respiratory failure or pulmonary edema. She was diagnosed with retinopathy of prematurity that did not severely impair her vision. However, strabismus and refractive errors are noted and have been corrected with surgery and glasses, respectively.

Due to her motor impairments, Tameka is unable to sit independently or walk. She uses a power wheelchair for mobility, which she operates with a joystick. When she began using her power chair, Tameka demonstrated visual-perceptual difficulties that caused her to veer to the left and bump into walls. A large orange line was painted in the middle of the hallway as a guide for Tameka when she drove her wheelchair. This cue assisted her in paying attention and improving her "driving" skills. Ankle foot orthoses

(AFOs) are worn to maintain proper positioning of Tameka's ankles and feet. Due to increased tightness in her hamstrings and calves, she underwent muscle lengthening surgery in September 2000. This is a process where the muscles are clipped to allow for stretching and lengthening. Periodically, Tameka receives botox injections that paralyze her rigid muscles and cause them to relax slightly. The effect of each injection lasts approximately 6 months.

Tameka's hand skills are poor due to low tone. She is unable to dress herself independently or write. She uses a portable word processor to complete any written work. Hand splints are utilized to maintain proper finger and wrist positioning. Tameka cannot straighten her arms completely to give a hug, but is able to hug with her arms bent. The grasp she maintains is tight and often difficult for her to release voluntarily. Tameka's favorite activity in occupational therapy is painting her therapist's fingernails. While Tameka is having fun, her therapist is improving Tameka's grasp on objects and her fine motor skills.

Tameka demonstrates poor oral motor skills that result in feeding issues. Due to a history of aspiration, her food is chopped and her liquids are slightly thickened. She uses a scoop dish, curved spoon, feeding platform (to raise her bowl), and two-handled cup to improve her self-feeding skills.

Tameka receives individual speech and language therapy two times per week and therapy within her classroom setting one time per week. Speech skills are affected by dysarthria. Her speech is characterized by imprecise sound production and final consonant deletion. Vocal quality is normal except for occasional breathiness. Intelligibility of speech is judged to be fair to good and has improved over the past few years.

Receptive language skills are on a 4 to 4.5 year level. Tameka demonstrates difficulty following complex directions and understanding quantity concepts, passive voice sentences, and part/whole relationships. She requires the repetition of oral directions. Tameka is distracted by noises outside of her classroom and requires frequent redirection to task. Expressive language skills are on a 2.5 to 3 year level and are negatively affected by dysarthria, which influences the length and syntax of her sentences. Tameka demonstrates difficulty using prepositions and answering "wh" questions. Her conversational speech is characterized by sentences of four to five words in length, which frequently begin with "I" (i.e., "I want that toy," "I go my house"). She is able to ask answer simple questions and maintain eye contact. Topic maintenance skills are poor. Vocabulary skills coincide with Tameka's language skills.

Tameka receives services in a special education classroom with one teacher, one teacher's aide, and seven children with disabilities. She learns math, reading, writing, and English, but at a much slower pace than her nondisabled peers. Tameka learns most successfully through functional activities in the classroom and appears to have difficulty grasping abstract concepts. She is learning to spell and completes all of her written homework and class work on her word processor.

Tameka requires the assistance of a teacher's aide for toileting and for food setup in the cafeteria. She suffers from chronic asthma and receives nebulization treatments (the process by which medication is administered in a mist form through the nose and mouth) three times per day.

Family support is limited. Tameka's mother frequently misses her daughter's meetings and often fails to give Tameka her glasses. Communication between home and school is poor.

Tameka is an outgoing and determined child. She has become very independent and often says, "I can do it myself." She appears unaware of her differences and has developed a positive self-concept. Tameka attends music and art classes with her nondisabled peers. They accept her because she is so friendly and willing to participate. Her peers are anxious to carry Tameka's books or hand her project supplies. The children enjoy sitting next to Tameka and gladly oblige when she asks them to hold her hand. When Tameka becomes excited, the muscles in her extremities tighten, resulting in arm and leg extension.

Tameka demonstrates typical characteristics of a child with CP. Her gross and fine motor skills, vision, speech, language, attention, pragmatics, and feeding skills are all affected by the disorder. She is part of a special education classroom due to her co-occurring developmental delay. Tameka receives physical, occupational, and speech and language therapies and is followed by an orthopod. Her impairments will not progress, but Tameka will require intervention for the remainder of her life to maintain her skills.

Case Study 2: The Effects of CP on an Adolescent

Donny is a 16-year-old male who presents with spastic quadriplegia and severe to profound mental retardation. He has received special education services in a self-contained classroom since age 3. In addition, speech-language therapy, physical therapy, and occupational therapy are provided on a consultative basis.

Donny's motor skills are severely impaired. He has limited use of his upper and lower extremities bilaterally due to high muscle tone. Donny uses a manual wheelchair and is dependent for mobility. His physical therapist attempted training with a power chair, but she was unable to identify a body part that would consistently operate the controls. To allow Donny the opportunity to bear weight and stretch his hamstring and calf muscles, he is often placed in a prone stander. This device allows him to stand up while straps support his back and legs. However, he can stay in this device for only 20 minutes before fatigue sets in.

Donny's hand skills are poor. Due to high muscle tone, he is unable to grasp an object for more than 10 seconds. Therefore, he is unable to feed or dress himself, or complete simple craft activities. Donny's teacher uses adapted equipment to allow him to participate in classroom activities. When Donny is required to cut paper, his teacher attaches battery-powered scissors to a communication switch. Donny's activation of the switch powers the scissors as his teacher guides them over the paper. This technique provides Donny with control over the situation and allows him to participate in the activity.

Donny's oral motor skills are weak. He demonstrates an open mouth posture and high tone in his cheeks and tongue. He uses his tongue to mash the food against his hard palate. He does not lateralize the food or chew. His occupational therapist began placing small pieces of toast on Donny's molars to encourage chewing. Donny has eaten regular chopped foods for most of his life. His SLP began to observe coughing and a wet vocal quality after Donny ate. Donny was referred for a modified barium swallow (MBS), a test that utilizes barium-coated food and x-ray machines to observe the patient's swallow. The results of the MBS showed that Donny was aspirating regular textured foods and thin liquids. Therefore, he was put on a pureed diet with thickened liquids. Since his diet modifications, Donny's coughing has decreased and vocal quality has improved.

Donny is dependent on others for toileting and bathing. He is unable to indicate that he has to go to the bathroom, so he wears adult diapers throughout the day. A bath chair, a chair with supports that sits in the bathtub, is used to assist Donny's mother in bathing him. However, since Donny entered his teenage years, it has become more difficult for his mother to lift him in and out of his bath chair. Eventually, she will require human or mechanical assistance in transporting her son in and out of his chair.

Speech skills are limited. Due to weak oral musculature and high tone, Donny is able to produce only one word ("yeah") and vocalizations. He has used a communication device since 1996. At the time, the device was programmed with four pictures that allowed Donny to communicate basic wants and needs. With daily practice and encouragement, he now has 20 pictures per page. Donny is able to navigate independently throughout the various pages on his device using visual scanning and a switch that he accesses with his head. His doctors initially gave Donny the diagnosis of severe to profound mental retardation. However, use of the communication device has allowed Donny to display his cognitive skills accurately. He has begun sight reading words, telling the weather, making choices, and reporting sports scores. Use of the communication device has increased Donny's participation in social and academic classroom activities.

Standardized testing reveals that Donny's receptive language skills are on a 3 to 3.5 year level. However, informal observations suggest that these skills are higher. As previously stated, Donny is able to use his communication device to identify letters and colors and to make decisions. Due to physical limitations, he is not able to complete many of the items on standardized tests accurately. Therefore, observing Donny's functional comprehension of language appears to be the most effective way to obtain information regarding his strengths and needs. Expressive language skills are on a 6 month to 1 year level and are negatively affected by Donny's poor speech skills.

Donny receives special education services in a self-contained classroom that consists of 10 students, one special educator, and three teacher's assistants. While positioning, toileting, and eating occupy a large portion of his day, Donny also receives instruction on current events, sequencing, colors, numbers, and spelling. He appears to enjoy learning and likes to use his communication device to be the first student to answer a question. When Donny is age 21, he will graduate from his school. However, the transition process has already begun so that Donny will have a smooth transition to his next placement. He will either attend an adult day program or be employed at a sheltered workshop where he can complete simple computer activities.

Donny has a great deal of family support. His mother is a single parent who gave birth to Donny when she was 16 years old. She receives assistance from family members, but prefers to be her son's main care provider. Donny's mother is a strong advocate for her son, as she attends all of his meetings and verbalizes concerns. Though her literacy skills are limited, she learned how to program Donny's communication device so that he could share his home experiences with classmates. Financially, Donny's mother relies on her son's social workers to assist in securing funds for a wheelchair ramp, bath chair, and accessible van. Donny has a strong relationship with his mother and squeals with joy when her name is mentioned.

Donny is an outgoing and friendly teenager. He likes to listen to rock music, report the baseball scores, and use his friendly smile to flirt with girls. Like any teenager, Donny is emotional and becomes upset when his routine is interrupted. He enjoys private time in his room as much as socializing with friends. As his verbal abilities have increased through the use of his communication device, so has his interaction with others. His mother hopes that one day Donny will be able to be a greeter at a department store. She feels that he can use his communication device and welcoming brown eyes to greet the customers as they enter the store. Donny's strong personality and determination will assist him as he prepares to transition to adulthood.

Though Donny's CP affects his mobility, speech, feeding skills, and independence, he is just like any other teenager. Adapted equipment, supportive family, intensive therapy, and caring teachers have given Donny a strong foundation for the future. His determination and easygoing personality will assist him in living a happy and satisfying life.

REVIEW QUESTIONS

1. What information would you give parents of a child with CP and dysarthria to convince them that use of an AAC device would encourage rather than discourage natural speech production?

2. Discuss why a high incidence (75 percent) of MR co-occurs with CP.

3. Compare and contrast characteristics of apraxia and dysarthria. What are the main differential diagnoses?

4. Though CP cannot be cured, discuss the various types of intervention that would inhibit the decline of motor skills.

5. When assessing a child with CP, do you think it is most beneficial to compare the child's skills with those of same age nondisabled peers (through standardized testing) or to use informal testing to gain knowledge of functional skills? Why?

6. Why after age 5 does a child receive a diagnosis of TBI rather than CP after an injury?

7. Discuss the pros and cons of letting a child with spastic quadriplegia who has severe motor involvement and normal cognitive skills attend an included or regular school classroom rather than a special needs school or classroom.

8. How would poor trunk control, weak oral motor skills, and poor hand skills negatively affect a child with CP's ability to feed himself or herself?

REFERENCES

Anderson, S. (1991). Daily care. In E. Geralis (Ed.), *Children with cerebral palsy: A parents' guide* (pp. 91–131). Bethesda, MD: Woodbine House.

Arvedson, J. C. (1993). Management of swallowing problems. In J. C. Arvedson & L. Brodsky (Eds.), *Pediatric swallowing and feeding* (pp. 327–387). Clifton Park, NY: Delmar Learning.

Bach, J. R., & Ishikawa, Y. (2000). Respiratory insufficiency: Pathophysiology, indications, and other considerations for intervention. In D. C. Tippett (Ed.), *Tracheostomy and ventilator dependency* (pp. 47–64). New York: Thieme.

Bernstein, D. K. (1993). Language development: The school age years. In D. K. Bernstein & E. T. Tiegerman (Eds.), *Language and communication disorders in children* (pp. 123–145). New York: Macmillan.

Blacklin, J. S. (1991). Your child's development. In E. Geralis (Ed.), *Children with cerebral palsy: A parents' guide* (pp. 175–208). Bethesda, MD: Woodbine House.

Brookshire, R. H. (1997). *Introduction to neurogenic communication disorders.* St. Louis, MO: Mosby.

Carter, C. R., Yorkston, K. M., Strand, E. A., & Hammen, V. L. (1996). Effects of semantic and syntactic context on actual and estimated sentence intelligibility of dysarthric speakers. In D. A. Robin, K. M. Yorkston, & D. R. Beukelman (Eds.), *Disorders of motor speech* (pp. 67–87). Baltimore: Paul H. Brookes.

Dikeman, K. J., & Kazandjian, M. S. (2003). *Communication and swallowing management of tracheostomized and ventilator-dependent adults* (2nd ed.). Clifton Park, NY: Delmar Learning.

Driver, L. E. (2000). Pediatric considerations. In D. C. Tippett (Ed.), *Tracheostomy and ventilator dependency* (pp. 193–235). New York: Thieme.

Duffy, J. R. (1995). *Motor speech disorders.* St. Louis, MO: Mosby.

Foltz, L. C., DeGangi, G., & Lewis, D. (1991). Physical therapy, occupational therapy, and speech and language therapy. In E. Geralis (Ed.), *Children with cerebral palsy: A parents' guide* (pp. 209–260). Bethesda, MD: Woodbine House.

Gerring, J. P., & Carney, J. M. (1992). *Head trauma: Strategies for educational reintegration.* Clifton Park, NY: Delmar Learning.

Gersh, E. S. (1991). What is cerebral palsy? In E. Geralis (Ed.), *Children with cerebral palsy: A parents' guide* (pp. 1–32). Bethesda, MD: Woodbine House.

Glennen, S. L. (1997). Introduction to augmentative and alternative communication. In S. L. Glennen & D. C. Decoste (Eds.), *Handbook of augmentative and alternative communication* (pp. 3–19). Clifton Park, NY: Delmar Learning.

Hall, P. K., Jordan, L. S., & Robin, D. A. (1993). *Developmental apraxia of speech.* Austin, TX: Pro-Ed.

Love, R. J., & Webb, W. G. (1996). *Neurology for the speech-language pathologist.* Boston: Butterworth-Heinemann.

Magill-Evans, J. E., & Restall, G. (1991). Self-esteem of persons with cerebral palsy: From adolescence to adulthood. *American Journal of Occupational Therapy, 45,* 819–825.

Miller, F., & Bachrach, S. J. (1995). *Cerebral palsy: A complete guide for caregiving.* Baltimore: Johns Hopkins University Press.

National Information Center for Children and Youth with Disabilities. (1997). *General information about cerebral palsy.* Retrieved October 21, 2001, from http://www.kidsource.com/NICHCY/index.html.

Pellegrino, L., & Dormans, J. P. (1998). Definitions, etiology, and epidemiology of cerebral palsy. In J. P. Dormans & L. Pellegrino (Eds.), *Caring for the children with cerebral palsy* (pp. 3–30). Baltimore: Paul H. Brookes.

Pellegrino, L., & Dormans, J. P. (1998). Making the diagnosis of cerebral palsy. In J. P. Dormans & L. Pellegrino (Eds.), *Caring for the children with cerebral palsy* (pp. 31–54). Baltimore: Paul H. Brookes.

Pellegrino, L., & Meyer, G. (1998). Interdisciplinary care of the child with cerebral palsy. In J. P. Dormans & L. Pellegrino (Eds.), *Caring for the children with cerebral palsy* (pp. 55–70). Baltimore: Paul H. Brookes.

Pincus, D. (2000). *Everything you need to know about cerebral palsy.* New York: Rosen.

Solot, C. B. (1998). Promoting function: Communication. In J. P. Dormans & L. Pellegrino (Eds.), *Caring for the children with cerebral palsy* (pp. 347–389). Baltimore: Paul H. Brookes.

Trachtenburg, S. W., & Rouse, C. F. (1998). The family. In J. P. Dormans & L. Pellegrino (Eds.), *Caring for the children with cerebral palsy* (pp. 429–445). Baltimore: Paul H. Brookes.

Trauner, D. A. (1988). Learning disabilities. In W. C. Wiederholt (Ed.), *Neurology for the non-neurologists* (pp. 309–319). Philadelphia: W. B. Saunders.

United Cerebral Palsy Association. (2001). *Education.* Retrieved October 21, 2001, from http://www.ucpa.org.

Vigil, A., & van Kleeck, A. (1996). Clinical language teaching: Theories and principles to guide our responses when children miss our language targets. In M. D. Smith & J. S. Damico (Eds.), *Childhood language disorders* (pp. 64–96). New York: Thieme Medical.

Yorkston, K. M., Beukelman, D. R., & Bell, K. R. (1988). *Clinical management of dysarthric speakers.* Austin, TX: Pro-Ed.

PART II

Developmental Brain Differences

Chapter 3

Attention Deficit/Hyperactivity Disorder

Lisa Schoenbrodt, Ed.D., CCC-SLP

CHAPTER OBJECTIVES

Upon completing this chapter, the reader should be able to:

1. Define ADD and ADHD
2. Understand the organic bases of attention deficits in children and adolescents
3. Propose additional characteristics to enhance the accepted definitions of ADD and ADHD
4. Understand coexisting conditions associated with ADHD
5. Define Tourette syndrome and identify associated characteristics
6. List the components of a multidisciplinary evaluation for both children and adolescents
7. Present pros and cons associated with interventions for ADHD

INTRODUCTION

Attention deficit/hyperactivity disorder (ADHD) is diagnosed in roughly one student in every classroom, or at a rate of 4 to 5 percent. While the focus of the disorder is on behavioral characteristics of inattention, overactivity, and impulsivity, speech and language characteristics secondary to these may exist. **Speech-language pathologists** (SLPs) and other service providers to this population must be aware of the characteristics that present and the many comorbid disorders that may exist in order to provide the most effective assessment and intervention. The purpose of this chapter is to provide information regarding the organic bases of the disorder, as well as all characteristics, including speech language, and current assessment and intervention approaches.

ADHD is one of the most widely researched areas in childhood and adolescence. The disorder accounts for as many as 40 percent of referrals to child behavioral clinics, and roughly one child in every classroom is identified as hyperactive. According to Barkley (1998), the ratio of males to females diagnosed with ADHD is 3:1. The prevalence rate is related to the fact that other disruptive problems such as oppositional defiant disorder and conduct disorder may coexist in boys, making them more identifiable based on those characteristics. Goldstein (1999) reported that ADHD is a disorder in which the severity of the child's problems results from his or her temperament and the demands of the environment in which the child interacts, indicating a "biophysical" problem. In other words, while biology is clearly involved in the nature of this disorder, the child's environment plays a large role in the level of complaints that arise and the severity of the disorder. As a result, many researchers suggest that ADHD is not a single behavioral disorder but rather a cluster of behavioral problems that are unique to this population.

Etiology

Certain chemicals in the brain permit nerve cells to transmit information. These chemicals, known as neurotransmitters, may be deficient in persons with ADHD. The pathophysiology of ADHD implicates two neurotransmitters in particular: dopamine (DA) and norepinephrine (NE). Dopamine is involved in risk taking, impulsivity, mood, and reward behaviors. Norepinephrine is implicated in attention, arousal, and mood (Dopheide, 2001). Two genes regulate dopamine and, by extension, are associated with ADHD. One gene is the dopamine transporter (DAT1) gene, and is involved in the removal of dopamine from the synapse. The other gene, known as the DRD4 or dopamine receptor gene, determines how sensitive the neurons are to the dopamine. Studies of the brain indicate people with ADHD may have a deficiency in the dopamine receptor gene and an "overexpression" of the dopamine transporter gene (Barkley, 2000; Cook, Stein, Krasowski, Cox, Olkon, Kieffer, et al. 1995; Dopheide, 2001; Swanson & Castellanos, 2001). While current research appears to indicate neurotransmitters are involved in the pathophysiology of ADHD, more research is needed to be conclusive.

In addition to the theory of neurotransmitter involvement, studies have revealed decreased brain activity in the frontal lobe of persons identified with ADHD. The frontal lobe plays a key role in **executive function** and is involved in developing plans and organizing ideas. The frontal lobes are also involved in inhibiting behaviors necessary for attention (e.g., maintaining focus without being distracted by irrelevant stimuli in the environment).

Many studies using electroencephalograph (EEG) analysis also indicate significantly lower brain electrical activity in children with ADHD as compared to those without ADHD (Barkley, 2000; Barababsz & Barababsz, in press). Studies utilizing magnetic resonance imaging (MRI) of brain anatomy reported that children with ADHD had brain volumes that were smaller than normal in the anterior superior and anterior inferior regions. Specifically, deficits were located in the right anterior frontal, caudate, and globus pallidus regions (Castellanos, Giedd, Marsh, Hamburger, Vaituzus, Dickstein, et al., 1996; Fillipek Semrud-Clikeman, Steingard, Renshaw, Kennedy, & Biederman, 1997). More recent studies utilizing positron emission tomography (PET) scans indicated that children with ADD and ADHD showed reduced activity in the left side of the frontal region. In addition to deficiencies in brain structure and neurotransmitters, literature supports the influence of genetics and environment on the etiology of ADHD/ADD (Faraone, Biederman, Mennin, & Russell, 1998).

Genetics

Studies have been conducted comparing the prevalence of ADHD in first-degree relatives (mothers, fathers, siblings) of children with ADHD to the prevalence in family members of children without ADHD. According to those results, over 25 percent of first-degree relatives of children with ADHD also have ADHD versus only 5 percent in the families of children without ADHD (Faraone et al., 1998). Even more persuasive are results from twin studies or the habitability of ADHD, which reported that ADHD is inherited in 80 percent of the cases.

Faraone (2000) reported that the inconsistent results regarding the dopamine transporter and receptor gene create an argument that ADHD may involve several disorders having different genetic and nongenetic etiologies. His work supports the ideas presented by Eaves, Silberg, and Hewitt (1993), who offered two approaches to the genetic analysis of ADHD. The first is the categorical approach, which views ADHD as a distinct condition. The second is the dimensional approach, which characterizes ADHD as a continuous trait. In this model, some people exhibit few to no symptoms of ADHD while others fall along the moderate to severe portions of the continuum. Faraone (2000) suggests that of the two, the dimensional model is better and explains the genetic heterogeneity of the disorder. He bases his idea on the results of prior twin studies that support the argument that a set of genes influences symptoms in persons with ADHD. Someone who has many of these genes will develop ADHD, while someone with fewer genes may have little to no symptoms or fall somewhere in between on the continuum. Studies on a larger scale are needed to continue to support this hypothesis. The final factor that may affect the etiology of ADHD is the child's environment.

Environment

Exposure to toxins during pregnancy, through, for example, smoking, alcohol use, or cocaine abuse, has been linked to abnormalities in the development of the caudate nucleus and the frontal regions of the brain in children. Milberger, Biederman, Faraone, Murphy, and Tsuang (1995) found a significant relationship between the number of cigarettes smoked during pregnancy and the child's risk for developing ADHD. Children exposed to alcohol in utero face similar problems. Children born to alcoholic mothers are more likely to display hyperactive and inattentive behaviors.

Exposure to lead may also be associated with a greater risk for the development of hyperactive and inattentive behaviors. The risk is greater when children are exposed to lead between 12 and 36 months of age. Barkley (2000) reported that high levels of lead in the body injure brain tissue and may cause ADHD.

While not a primary cause, family environment adversity factors are loosely linked to increased rates of ADHD (Dopheide, 2001). Children with ADHD may have more disorganization in their family life which may, in turn, be related to the heredity issue discussed earlier. For example, the child with ADHD may have a parent with ADHD or other psychological or psychiatric problems, which may create more stress in the environment when compared to the child without ADHD. The studies supporting this issue point to the existence of a small subgroup composed of children with serious problems with aggression, defiance, and antisocial behavior. The parents of this subgroup reportedly had more problems with drug abuse, antisocial behavior, and depression. The researchers further contend that the child's ADHD was not the cause of the family problems, which instead were a result of antisocial, defiant behavior (Barkley, 2000).

Many reviews of studies evaluate the etiological factors of ADHD. While more research needs to be conducted for results in this area to be conclusive, the research reported in the previous section shows that ADHD is the result of abnormalities in brain development that are more related to factors involving heredity than those involving environment. With these etiological factors identified, the definition of ADHD can be explored.

DEFINING ADHD

The term *attention deficit disorder* (**ADD**) was originally proposed by the American Psychiatric Association (APA) as a substitute for the term *minimal brain dysfunction* (APA, 1980). The terminology was changed to attention deficit/hyperactivity disorder (ADHD) in 1987. Medical researchers used the term *minimal brain dysfunction* to include a cluster of symptoms including specific learning deficits, hyperkinesis, impulsivity, and short attention span as confirmed by examination of equivocal neurological signs and an EEG that was either borderline abnormal or abnormal. The medical model focused on biological deficits, whereas educational researchers focused on academic and language difficulties and characterized children as having a learning disability.

The publication of the third edition of the *Diagnostic and Statistical Manual of Mental Disorders* (DSM-III) in 1987 represented a significant advance in the establishment of a valid diagnoses of hyperactivity (ADD). The term *ADD* was developed because investigators believed that factors relating to attention, rather than activity levels, were the major symptoms of the disorder (Cantwell, 1983; Douglas & Peters, 1979). DSM-III differentiated between two subtypes of ADD based on the presence or absence of symptoms of hyperactivity, though no clear distinctions were made regarding the two subtypes: attention deficit disorder with hyperactivity (ADHD) and attention deficit disorder without hyperactivity (Epstein, Shaywitz, Shaywitz, & Woolston, 1991). DSM-III-R (1987) added further confusion to the differentiation, focusing on ADHD and classifying attention deficit without hyperactivity in the category of undifferentiated ADD.

The current **DSM-IV-TR** (2000) identifies the diagnostic criteria for attention deficit/hyperactivity disorder as symptoms in the areas of inattention, hyperactivity, and impulsivity that have persisted for at least 6 months and "to a degree that is maladaptive and inconsistent with developmental level" (p. 87). The manual also states that some symptoms must be present before the child is age 7 and in two or more settings, such as at school, at home, in the community, or at work. In addition to the above, the DSM-IV-TR defined Attention Deficit/Hyperactivity Disorder Not Otherwise Specified as a category for disorders that have symptoms similar to ADHD, but do not meet the criteria. The manual identifies the following examples:

1. Individuals whose symptoms and impairment meet the criteria for ADHD, predominantly inattentive type, but whose age at onset is 7 years or older.
2. Individuals with clinically significant impairment who present with inattention and whose symptom pattern does not meet the full criteria for the disorder but have a behavioral pattern marked by sluggishness, daydreaming, and hypoactivity.

The DSM-IV-TR manual specifies the criteria for ADHD, which is applied in many settings. Goldstein and Goldstein (1998) propose that while the criteria are important, it is equally as prudent to use a more "practical" definition that focuses on the characteristics of the behavior of these children. Their definition includes the following five components:

1. Impulsivity: Impulsivity implies a lack of reflection in behavior that may be demonstrated through verbally blurting out and interrupting, physical irritation of others, answering without thinking on educational measures, and a tendency to shift excessively from one activity to another. Impulsive children also tend to use less mature and/or systematic strategies rather than reflective strategies (Schoenbrodt & Smith, 1995).

2. Inability to sustain attention: The most frequently noted characteristic of ADHD is the inability to sustain attention and effort for tasks. Indicators of distractibility can include difficulty in persevering in schoolwork, frequent daydreaming, and overreaction to external events (Cantwell, 1977; Routh, 1980). ADHD almost always involves shortness of attention span that often persists into adulthood. A child who demonstrates a short attention span typically cannot attend to any academic task for more than a few seconds at a time. As new information is given, the child's attention to the relevant task breaks down and momentarily fixates on something else. The child's thought patterns are too loose and poorly organized to allow enough concentration to finish the task. According to Goldstein (1999), from a neuropsychological viewpoint attention is an executive function that includes self-regulation, planning, execution, maintenance, and sustained mental effort.

3. Overactivity or overarousal: Though distractibility is a primary characteristic of ADHD, overactivity tends to be the most obvious symptom, characterized by intense and undirected energy, fidgetiness, the inability to remain seated, and sometimes a reduced need for sleep. Children with ADHD may also experience many academic difficulties directly related to the overactivity. Holborrow and Berry (1986) reported that seven times as many hyperactive children were described as having a great deal of difficulty in all academic areas as compared to their nonhyperactive peers. Goldstein (1999) reported that when compared to their peers, hyperactive children move with a greater speed and intensity in relation to their extreme emotions.

4. Difficulty with gratification: Children with ADHD often require immediate and frequent meaningful rewards. These children have difficulty waiting for long-term rewards and thus may perform better with more frequent, brief rewards.

5. Emotions and social skills: Children with ADHD are described as being "on an emotional roller coaster." When these children are happy, they are extremely happy, and when they are angry or unhappy, they become so distressed that they have problems controlling their emotions. Because of this, children with these problems have difficulty accepting responsibility for their emotional behavior and frequently project blame onto others. As a result, many children with ADHD also demonstrate poor social skills.

A child who exhibits characteristics of ADHD often does not fit well into groups. The child is often less mature than most of his or her peers. Outbursts of anger and lack of self-control occur frequently. The child is viewed as immature, irritable, disruptive, demanding, and uncooperative by teachers and peers. These children also have difficulty in establishing and maintaining satisfactory social relationships.

Five hypotheses have been generated regarding the relationship between social skills deficits and children with ADHD: (a) social skills deficits and academic deficits result from the same neurological dysfunction; (b) learning problems prevent the development of social skills; (c) children fail to acquire social skills due to the lack of opportunity in the environment; (d) a dysfunctional family system causes decreased opportunities for social interaction; and (e) a clear overlap between learning disabilities and hyperactivity exists (Forness & Kavale, 1991).

COMORBIDITY

One of the problems with identifying ADD/ADHD is that the condition coexists with many other conditions and syndromes. In some cases, ADHD behaviors are involved in the condition; in other cases, ADHD characteristics are part of the condition. For this reason, it is important to understand comorbidity syndromes and medical and behavioral conditions that exist with ADHD. Flick (1998) describes the coexistence of ADHD associated with medical conditions and psychological conditions. The importance of recognizing these characteristics in diagnosing ADHD cannot be overstated. The fact that ADHD is one of the most common childhood disorders may be due to its coexistence with so many other syndromes as a primary or secondary characteristic. Many of the disorders that coexist with ADHD are described in other chapters. One low-incidence disorder not described elsewhere in the text and requires discussion is Tourette's syndrome.

TOURETTE'S SYNDROME

Tourette's syndrome (TS) is a neurological disorder that is named for the French neurologist, Georges Gilles de la Tourette, who first described the disease in 1885. Pedigree and twin studies support the idea that TS is an organic disorder that is hereditary (Comings, 1990). Biological and neuropsychological studies using positron emission tomography (PET) scans, electroencephalographic (EEG) studies, evoked potentials, and neurotransmitters confirm that TS has a biological basis. These studies implicate any of or all of the following: asymmetries of the basal ganglia and caudate nucleus, increases in metabolic activity in the frontal cortex, deficits in the reticular activating system, and hyperactivity, hypersensitivity, or both of the dopamine neurons, or receptors (Comings, 1990; Jankovic, 2001). The disorder is the most severe of the continuum of tic disorders. Tic disorders represent a clinical spectrum ranging from the mild transient tic to the more severe Tourette's syndrome (Singer & Walkup, 1991).

Tics are the most common involuntary movement disorder of childhood, existing in 4 to 5 percent of the school-age population. **Tics** are defined as involuntary, rapid, and repetitive movements that occur suddenly and irregularly. Tics generally involve motor movement or phonic or vocal productions that include the muscles of the head, neck, and shoulders. Tics are typically described in terms of their location, frequency, duration, and intensity. Tics are also characterized in terms of their level of complexity—that is, whether they are considered "simple" or "complex." These descriptors are used in several classification systems in describing tic disorders. These classification systems include (a) the American Psychiatric Association's *Diagnostic Statistic Manual*; (b) the World Health Organization's International Classification of Disease and Related Health Problems (ICD-10); and (c) the Classification of Tic Disorders (CTD) from the Tourette's Syndrome Classification Group. The most commonly used definitions are those that are found in the DSM-IV-TR (APA, 2000). Transient tic disorder is classifed by single or multiple motor and/or vocal tics that occur several times a day with a duration of no more than 12 consecutive months and an onset prior to 18. Chronic motor or vocal tic disorder is defined as single or multiple motor or vocal tics that occur frequently each day for a period of no more than 1 year with no tic-free period of more than 3 months. Finally, Tourette's syndrome includes the same symptoms as chronic tic disorder but involves multiple motor and one or more vocal tics that are present.

While the APA classification system is used most often, the classification system provided by the Tourette's Syndrome Classification Study Group provides five additional categories that make the characteristics more discrete in order to avoid cases being identified in "not otherwise specified" or mistakenly in another category. The additional categories include: definite single tic disorder, nonspecific tic disorder, definite tic disorder-diagnosis deferred, probable TS, and probable multiple tic disorder. The importance to the reader, as a future researcher or clinician, is to be aware that more than one classification system does exist and may be employed in research studies and for diagnostic purposes.

Typically, transient tic disorder includes tics involving one muscle group and lasts less than 1 year. These tics often begin during the school years with the prognosis being good for spontaneous remissions with no medical or psychological intervention necessary. Tics may include motor tics or vocal tics involving one muscle group, such as nose puckering, eye blinking, humming, and other throat noises. A child who exhibits these symptoms for more than 1 year and who has accompanying attention, learning, or behavior problems should be referred for a complete multidisciplinary assessment.

Chronic tic disorders differ from transient tic disorders in the duration of tics (usually over many years) and in the unchanging nature of the tics. Chronic tics may persist in the same state for years. Chronic multiple (motor or vocal) tic disorders are characterized by the presence of tics for more than 12 months that are either motoric or vocalic in form (Singer & Walkup, 1991). The final category, Tourette's syndrome, involves both motoric and vocalic tics that are considered chronic and debilitating. It is worth noting that several researchers stated that the APA definition does not adequately portray the range of behavioral problems that may accompany or exist concomitantly with TS. These behavioral problems include academic problems, attention deficits, obsessive-compulsive disorder, and other psychiatric disorders (Bruun, Cohen, & Leckman, 1990; Singer & Walkup, 1991; Wodrich, Banjamin, & Lachar, 1997).

Characteristics of Children with Tourette's Syndrome

Tics are the single common characteristic in children diagnosed with TS. Tics are, as stated in many definitions, sudden, rapid, recurrent, stereotypical types of movements involving various muscle groups. Tics can involve movement, as in motor tics, or sounds, as in phonic or vocal tics (Jankovic, 2001). Motor tics can take a variety of forms from simple to complex. Simple tics involve a limited number of muscle groups and may include eye blinking, head jerking, or limb jerking. According to Jankovic (2001), a further delineation of simple tics is as follows: (a) clonic tics, which cause a single group of muscles to produce a sudden, jerking movement; (b) dystonic tics, which involve a single muscle group that may produce a slowing of movement and an abnormal posture; and (c) tonic tics, which involve an isometric concentration of a single muscle group. Complex motor tics, on the other hand, involve several muscle groups. Complex motor tics include jumping, finger snapping, hitting of self or others, making obscene gestures (copropraxia), and imitating other's gestures (echopraxia) (Jankovic, 2001; Roddy, 1989).

Vocal tics also vary in individuals diagnosed with TS in the form of simple to complex as described above. Vocal tics include a continuum from noises produced in the throat to the shouting of syllables, words, and phrases. Complex vocal tics may include throat clearing, barking, stuttering, echolalia, palilalia, and coprolalia. The latter three types of tics are less common. **Echolalia** involves the repetition of the last word or phrase of another person. **Palilalia** includes the repetition of one's own last word or phrase. Finally, **coprolalia,** the counterpart to copropraxia, involves the speaking of obscenities. These two were once thought to be distinguishing characteristics of individuals with TS, and are often exploited in the media in reference to the syndrome. However, in actuality, coprolalia and copropraxia occur in only 10 percent of individuals diagnosed with TS.

Tics can be diagnosed as mild, moderate, or severe, based upon the complexity and the degree of impairment or disruption to the child's daily activities. It is also important to note that tics wax and wane, causing a great deal of variability in the frequency and severity over time. Tics can become worse during periods of stress, excitement, and fatigue. In addition, tics can change form over a period of time. New tics may develop as old ones disappear. Controlled studies of individuals with TS indicate that the tics do not necessarily diminish during sleep. Therefore, sleep interruptions result and can lead to other problems in children such as enuresis (Glaze, Frost, & Jankovic, 1983).

Another important fact to note about tics is that they are involuntary. A child may be able to make a conscious effort to suppress a tic temporarily and be successful. However, this suppression creates a buildup of stress that the child must release, which may cause a flurry of tic activity. Tics are also often preceded by sensations that are relieved only after the tic has been released. Many individuals with TS have reported that the release of the one tic may not be enough to satisfy the sensation. Therefore, one may need to continue to repeat a tic until the urge is satisfied. In addition, because tics involve muscle groups, individuals with TS report pain, stiffness, and exhaustion in muscles due to constant, jerky movement of muscle groups.

While TS was once thought to be very rare, the prevalence is between one and eight cases in 1000 boys, with males being affected three times as often as females (Leckman & Cohen, 1999). Studies reported that the average age of onset of tics is 5 with an increase in the severity of tics by age 10 and a dissipation of tics by age 18. Individuals with more severe tics may have persistent difficulty into adulthood. However, for many individuals with TS, the tics may disappear or the severity may decrease dramatically (Leckman et al., 1998). Unfortunately for many individuals with TS, it is not the tics that continue to cause as many problems as the learning and psychiatric conditions that coexist with this syndrome.

Associated Psychiatric and Learning Disorders

Learning Disabilities

Studies examining the coexistence of learning disabilities in children with TS show estimates ranging from 23 to 50 percent (Abwender et al., 1996; Schuerholz, Baumgardner, Singer, Reiss, & Denekla, 1996). Because of this range in estimate, it is important that children diagnosed with TS be monitored frequently for signs of underachievement and/or a possible learning disability. The need for evaluation is substantiated regardless of the age of onset or the diagnosis of TS.

The learning disabilities that are typically associated with individuals with TS are those that are not language based. That is, the learning disabilities are manifested in the areas of written language (organizational skills), arithmetic (in actual visual perception of calculation of math problems), and reading. A large number of children with TS experience visual-motor integration problems that directly affect the areas described (Bronheim, 1991; Matthews, 1988). Tasks that require children to visualize the material, process the information, and then transfer that information to paper is daunting. Lengthy assignments can also produce frustration, particularly when there is a time limit. **Dysgraphia,** or difficulty producing legible handwriting, may also exist, which may contribute to deficits with written language. Writing to a prompt is a typical activity in elementary, middle, and high school. This task involves the comprehension of the prompt, the preparation of an outline to guide the organization of events, the development of a plot or theme, and resolution. Children with organizational problems associated with executive functioning will experience frustration in planning and executing these activities, particularly in a timed situation.

Reading deficits are also noted as a learning disability in children with TS. Comings (1990) reported that dyslexia does exist in this population. Difficulties do not exist in the input of sensory information, but in the proper storage of images of words into the memory. Words are stored without a complete set of phonetic clues, making word recall difficult. A related problem exists in children suffering from blocking. They cannot read fluently because they get stuck on sentences or words. The compulsive need to start at the beginning, repeat a word, count the words in a sentence, and the like can interfere with the child's ability to read. While this type of blocking is related to a secondary problem involving obsessions and compulsions, it does affect the ability to read.

Interpersonal problems in pragmatics and social skills can also be affected. The question of whether these problems are due to the overt expression and reaction of others to tics depends upon each individual. If words are repeated, as in echolalia, or if the tics are explosive, the listener can become distracted and disengaged in the conversation. Stuttering may also co-occur as a speech difficulty or in the form of a tic. The stuttering, which may take the form of loud and pressured speech, may also affect interpersonal communication (Comings & Comings, 1987). Because there are so many factors affecting pragmatic skills, it is important that a thorough evaluation be completed to determine the degree of impairment in each individual, and whether or not the symptoms exist as tics as opposed to specific communication disabilities. In addition to these factors, other psychiatric problems, such as attention deficit/hyperactivity disorder, affect learning and interpersonal communication skills in individuals with TS.

Tourette's Syndrome and Attention Deficit/Hyperactivity Disorder

The comorbidity rates of TS and ADHD vary across studies, with estimates ranging from 55 to 94 percent, depending upon the method of instrumentation used. For example, Sverd et al. (1988) used parent and teacher rating forms as well as structured interviews to identify TS in a psychiatric setting. Another study conducted by Park, Como, Cui, and Kudan (1993) found that 55 percent of the population was affected when interviews and neuropsychological assessment information were used. Walkup, Leckman, Price, Hardin, Ort, and Cohen (1988; as cited in Leckman & Cohen, 1999) reported the coexistence of TS and ADHD may account for other psychiatric problems seen in children, including depression, anxiety, and behavioral disorders. Short attention span, distractibility, impulsivity, and hyperactivity are the characteristics frequently noted in this population. The attentional difficulties may precede the onset of symptoms of TS and worsen as the tics develop. Children with TS may actually be referred for symptoms of ADHD rather than the tics prior to the diagnosis of TS. Comings and Comings (1987) reported that children are diagnosed with TS an average of 2.4 years after the ADHD symptoms are documented. Comings (1990) reported more behavior problems in the form of conduct disorders in children with coexisting TS and ADHD than in those with pure ADHD. In addition, the more severe the TS, the more pronounced the ADHD will be. The characteristics and treatment issues surrounding ADHD are discussed in Chapter 4. What is important to note is that stimulant medication that is used to treat ADHD may exacerbate tics for some children with TS (Castellanos et al., 1997). For these children, alternative medications may be prescribed.

For many children with TS and ADHD, the symptoms of ADHD may be more disabling than the tics. In these instances, behavioral and educational approaches may be considered first to control the ADHD. When these approaches are not effective, trial dosages of pharmacological treatments are recommended in controlled contexts. If the child improves overall and the tics do not worsen significantly, the medication is continued. However, if the ADHD improves, but the tics worsen, the medication is discontinued and an alternative medication is recommended for a trial period (Singer & Walkup, 1991). According to Jankovic (2001), difficulties in paying attention may be due to coexisting ADHD or to the "uncontrollable intrusions of thoughts or obsessive fixation of attention on irrelevant objects or topics, or the mental concentration that is exerted in an effort to suppress tics and premonitory urges, and of the sedative effects of the medications used to treat Tourette's syndrome" (p. 1186). Obsessive-compulsive disorder is another psychiatric condition that coexists with TS.

Tourette Syndrome and Obsessive-Compulsive Disorder

There are many studies that support the idea that TS and obsessive-compulsive disorder (OCD) are associated disorders. Research suggests that there is not only a genetic vulnerability to either TS or OCD, but a familial relationship as well (Como, 1993). Characteristics of OCD include the presence of recurrent behaviors, thoughts, or both that intrude on the consciousness. These symptoms are involuntary and distressing to the child. The characteristics can become debilitating when they cause significant impairment. Compulsions consist of the behaviors carried out in response to the obsessions. Possible compulsive behaviors include repeated hand washing, counting rituals, cleaning objects, and checking things frequently, such as windows or door locks. Obsessions may include fears of contamination with dirt or germs, fears of loved ones being harmed, and other thoughts or images that intrude on consciousness (Singer & Walkup, 1991).

Singer and Walkup (1991) noted that there is an overlap among compulsive behaviors, complex tics, and obsessive thoughts. For example, a recurring desire to touch an object or a part of the body may be either a complex motor tic or a compulsive behavior. Like tics, OCD symptoms wax and wane. These symptoms worsen when there is stress or fatigue, and cannot be consciously controlled.

Tourette Syndrome and Behavioral Disorders, Anxiety, and Depression

Conduct disorder co-occurs frequently in children with TS. Several types of behavior problems have been identified: aggressiveness, lying, stealing, starting fires, vandalism, and fighting. (There are others.) Behavior problems may in part be a response to having a stigmatizing disorder, may be secondary to the accompanying diagnosis of ADHD, may be genetically inherited, or may not be attributable to the TS at all (Comings, 1990; Singer & Walkup, 1991). Other associated disorders, anxiety, depression, bipolar disorder, and thought disorders may all be coexisting in the population of TS. All of the above are described earlier in this chapter in the context of psychiatric disorders and speech and language correlates. What is important to remember in the population with TS is that the accompanying psychiatric and behavior problems may be manifested in the family pedigree and not be recognized as a genetic link to TS, thereby making a definite diagnosis difficult. Proper diagnosis is critical in the context of a multidisciplinary evaluation. In the case of TS, the neurologist is a critical part of this team for proper assessment and diagnosis.

DEVELOPMENTAL CHARACTERISTICS OF ADHD

It was once believed that children's problems with attention, overactivity, impulsivity, and excitability remitted at puberty. However, current research reveals that while overactivity tends to decrease between the ages of 12 and 16, many of the associated problems persist. Follow-up studies have tracked behavioral difficulties into adolescence and adulthood, which means that the characteristics of ADHD change from early childhood into adulthood.

Preschool Children and Toddlers with ADHD

According to Barkley (2000) and Flick (1998), mothers of children with ADHD report that they noticed that their child had ADHD from early infancy, and sometimes before birth. By age 4, 40 percent of children identified have enough difficulty with inattention to be a concern to teachers and parents. Barkley (2000) reported that many of these children will have symptoms that subside in several months. Even those children with a more severe diagnosis may have the same severity of symptoms by late childhood or early adolescence. The combination of the severity of symptoms and the length the symptoms persist determines which children may be more likely to show a "chronic" course of ADHD.

Parents of preschoolers with ADHD reported that their children are much more active than their peers, often describing them as "driven by a motor." Other reported characteristics include rapid mood changes, restless behavior, temper tantrums, poor sleep patterns, low tolerance for frustration, low adaptability to situations, and short attention span. These children are also more likely to have more speech and language problems and difficulty with motor coordination.

School-Age Children

As the preschool child matures and enters school, the ADHD behavior pattern becomes increasingly worse, due in part to the social demands placed on children between preschool and adolescence. These problems also intensify as classroom demands for focused behavior on tasks increases, since these children have more difficulty paying attention in class and focusing their efforts on the assignment or on the teacher, and following through with tasks. Demands at home also increase, particularly for completing homework assignments. Parents report many problems in getting their children to follow through with chores at home and with completing school assignments.

Another problem that begins to compound at this age is difficulty in developing appropriate social skills. Many of these children have problems fitting in with the crowd because they have difficulty, for example, waiting in line for a turn. They may appear pushy and verbally aggressive when playing games and insist it is their turn. Many children will shy away from the child with ADHD because of these faulty skills. In addition to lacking social "friendship-making" skills, these children may also display difficulty with basic pragmatic skills. Given their negative experiences, children with ADHD lack the opportunity to practice correct conversational skills. This lack of positive feedback gives these children even less of an opportunity to practice these essential skills in a naturally reinforcing atmosphere. All these compounding difficulties may lead to an increased risk that the school-age child will develop antisocial behaviors that may ultimately lead to symptoms of conduct disorder and social conflict. In fact, Barkley (2000) reports that 30 to 50 percent of ADHD children between ages 7 and 10 are likely to develop symptoms of antisocial behavior and conduct disorder before they reach adolescence.

Adolescence

While overactivity may subside by adolescence or adulthood, this characteristic is often replaced by a feeling of restlessness. Before the 1970s, many studies reported that children outgrow ADHD by adolescence. More recent research reveals the contrary. Barkley (2000) reported that 70 to 80 percent of children clinically diagnosed with ADHD will continue to display these behaviors. In addition, he reports that 25 to 35 percent of this group may display antisocial behavior or conduct disorder. Many adolescents with ADHD will experiment with drugs and/or alcohol, and have difficulties in school (including being retained, suspended, or expelled). These adolescents are also more susceptible to peer pressure and will demonstrate more risk-taking behaviors. As a result, they may be more likely to engage in sexual relationships early on, resulting in teen pregnancy and an increased risk of contracting sexually transmitted diseases. Unfortunately, a large majority of adolescents will continue these behaviors into adulthood.

ADHD in Adults

Adults with ADHD may exhibit adult antisocial personality disorder and antisocial behavior may exist. Barkley (2000) reports that 10 to 20 percent of children diagnosed with ADHD reach adulthood free of any additional psychiatric diagnosis. In general, adults demonstrate difficulty in the workplace in remaining organized, working independently, and meeting deadlines. While the prognosis for remission of all symptoms of ADHD is dim, many interventions are used to help individuals with ADHD compensate for deficiencies resulting from these symptoms. However, before appropriate interventions can be explored, a thorough assessment of ADHD that meets the clinical criteria outlined by DSM-IV-TR must be undertaken.

ASSESSMENT OF ATTENTION DEFICIT/HYPERACTIVITY DISORDER

The speech-language evaluation should be part of a multidisciplinary evaluation that assesses all aspects of the functioning of the ADHD student, and which may involve professionals. This professional team should include a developmental pediatrician or physician, a psychologist or neuropsychologist, an SLP, teachers and specialists from the school, and parents. The team may also include a psychiatrist, counselors, and others with particular expertise in assessment of children with ADHD. All members of the team should be familiar with the student. In-depth testing should include a neuropsychological or psychological evaluation, academic assessment, speech-language evaluation, behavioral observations, and an in-depth developmental case history. Information should be obtained from both the home and school environments.

Neuropsychological Assessment

A wide range of functions is assessed as part of a neuropsychological evaluation. The assessed categories allow the neuropsychologist or psychologist to rule out comorbid disorders and syndromes, and to include ADHD/ADD as the final diagnosis. The functions that are addressed include:

- Ability, which is assessed through intelligence scales such as the Wechsler Intelligence Scale for Children-III or the Kaufman Brief Intelligence Test (KBIT)
- Achievement, which is measured through tests that evaluate reading, math, spelling, reading comprehension, numerical operations, listening comprehension, oral expression, and written expression, such as the Wechsler Achievement Test, the Woodcock-Johnson Psychoeducational Battery, and the Peabody Individual Achievement Test
- Executive control, which is assessed through measures that evaluate motor speed and mental flexibility
- Visual-motor skills
- Motor skills
- Memory functions
- Attentional skills, which are measured through the use of a continuous performance test such as the Gordon Diagnostic System or the Test of Variables of Attention (TOVA)

- Self-concept and self-esteem, which are measured by instruments such as the Self-Esteem Index or the Multidimensional Self-Concept Scale
- Social skills, which are measured by direct observation or the Social Skills Rating System
- Visual-spatial skills
- Language skills
- Behavioral-emotional assessment, which is measured by parent/teacher checklists

LANGUAGE IMPAIRMENTS IN CHILDREN WITH ADHD

No clear causal relationship has been established between ADHD, ADD, and language impairments (LI). However, descriptive studies consistently link ADHD and ADD with LI. Benner, Nelson, and Epstein (2002) reviewed the current research on the language skills of children with emotional and/or behavioral disorders (EBD). Studies consistently showed that reading and language were the most difficult academic areas for children with EBD. The language problems in particular were associated with lower academic achievement, psychiatric and reading problems, and grade retention (Beitchman, Cantwell, Forness, Kavale, & Kauffman, 1998; Tomblin, Zhang, Buckwalter, & Carts, 2000).

The relationship between communication, speech and language problems, and antisocial behaviors (including ADHD) have been reviewed in the literature with the following conclusions:

1. Children who had receptive language problems are at a higher risk for antisocial behavior than children with purely speech deficits. The receptive problems frequently go undetected and make these children more at-risk for developing reading problems.
2. Longitudinal studies showed that there is a strong relationship between language disorders and antisocial behaviors that increases as the children age (Baker & Cantwell, 1987; Stevenson, Richman, & Graham, 1985).
3. The language disorders create problems in interpersonal relationships, particularly in the area of language use or pragmatics. These children with EBD and LI tend to use more physical actions to solve problems as opposed to verbal communication because they lack the language skills for effective communication (Fujiki, Brinton, Morgan, & Hart, 1999; Gallagher, 1999).

Benner, Nelson, and Epstein's (2002) review confirmed the above, showing that children with EBD demonstrated problems in the areas of pragmatic, receptive, and expressive language. They also found that the deficits would stabilize or increase over time. The authors suggested that further research is needed to identify the processes underlying language deficiencies in children with EBD. They also contended that children with EBD should be evaluated for language deficits, as 40 percent of children with EBD have language problems that go undiagnosed (Cohen et al., 1998). This missed diagnosis may cause children with EBD and LI to have difficulty learning in the academic setting and difficulty communicating effectively with peers.

In addition to the co-occurrence of EBD (including ADHD/ADD) and LI, is the documented co-occurrence of auditory processing disorder (APD) and LI (Tallal & Piercy, 1973; Tallal et al., 1990), and APD and ADHD/ADD (Katz, 1992; Pillsbury, Grose, Coleman, Conners, & Hall, 1995; Riccio, Hynd, Cohen, & Gonzales, 1993; Riccio, Hynd, Cohen, & Molt, 1996). While there is overlap in the behavioral characteristics of APD and ADHD/ADD, current research concludes that each is a distinct clinical disorder (Chermak, Hall, & Musiek, 1999). Chermak, Hall, and Musiek (1999) define **auditory**

processing disorder as a deficiency in "one or more of the central auditory processes responsible for generating the auditory evoked potentials and the behaviors of sound localization and lateralization, auditory discrimination, auditory pattern recognition, temporal processing, auditory performance with competing acoustic signals, and auditory performance with degraded acoustic signals" (p. 290).

A person with APD has difficulty understanding spoken language when there is competing background noise. Children with APD may have problems paying attention, become easily distracted, have problems following through on complex directions, and have problems understanding conversation. Chermak and Musiek (1997) reported that the prevalence of APD in children is 2 to 3 percent.

The authors state that there is a difference in the types of attention deficits that are seen in ADHD, ADD, and APD. Attention deficits associated with ADHD may be related to sustained attention whereas selective attention and information-processing speed may be related to ADD. Selective and divided auditory attention deficits are characteristics of APD (Chermak, Hall, & Musiek, 1999; Chermak & Musiek, 1997). Researchers also state that the deficits in rule-governed behavior associated with ADHD may lead to problems initiating, sustaining, or inhibiting responses (Barkley, 1990; Haenlein & Caul, 1987; Zentall, 1985). These problems may be related to self-control problems, social skills deficits, and language disorders related particularly to language use (initiating, maintaining, and turn-taking conversational discourse) that are often observed in children with ADHD (Augustine & Damico, 1995).

The student with self-control problems and/or antisocial behavior may be verbally and physically aggressive, disruptive to others, and easily angered. In addition, attention-seeking behaviors may be accompanied by the tendency to violate rules and blame other people. This student may also seek aggressive solutions to problems. For example, in response to being teased, the student may choose to strike out physically at his or her peer rather than choosing a nonviolent alternative.

Speech and Language Assessment in the Child with ADHD

A basic language assessment battery for the child with ADHD should consist of the following:

- History and data review
- A comprehensive language evaluation, such as the Clinical Evaluation of Language Fundamentals-Revised (CELF-R), the Comprehensive Assessment of Speech and Language (CASL), the Test of Language Development (TOLD)—primary or intermediate, the Woodcock Language Proficiency Battery, or the Detroit Test of Learning Aptitude
- Normed supplementary batteries as needed for probing language and auditory processing
- Social skills checklists and observations
- Audiological evaluation for assessment of the auditory system and auditory perceptual abilities

The tests mentioned throughout the assessment section are examples of tools in each area and not an exhaustive list. Students should be aware that when deciding upon the use of an assessment tool, the most recent revision should be used.

Pate (1993) outlined some basic behavioral guidelines for completing an assessment: outline the routine and set clear rules that allow for some flexibility; allow the student choices in where to sit in the testing area; plan breaks in the testing session; be prepared to restrain hands when pointing responses are involved; and have a system prepared to double-score responses. In addition to these guidelines, Pate posed four questions to be answered from the assessment data: What age-appropriate skills does the child need? What age-appropriate skills does the child have? What new skills can be acquired through intervention? What options are available for collaborative support? The answers to these questions will lead to the development of a functional, successful intervention plan for the student with ADHD.

INTERVENTION

A number of interventions have been applied to the characteristics of hyperactivity. These interventions have emanated from several views, including the biophysical, behavioral, and cognitive-behavioral models.

Biophysical

The biophysical model focuses on the concept of disease. Two of the typical treatment alternatives include pharmocotherapy (drug interventions) and diet-related treatments.

Pharmacotherapy

Stimulant medication is both the most common and the most controversial treatment choice for children in the United States (NIH, 1998). The medication most frequently used is methylphenidate (Ritalin), while Dexedrine and Cylert are also frequently used. These medications are part of a class of drugs known as stimulants. Other medications in this category include antidepressants, which may be used when there are comorbid characteristics of anxiety. Of these medications, Ritalin appears to be used about 10 times more frequently than the others because the effect on growth is less marked (Gadow, 1986; NIH, 1998).

Stimulant medication is effective in reducing overactivity for short periods of time. Barkley (2000) reported that 75 percent of children with hyperactivity showed a positive response to stimulant therapy. Ottenbacher and Cooper (1982) reviewed 61 studies relevant to the drug treatment of children with hyperactivity and found that stimulants did change the behaviors and performance of hyperactive children. The greatest effect was on behavioral measures of performance; in contrast, the smallest effects were on academic achievement measures of IQ. Many factors can limit the efficacy of treating ADHD with stimulant medication: (a) stimulant medication must be closely prescribed, monitored, and withdrawn under a physician's treatment; (b) long-term studies of stimulant effects have shown maintenance of behaviors over a period of time; (c) stimulant medication is not appropriate for all children with ADHD; and (d) moderate doses of stimulant medication carry possible side effects of insomnia, anorexia, headache, nausea, moodiness, stomachache, and irritability (Barkley, 2000).

In summary, while stimulant medication has been shown to enhance self-control, interpersonal behavior, and academic performance short term, the possible side effects of stimulant medication, as well as the variability of generalization and maintenance across time and settings, make this a discouraging choice for many parents and educators.

Dietary Interventions

Dietary and nutritional approaches to controlling hyperactivity offer another form of treatment for children with ADHD. These approaches rely on the premise that overactivity is related to the digestion of food substances containing such items as refined sugars and salt compounds. Thus by eliminating such products from the diet of hyperactive children, it is presumed that overall behavior should improve.

One of the more well-known food plans is the Kaiser Permante (K-P) diet, which was originally described by Feingold in 1975. Feingold proposed that the elimination of foods containing artificial colors, flavors, and salicylates (a salt compound found in apples, cherries, oranges, and peaches) could result in the remission of symptoms for 30 to 50 percent of hyperactive children. Nonetheless, many studies fail to find positive results for dietary control. Those reporting positive results document improvement rates similar to those found in placebo conditions (Connors, 1980).

Behavioral Interventions

The behavioral model emphasizes the analysis and control of the environment, relying on the fundamental assumption that all behavior is learned. Behavior modification is very effective in the short term, and in the long term may be more effective than drug treatment in controlling impulsivity, interpersonal behavior (including self-control skills), and academic performance.

Behavioral treatment programs for the control of hyperactive behavior typically involve the strengthening and/or weakening of behaviors. For example, Ross and Ross (1982) reported the successful use of differential training and modeling to modify the impulsivity of a 6-year old hyperactive boy. Results indicated a substantial behavioral improvement in the home environment. Improvements were also noted when the procedure was extended to the school environment.

Treatment programs to control hyperactive behaviors involve strengthening or weakening target behaviors through the delivery of reinforcers and punishers. Reinforcement refers to a reward given following an increase in the frequency or intensity of the target behavior. Praise or rewards must increase the strength of a target behavior in order to be considered a positive reinforcer. Therefore, selecting effective reinforcers that possess the best outcome for increasing behavior is important. Typical reinforcers used included edibles, praise and attention, performance feedback, tokens, and contingency contracting.

Edibles are used with a variety of populations. Typical edible reinforcements include such items as candy, ice cream, and gum. An obvious disadvantage to using edibles is that transporting these items to and from the classroom is difficult and that sugars and other additives in some foods may actually contribute to the negative behavior.

Praise and attention are examples of social reinforcers that can be easily administered by parents and teachers in all settings. In order for praise and attention to be effective, delivery should take place immediately following the target behaviors. Walker (1979) reported that this type of reinforcement is most effective if delivered immediately and that the statements of praise should be varied but also descriptive of the target behavior. An important point to mention is that children with ADHD seldom receive much praise. Their interactions with parents, teachers, and peers are often negative and involve a great deal of verbal disapproval. For this reason, it important that these children receive some positive verbal reinforcement every day.

Feedback is defined by Kazdin (1975) as the knowledge of the results of one's efforts toward the attainment of a goal and can prove a powerful reinforcer. Jens and Shores (1969) showed that charted feedback is effective in reinforcing the effects of behavioral programming in children with ADHD. Another type of reinforcement is tokens, which can take a variety of forms, including chips, checkmarks, stickers, or tickets. Tokens can be used to purchase a variety of reinforcers, thus helping avoid satiation of reinforcers for children with ADHD. In addition, tokens can also be used effectively in shaping nonimpulsive behaviors (Alberto & Troutman, 1986). Shaping involves the reinforcement of successive approximation to the desired goal and reinforcing the behavior in the direction of attaining the goal. If using tokens to aid in shaping behavior, the reinforcement, or the shaping, should begin with acceptance of approximations of the behavior. If teachers or parents wait for a large behavior change rather than small approximations, shaping may never take place (Robin, 1992). While many advantages are associated with the use of tokens, one major problem is record keeping, which requires a great deal of instructor or parent time.

Contingency contracts are written agreements that specify relationships between appropriate child behaviors and the positive consequences to be given. Contingencies in the contract must be the direct result of consultation between the child-parent-teacher triad. In addition, positive and negative consequences must be specified in advance, making the child responsible for knowledge of all aspects of the contract. Contingency contracts are beneficial to impulsive children because positive and aversive consequences are stated in advance; thus teacher or parental responses to situations cannot be viewed as unfair or arbitrary. Some disadvantages of this type of management include the time and energy to set up and implement the contract, as well as problems in defining the behaviors that are established in the contract (DuPaul, Eckert, & McGoey, 1997; Frazier & Merrell, 1997).

Punishment can also be used to manage the behavior of children with ADHD. Typical punishments include reprimands, response-cost, and time-out. A reprimand is defined as an expression of disapproval directed toward a behavior. Studies of reprimands showed that they can effectively control the behavior of an ADHD child when combined with praise for appropriate behavior (Axelrod, 1971). Reprimands may not have a strong lasting effect on behavior consistency and the delivery of the punishment is difficult (Frazier & Merrell, 1997).

Response-cost, a formal system of penalties applied to the occurrence of inappropriate behaviors, usually involves the removal of points or tokens, or sometimes the loss of privileges (Kazdin, 1972). Outcome studies indicate that response-cost contingencies add a more direct focus on problem-solving training (Urbain & Kendall, 1980). Other research argues that this technique may be ineffective unless it is administered in a clear and consistent manner (Frazier & Merrell, 1997).

Time-out is defined as the contingent removal of the opportunity to earn positive reinforcement (Craighead, 1982). During time-out, a child is placed in a restricted environment following disruptive behavior and remains in isolation for a minimum time period. Return to the classroom is contingent upon the passage of the time period in addition to exhibition of appropriate behavior. In order to achieve maximum benefits with time-out, the child should not have access to reinforcers. Unfortunately, removing all reinforcing events is difficult in a classroom with students with ADHD. Time-out areas may possess a variety of reinforcers. In addition, the teacher or therapist who is monitoring the time-out needs to be aware that the time-out experience itself can become a positive way of gaining attention. For example, the child may purposely act out in order to go to time-out to receive attention from the teacher or to avoid activities that are boring or too difficult (DuPaul, Eckert, & McGoey, 1997; Frazier & Merrell, 1997).

Though behavioral programs can effectively control some behaviors, the use of behavioral procedures alone does not result in a more reflective child. In addition, significant evidence argues that behavioral management programs do not generalize across settings or over time (Abikoff, 1991; DuPaul, Eckert, & McGoey, 1997). In the past, behavior therapists have attempted to change behavior through nonverbal methods, whereas cognitive-behavioral therapists utilized speech as an instrument of change. Combining traditional behavioral techniques with cognitive training may prove an effective alternative form of treatment for children with ADHD.

Cognitive-Behavior Modification

Cognitive-behavioral modification (CBM) refers to a general category of intervention techniques that attempt to modify behavior by altering the thought patterns of individuals (Abikoff, 1991; Radcliff, 2000). CBM combines the manipulation of environmental changes with an individual's self-control processes, which may include self-instruction, self-monitoring, and/or self-reinforcement in order to create a more durable and prolonged change in behavior through the manipulation of the child's mediational cognitions (Meodor & Ollendick, 1984). CBM has been referred to as a means for developing generalized problem-solving methods or algorithms (Hall, 1980). CBM interventions place emphasis on self-control. Self-monitoring and self-assessment are frequently used strategies to aid in self-control, but are effective only when children are taught to become aware of their own behavior and the strategies they use for problem solving. Consequently, metacognitive training is a critical component to CBM interventions.

Cognitive-Behavior Modification with Children with ADHD

Cognitive-behavioral techniques are currently used with children exhibiting any of a variety of disorders, but children with ADHD were among the first groups to benefit from such methods (e.g., Kagan, Pearson, & Welch, 1966; Palkes, Stewart, & Kahana, 1968). In fact, cognitive-behavior training procedures are now popularly used in combination with pharmacological interventions.

The overall goal of CBM is to develop self-control skills and reflective problem-solving skills, both of which are thought to be deficient in children with ADHD. These deficiencies appear to account for difficulties in children's abilities to regulate inattentive, impulsive, and inappropriate interpersonal behaviors. CBM can provide children with the ability to regulate behavior more appropriately, and thus enhance social and academic performance (Abikoff, 1991).

Self-talk and modeling are core components of CBM (Lloyd, 1980; Whalen & Henker, 1987, 1991). With the child involved as an active participant in the intervention program, results will assumingly generalize and be maintained with greater frequency and regularity (Meichenbaum & Asarnow, 1979). While CBM can employ a number of different treatment procedures and approaches, verbal self-instruction and problem-solving training are used most often with this population.

Verbal Self-Instruction

Early research by Luria (1961) and Vygotsky (1962) identified the importance of the relationship between internal verbalizations and overt behavior. Their research relied on the assumption that children assume control over their behavior by internalizing self-directed verbal commands (O'Brien & Obrzut, 1986). This work resulted in the proposal of a theoretical model in which behavior is directed first by the speech of others, next by the child's own overt speech, and finally by the child's own covert or inner speech.

Meichenbaum and Goodman's (1971) prototypic self-instruction training package was influenced by the work of Luria and Vygotsky. Their now classic self-instructional package combined modeling, overt and covert rehearsal prompts, feedback, and social reinforcement. While many studies have demonstrated the effectiveness of verbal self-instruction, few showed the maintenance or generalization of this skill. Another major class of interventions within the realm of CBM, which was also shown to be effective, advocates a problem-solving approach to social difficulties. Some versions of self-instructional training have included problem solving, though few utilize verbal self-instruction.

Problem-Solving Interventions

The purpose of problem-solving training is to teach children to generate alternative solutions to interpersonal problems and to evaluate cause-effect relationships. Kneedler (1980) suggested that children exhibiting problems in social skills also have deficiencies in problem-solving skills. In problem-solving situations where there is an uncertainty in response, children with ADHD respond in an impulsive fashion (Whalen & Henker, 1991). Such children perform less efficiently in social skills than children who approach problem-solving situations in a careful, reflective manner. Moreover, studies of the problem-solving behavior of reflective and impulsive children (e.g., Hogg, Callias, & Pellegrini, 1986; Copeland, 1981; Whalen & Henker, 1991; Meodor & Ollendick, 1984) have indicated that impulsive children utilize less mature strategies than reflective children of the same age. In addition, longitudinal studies have demonstrated that impulsive children evidence a delayed pattern of strategic development between the ages of 7 and 9, a pattern seemingly unrelated to intellectual ability.

Many studies have identified stages or sequences of problem-solving behavior. In one such study, D'Zurilla and Goldfried (1971) defined problem solving as a behavioral process and outlined five stages of problem solving, including (a) developing a general orientation to possible problems; (b) developing the ability to identify the components of a problem; (c) developing alternative strategies to solve a problem; (d) evaluating the consequences of the solutions generated; and (e) evaluating the outcome and employing self-reinforcement. Outcome studies indicate that problem-solving interventions tend to be generally effective. Most notably, children exhibit improved performance in identifying a general schema for making personal decisions and applying this schema to solving novel problems. In fact, in studies where problem-solving interventions were used in comparison to medication, children with ADHD were more likely to attribute their successes to effort and ability rather than to the medication (Whalen & Henker, 1991). CBM strategies and programs that utilize both problem solving and verbal self-instruction were also developed for targeting deficient social skills, a prominent area of deficit for children with ADHD. These programs seek to increase self-control in social situations, which in turn can aid overall acceptance by adults and peers.

Social Skills Instruction

Social skills instruction is designed to increase interpersonal skills in critical life situations. Three general definitions of social skills exist. The first uses measures of peer acceptance or popularity to define children as socially skilled (Elliott & Gresham, 1987). From a behavioral perspective, social skills include those situationally specific behaviors that secure the probability of maintaining positive reinforcement depending on one's social behavior. Finally, social skills are also defined in terms of social validity: those behaviors that predict important social outcomes for children. Many impulsive children may know how to interact appropriately with adults, and less frequently, peers, yet cannot maintain this skill due to impulsivity in responding (Whalen & Henker, 1991). For this reason, children with ADHD are appropriate candidates for social skills training.

Most programs developed to teach social skills to students with ADHD employ the social skill deficit model, which assumes that changes in the child's behavior will result in changes in the way the child is perceived (Hymel, 1986). A review by Whalen and Henker (1991) investigated the social impact of stimulant medication for children with ADHD, determining that, on the whole, children with ADHD have serious and persistent social deficits that cause frequent conflicts in social situations. The children's pragmatic style of social exchange is characterized by deficits in initiating conversation, poor eye contact, and inappropriate conversational behavior, which is often perceived as immature, inappropriate, and intrusive. Children with ADHD may exhibit social learning disabilities that hamper them from achieving effective pragmatic skills. While medication did effectively reduce the disruptive nature of conversational speech, medication did not promote overall social competence.

In general, stimulant medication cannot increase the social skills that children with ADHD lack. Social skills programs, on the other hand, can teach children how to reduce inappropriate social behavior as well as how to establish and build friendships and social relationships. These programs are not short-term interventions, as social skills deficits can plague children with ADHD into adulthood. The most effective interventions will employ intensive training in social skills instruction that sufficiently allows for the use of peers and naturalistic environments.

Which Intervention Is the Best for the Child with ADHD?

The question as to which treatment is the best is highly debated in the literature. While this discussion presents some of the more frequently used and researched interventions, many more exist. The biggest controversy exists over the use and possible overprescription of medication. Recent studies suggest that even low dosages of stimulant medication produce the greatest improvement in academic and social adjustment (Jensen, Kettle, Roper, Sloan, Hoven, & Hector, 1999). Reviews of the literature regarding cognitive behavior modification have not produced studies evidencing long-term changes in behavior in the pediatric ADHD population. Abikoff (1991) reported that cognitive training cannot compete with stimulant medication in terms of overall effectiveness. His review also emphasizes CBM's failure to enhance the positive effects of stimulant medication.

Overall, many studies report that a combination of stimulant medication and a behavior modification program offers the optimal treatment plan for children with ADHD (Jensen et. al., 1999; Kollins, Barkley, & DuPaul, 2001; Swanson, Cantwell, Lerner, McBurnett, & Hanna, 1991; Whalen & Henker, 1991). However, researchers warn that the most visible effects of medication relate specifically to helping children with ADHD reduce overactivity and maintain attention for longer periods of time. In other words, the medication helps the child with ADHD achieve behaviors that permit learning to take place. If the child, however, has deficits in academic and/or social learning, medication alone will not compensate for this deficit. For example, an overactive child with a social skill deficit may appear better accepted by peers and adults once on medication because this child does not interrupt or touch or push others during a conversational exchange. If this same child has difficulty initiating and maintaining a conversation, however, medication will not solve the problem and social skill instruction is warranted. In summary, while the literature clearly supports the use of medication in the overall treatment of children with ADHD, whether alone or in combination with behavioral treatments, each child should be treated as an individual requiring careful evaluation in order to determine the best possible treatment plan.

PSYCHOSOCIAL ISSUES AND ADHD

Numerous issues surround the child with ADHD and his or her family. This chapter emphasizes the potential difficulties that parents and family members can encounter when dealing with children with ADHD. Most children with ADHD have difficulty following instructions from their parents. These children frequently become frustrated, interrupt conversations, and instigate sibling conflicts. This type of behavior, particularly when coupled with a controlling attitude, can make life at home difficult, often causing marital and family stress.

A major conflict that can arise between parents involves parenting style. Studies show significant differences in parenting styles in mothers and fathers. Children with ADHD generally appear to behave better for their fathers than their mothers. Several hypotheses have been offered to explain this finding. One theory holds that fathers tend to deliver behavioral consequences more quickly and may be more punitive than mothers (Parker, 1992). Another theory argues that children with ADHD spend more time with their mothers and have learned how to avoid or delay a negative response. Thus, if the father spends the same amount of time with the child as the mother, the child will react to the father as she or he does to the mother. These differences in behavior management can cause conflict between the parents and confusion for the child.

A recent study by Hankin, Wright, and Gephart (2001) reported on the related costs of ADHD upon the family unit. Their review indicated that the cost occurs across several domains, including: (a) family burden: including parent stress, marital difficulties, sibling conflicts, and depression and alcohol abuse in parents; (b) employer burden: including decreased work productivity in parents and increased absences from work due to incidents involving the child (e.g., trips to the emergency room, problems at school); and (c) burden on the health care system (which is not only a burden to the system but a financial burden to the family): including increased accidents due to higher rates of risk-taking behavior. Such burdens are very realistic for educators and practitioners to be aware of when counseling family members on the best methods for helping their child achieve success behaviorally, academically, and socially.

CONCLUSION

Children with ADHD present with a variety of characteristics that may prove challenging for family members and educators working with them. Such characteristics can affect the child's ability to function behaviorally, academically, and socially. While the criteria for diagnosis are clear, ADHD often exists comorbidly with other learning and behavioral disorders, leaving assessment and treatment procedures unclear. An assessment therefore should be multidisciplinary, incorporating and documenting input from specialists, educators, and family members. Upon diagnosis, numerous interventions are available, including biophysical, pharmacological, behavioral, cognitive-behavioral, and social skills methods. The type of intervention used depends upon the individual characteristics and needs of the child and the family. Finally, the characteristics of ADHD can prove to be debilitating to the child, causing numerous social problems and resulting psychosocial issues that challenge the family as well. In order to fully integrate services for the child with ADHD, interventions may also be needed to help family members cope with the child.

Case Study 1: JD's Case Study

JD was referred for a comprehensive evaluation by his elementary school due to educational concerns in attention and concentration, organization, work completion, academic progress, speech and language, and social skills. According to JD's mother, her pregnancy with JD was uncomplicated with a normal delivery and birth weight just under 7 pounds. Developmental milestones were reported to be within normal age range, with speech and language development being described as "slow." JD's medical background was positive for allergies and asthma.

JD's academic history was relatively uneventful up to this year, when he entered the fourth grade. His mother reported concerns in following multistep directions, decoding directions, and sustaining attention. The school reported academic concerns in the areas of reading comprehension, math calculation, and math reasoning (word problems). JD participates in a social skills group on a weekly basis with the school guidance counselor that focuses on friendship-making skills.

Results of formal and informal speech and language testing revealed that no problems existed in the areas of articulation, vocal resonance, quality, pitch, and intensity of speech. Language testing, however, revealed overall language skills to be in the below average to average range. Individual subtest scores on receptive and expressive language tests ranged from below average to the average range. Relative strength (average performance) was indicated in receptive vocabulary, acquisition of word classes, and auditory memory for sentences. Individual weaknesses (below average performance) were indicated in word retrieval, knowledge of synonyms and figurative language, expression of word definitions in multiple contexts, and sentence formulation. Informal evaluation revealed significant weaknesses in auditory processing, word retrieval, and language usage related to organization of verbal output.

In the area of language usage, JD used language to relate personal and general information and to socialize. He expressed personal information, including his first, middle, and last names, birth date, address, and phone number. He was able to use conversational skills for expressing wants and needs, initiating conversation, and expressing greetings and farewells. He demonstrated inconsistent ability to maintain the topic of conversation and frequently interjected off-topic and/or associative questions and conversational comments. JD exhibited difficulty responding in an organized, relevant manner, asking for help, and expressing feelings. JD indicated that reading was the easiest subject and the math was the hardest subject. Classroom teachers indicated that he has difficulty asking for help and looking at people when he is talking or listening. According to his mother, JD has difficulty speaking clearly when talking to school staff.

The multidisciplinary team established attention deficit/hyperactivity disorder based upon a psychological evaluation, speech and language assessments, classroom teacher and parent rating scales, informal observation, and an educational assessment. Weaknesses were particularly noted in the area of speech and language. Direct intervention was recommended as well as modifications in the classroom, such as preteaching vocabulary and concepts; reducing the rate, length, and complexity of oral input; providing visual organizers for verbal output; and providing instruction presented with visual cues and within meaningful contexts. A reevaluation was recommended in two months to determine whether modifications and direct therapy were meeting JD's needs.

Case Study 2: Heather's Case Study

Heather was referred for a multidisciplinary assessment by her elementary school due to education concerns in attention, speech-language, academic performance, and health. Heather's mother reported that she was the product of a full-term pregnancy and a delivery by c-section, which was uncomplicated. The birth weight was 8 pounds, 14 ounces, and Apgar scores were remembered to be normal. Developmental milestones for speech-language and motor skills were reported to have been achieved within normal limits.

Heather's mother describes her as not being able to hear complete directions or distinguish sounds. She has difficulty understanding, seems very forgetful, and is poorly organized. Her mother feels that she hears words in a jumbled way and cannot discern different sounds. She continually needs repetition of directions. She does not filter out extraneous noise and gets easily distracted. The mother feels it may be due to insecurity, focusing or processing problems, or stress related to family life. Multiple family stressors are noted, including numerous family moves, significant financial difficulties, death of a grandparent, and an older sibling with a disability. In addition, the family history is significant for depression and anxiety, substance abuse, and developmental delays.

Heather repeated kindergarten and attended private school until second grade. She is currently in fifth grade at age 11 years, 10 months. Current teacher concerns include that Heather does not seem to hear and process directions. This causes her to struggle following instructions and teacher directions. She also displays difficulty understanding spoken language, comprehending, and spelling. She appears to need constant approval and cannot hear in background noise. A prior audiological assessment revealed normal hearing bilaterally.

The current evaluation was performed over three sessions. Heather was cooperative and friendly with the examiner. She displayed very slow processing, verbal formulation, and task completion. She displayed obvious auditory processing deficits and continually asked for multiple repetition and clarification of oral directions and information. She was distracted by noises in the testing room, such as the humming of the computer.

Overall assessment results showed that articulation, voice, and fluency were within normal limits. Language scores were in the average range on formal testing. Overall composite scores of the formal testing did not reflect the degree of difficulty that Heather experiences in auditory processing, word retrieval, and language usage. Individual weaknesses were indicated in processing and recall of information of spoken paragraphs. Relative weaknesses were noted in comprehension of idiomatic language and inferences and pragmatic judgment. Heather demonstrates a speech or language impairment characterized by moderate deficits in auditory processing, word retrieval, and language usage. While overall scores in formal testing were in the average range, informal analysis revealed moderate deficits in the above areas. In addition, the impairment has an impact on Heather's school day in academic and nonacademic tasks. Heather's impairment impacts her ability to follow classroom directions, answer questions, participate in classroom discussions, and interact with peers and adults within the educational environment. She also has difficulty keeping up with the pace of conversation presented by peers and adults and may miss the jokes and innuendoes presented by peers. Speech-language therapy is recommended for direct and indirect services.

REVIEW QUESTIONS

1. What are the differences between ADD and ADHD?

2. Identify the characteristics of ADHD and explain how they affect a child's functioning at home and at school.

3. What are the pros and cons of interventions for ADHD?

4. What factors contribute to the etiology of ADHD? How are those factors related to intervention strategies?

5. Create a continuum of characteristics from elementary, school-age, middle school-age, and late adolescence.

6. Name two assessment strategies that are important with the ADD/ADHD population.

7. Describe the characteristics of a child with Tourette syndrome.

8. How does ADHD coexist with Tourette syndrome or vice versa?

9. What are the academic problems a child with Tourette syndrome and ADHD may exhibit at school?

REFERENCES

Abikoff, H. (1991). Cognitive training in ADHD children: Less to it than meets the eye. *Journal of Learning Disabilities, 24*, 205–209.

Abwender, D. A., Como, P. G., Kurlan, R., Parry, K., Fett, K., Cui, A. L., Plumb, S., et al. (1996). School problems in Tourette's syndrome. *Archives of Neurology, 53*, 509–511.

Alberto, P. A., & Troutman, A. C. (1986). *Applied behavior analysis for teachers* (2nd ed.). Cincinnati: Merrill.

American Psychiatric Association. (1980). *Diagnostic and statistical manual of mental disorders* (3rd ed.). Washington, DC: American Psychiatric Association.

American Psychiatric Association. (2000). *Diagnostic and statistical manual of mental disorders* (4th Ed.). Washington, DC: American Psychiatric Association.

Augustine, L. E., & Damico, J. S. (1995). Attention deficit hyperactivity disorder: The scope of the problem. *Seminars of Speech and Language, 16*, 243–258.

Axelrod, S. (1971). Token reinforcement programs in special classes. *Exceptional Children, 37*(5), 371–379.

Barababsz & Barababsz (in press). Stimulants. In J. S. Werry & M. G. Aman (Eds.). *Practitioners guide to psychoactive drugs for children and adolescents* (2nd ed.). New York: Plenum.

Barkley, R. A. (1998). Gene linked to ADHD verified. *The ADHD Report, 6*(3), 1–5.

Barkley, R. A. (2000). *Taking charge of ADHD: The complete authoritative guide for parents—revised edition*. New York: Guilford Press.

Beichtman, J. H., Cantwell, D. P., Forness, S. R., Kavale, K. A., & Kauffman, J. M. (1998). Practice parameters for the assessment and treatment of children and adolescents with language and learning disorders. *Journal of the American Academy of Child and Adolescent Psychiatry, 25*, 528–535.

Benner, G., Nelson, R., & Epstein, M. (2002). Language skills of children with EBD: A literature review. *Journal of Emotional and Behavioral Disorders, 10*(1), 43–62.

Bronheim, S. (1991). An educator's guide to Tourette syndrome. *Journal of Learning Disabilities, 24*(1), 17–22.

Brunn, R., Cohen, D., & Leckman, J. (1990). *A guide to the diagnosis and treatment of Tourette syndrome* (pp. 5–31). (Available from Tourette Syndrome Association [TSA], 42–40 Bell Boulevard, Bayside, NY 11361.)

Cantwell, D. P. (1977). Hyperkinetic syndrome. In M. Rutter & L. Hersov (Eds.), *Child psychiatry: Modern approaches*. London: Blackwell Scientific.

Cantwell, D. P. (1983). Diagnostic validity of the hyperactive child (attention deficit disorder with hyperactivity) syndrome. *Psychiatric Developments, 3*, 277–300.

Cantwell, D. P., Baker, L., & Mattison, R. (1986). Psychiatric disorders in children with speech and language retardation. *Archives of General Psychiatry, 37*, 423–426.

Castellanos, F. X., Giedd, J. N., Elia, J., Marsh, W. L., Ritchie, G. F., Hamburger, S. D., et al. (1997).

Controlled stimulant treatment of ADHD and comorbid Tourette's syndrome: Effects of stimulant and dose. *Journal of the American Academy of Child and Adolescent Psychiatry, 36*(5), 589–597.

Castellanos, F. X., Giedd, J. N., Marsh, W. L., Hamburger, S. D., Vaituzis, A. C., Dickstein, D. P., et al. (1996). Quantitative brain magnetic resonance imagining in attention deficit disorder. *Child Psychiatry and Human Development, 16,* 221–232.

Chermak, G. D., Hall, J. W., & Musiek, F. E. (1999). Differential diagnosis and management of central auditory processing disorder and attention deficit hyperactivity disorder. *Journal of the American Academy of Audiology, 10,* 289–303.

Chermak, G. D., & Musiek, F. E. (1997). *Central auditory processing disorders: New perspectives.* Clifton Park, NY: Delmar Learning.

Cohen, N., Davine, M., & Meloche-Kelly, M. (1989). Prevalence of unsuspected language disorders in a child psychiatric population. *Journal of the American Academy of Child and Adolescent Psychiatry, 28,* 107–111.

Comings, D. E. (1990). *Tourette syndrome and human behavior.* Durate, CA: Hope Press.

Comings, D. E., & Comings, B. G. (1987). A controlled study of Tourette syndrome: Attention deficit disorder, learning disorders, and school problems. *American Journal of Human Genetics, 41,* 701–741.

Como, P. G. (1993). Neuropsychological testing. In *Handbook of Tourette's syndrome and related tic and behavioral disorders* (pp. 221–243). New York: Marcel Dekker.

Connors, C. (1980). *Food additives and hyperactive children.* New York: Plenum.

Copeland, A. P. (1981). The relevance of subject variables in cognitive self-instructional programs for impulsive children. *Behavior Therapy, 12,* 520–529.

Craighead, W. E. (1982). A brief clinical history of cognitive behavioral therapy with children. *School Psychology Review, 11,* 5–13.

Dopheide, J. (2001). *Platform presentation of the American Pharmaceutical Association 148th Annual Meeting.* San Francisco, CA.

Douglas, V. I., & Peters, K. G. (1979). *Toward a clearer definition of the attention deficit of hyperactive children.* In G. Hale & M. Lewis (Eds.), *Attention and the development of cognitive style* (pp. 173–247). New York: Pergamon Press.

DuPaul, G., Eckert, T., & McGoey, K. (1997). Interventions for students with attention-deficit/hyperactivity disorder: One size does not fit all. *School Psychology, 26*(3), 369–381.

D'Zurilla, T. J., & Goldfried, M. R. (1971). Problem solving and behavior modification. *Journal of Abnormal Psychology, 82,* 10–16.

Eaves, L. J., Silberg, J. L., & Hewitt, J. K. (1993). Genes, personality and psychopathology: A latent class analysis of liability to symptoms of attention deficit hyperactivity disorder in twins. In R. Plomin & G. McClean (Eds.), *Nature, nurture and psychology* (pp. 285–303). Washington, DC: American Psychological Association.

Elliot, S., & Gresham, F. (1987). Children's social skills: Assessment and classification practices. *Journal of Counseling and Development, 66*(2), 96–99.

Epstein, M. H., Shaywitz, S., Shaywitz, B., & Woolston, J. (1991). The boundaries of attention deficit disorder. *Journal of Learning Disabilities, 24,* 78–86.

Faraone, S. V. (2000). Toward guidelines for pedigree selection in genetic studies of attention deficit hyperactivity disorder. *Genetic Epidemiology, 18,* 1–16.

Faraone, S. V., Biederman, J., Mennin, D., & Russell, R. L. (1998). Bipolar and antisocial disorders among relatives of ADHD children parsing familial subtypes of illness. *Neuropsychiatry & Genetics, 81,* 108–116.

Feingold, B. (1975). *Why your child is hyperactive.* New York: Random House.

Fillipek, P. A., Semrud-Clikeman, M., Steingard, R. J., Renshaw, P. F., Kennedy, D. N., & Biederman, J. (1997). Volumetric MRI analysis comparing subjects having attention-deficit hyperactivity disorder with normal controls. *Neurology, 48,* 589–601.

Flick, G. L. (1998). Learning strategies and social skills training for students with ADHD. *Reaching Today's Youth, 2*(2), 37–40.

Forness S. R., & Kavale, K. (1991). Social skills deficits as primary learning disabilities: A note on problems with the ICLD diagnostic criteria. *Learning Disabilities Research and Practice, 6,* 44–49.

Frazier, M., & Merrell, K. (1997). Issues in behavioral treatment of attention-deficit/hyperactivity disorder. *Education and Treatment of Children, 20*(4), 441–461.

Fujiki, M., Brinton, B., Morgan, M., & Hart, C. (1991). Withdrawn and sociable behavior of children with language impairment. *Language, Speech, and Hearing Services in the Schools, 30,* 183–195.

Gadow, K. D. (1986). *Children on medication:* Volume 1. *Hyperactivity, learning disabilities, and mental retardation.* Boston: Little, Brown.

Gallagher, T. M. (1999). Interrelationships among children's literature, behavior, and emotional problems. *Topics in Language Disorders, 19*(2), 1–15.

Glaze, D. G., Frost, J. D., & Jankovik, J. (1983). Sleep in Gilles de la Tourette's syndrome: Disorder of arousal. *Neurology, 33,* 586–592.

Goldstein, S. (1999). Attention-deficit/hyperactivity disorder. In S. Goldstein & C. R. Reynolds (Eds.), *Handbook of neurodevelopmental and genetic disorders in children* (pp. 154–184). New York: Guilford Press.

Goldstein, S., & Goldstein, M. (1998). *Understanding and managing attention deficit hyperactivity disorder in children: A guide for practitioners* (2nd ed.). New York: Wiley.

Haenlein, M., & Caul, W. F. (1987). Attention deficit disorder with hyperactivity: A specific hypotheis of reward dysfunction. *Journal of the American Academy of Child and Adolescent Psychiatry, 26,* 356–362.

Hall, R. (1980). Cognitive behavior modification and information processing skills of exceptional children. *Exceptional Education Quarterly, 1*(1), 9–15.

Hankin, S., Wright, P., & Gephart, D. (2001). The burden of attention-deficit/ hyperactivity disorder. *Behavioral Health Trends, 13*(4), 7–15.

Hogg, C., Callias, M., & Pellegrini, D. (1986). Treatment of a 7-year old hyperactive boy with educational problems. *Behavioral Psychotherapy, 14,* 145–161.

Holborrow, P., & Berry, P. A. (1986). A multinational, cross-cultural perspective in hyperactivity. *American Journal of Orthopsychiatry, 56*(2), 320–322.

Hymel, S. (1986). Interpretations of peer behavior. Affective bias in childhood and adolescence. *Childhood Development, 57,* 431–445.

Jankovik, J. (2001). Tourette's syndrome. *New England Journal of Medicine, 354*(16), 1184–1192.

Jens, K., & Shores, R. (1969). Behavior graphs as reinforcers for work behavior of mentally retarded adolescents. *Educational Training of Mentally Retarded, 4*(1), 21–27.

Jensen, P., Kettle, B., Roper, M., Sloan, M., Hoven, C., Hector, R., et al. (1999). Are stimulants over-prescribed? Treatment of ADHD in four U.S. communities. *Journal of the American Academy of Child and Adolescent Psychiatry, 38*(7), 797–804.

Kagan, J., Pearson, L., & Welch, I. (1966). Conceptual impulsivity and inductive reason. *Child Development, 37,* 583–594.

Katz, J. (1992). Classification of auditory processing disorders. In J. Katz, N. A. Stecker, & D. Henderson (Eds.). *Central auditory processing: A transdisciplinary view* (pp. 81–92). St. Louis: Mosby Year Book.

Kazdin, A. E. (1972). *Behavior modification in applied settings.* Chicago: Dorsey Press.

Kazdin, A. E. (1975). *Behavior modification in applied settings.* Chicago: Dorsey Press.

Kazdin, A. E. (2000). *Behavior modification in applied settings* (6th ed.). New Haven: Yale University Press.

Kneedler, R. D. (1980). The use of cognitive training to change social behaviors. *Exceptional Education Quarterly, 1*(1), 65–73.

Kollins, S. H., Barkley, R. A., & DuPaul, G. J. (2001). Use and management of medication for children with attention deficit hyperactivity disorder (ADHD*). Focus on Exceptional Children, 33,* 1–24.

Leckman, J. F., & Cohen, D. J. (1999). *Tourette's syndrome: Tics, obsessions, compulsions.* New York: Wiley.

Leckman, J. F., Zhang, H., Vitale, A., et al. (1998). Course of tic severity in Tourette syndrome: The first two decades. *Pediatrics, 102,* 14–19.

Lloyd, J. (1980). Academic instruction and cognitive behavior modification: The need for attack strategy training. *Exceptional Education Quarterly, 1*(1), 53–64.

Luria, A. (1961). *The role of speech in the regulation of normal and abnormal behaviors.* New York: Liveright.

Matthews, W. (1988). Attention deficits and learning disabilities and children with Tourette syndrome. *Psychiatric Annals, 18*(7), 217–219.

Meichenbaum, D., & Asarnow, J. (1979). Cognitive behavioral modification and metacognitive developmental implications for the classroom. In P. C. Kendall & S. D. Hollen (Eds.), *Cognitive behavior interventions: Theory, research, and procedures.* New York: Academic Press.

Meichenbaum, D., & Goodman, J. (1971). Training impulsive children to talk to themselves: A means of developing self-control. *Journal of Abnormal Psychology, 77,* 115–126.

Meodor, A., & Ollendick, T. H. (1984). Cognitive behavior therapy with children: An evaluation of its efficacy and clinical utility. *Child and Family Behavior Therapy, 6*(3), 25–44.

Milberger, S., Biederman, J., Faraone, S., Murphy, J., & Tsuang, M. (1995). Attention deficit hyperactivity disorder and comorbid disorders: Issues of overlapping symptoms. *American Journal of Psychiatry, 152,* 1793–1799.

Neuwirth, S. (1996). Attention deficit hyperactivity disorder. *Decade of the Brain* (NIH Publication No.96–3572). Washington, DC: U.S. Department of Health and Human Services.

NIH Consensus Statement. (1998). *Diagnosis and Treatment of Attention Deficit Hyperactivity Disorder, 16*(2), 1–37.

O'Brien, M. A., & Obrzut, J. E. (1986). Attention deficit disorder with hyperactivity: Review and implications for the classroom. *Journal of Special Education, 20*(3), 281–295.

Ottenbacher, K., & Cooper, H. (1982). The effect of class placement on the social adjustment of mentally retarded children. *Journal of Research and Development in Education, 17*(2), 1–14.

Palkes, H., Stewart, M. S., & Kahana, B. (1968). Porteus maze performance of hyperactive boys after training in self-directed verbal commands. *Child Development, 39*, 817–826.

Park, S., Como, P. G., Cui, L., & Kudan, R. (1993). The early course of the Tourette's syndrome clinical spectrum. *Neurology, 43*, 1712–1715.

Parker, R. (1992). *The ADD handbook for schools*. Plantation, FL: Impact Publications.

Pate, S. (1993). *Language assessment and intervention*. Presentation at the annual convention of the Council for Learning Disabilities, Baltimore, MD.

Pillsbury, H. C., Grose, J. H., Coleman, W. L., Conners, C. K., & Hall, J. W. (1995). Binaural function in children with attention deficit hyperactivity disorder. *Arch Otolaryngology, Head and Neck Surgery, 121*, 1345–1350.

Riccio, C. A., Hynd, G. W., Cohen, M. J., & Gonzales, J. J. (1993). Neurological basis of attention deficit hyperactivity disorder. *Exceptional Children, 60*, 118–124.

Riccio, C. A., Hynd, G. W., Cohen, M. J., & Molt, L. (1996). *The Staggered Spondaic Word Test*: Performance of children with attention deficit hyperactivity disorder. *American Journal of Audiology, 5*, 55–62.

Robin, P. M. (1992). A comparison of behavior and attention functioning in children diagnosed as hyperactive or learning disabled. *Journal of Abnormal Child Psychology, 20*, 65–82.

Roddy, S. (1989). Bad habit, simple tic, or Tourette syndrome? *Contemporary Pediatrics, 6*, 22–35.

Ross, D. M., & Ross, S. A. (1982). *Hyperactivity: Current issues, research, and theory* (2nd ed.). New York: Wiley.

Routh, D. K. (1980). Developmental aspects of hyperactivity. In C. K. Whalen & B. Henker (Eds.), *Hyperactive children: The social ecology of identification and treatment*. New York: Academic Press.

Schoenbrodt, L., & Smith, R. A. (1995). *Communication disorders and interventions in low incidence pediatric populations*. Clifton Park, NY: Delmar Learning.

Schuerholz, L. J., Baumgardner, T. L., Singer, H. S., Reiss, A. L., & Denckla, M. B. (1996). Neuropsychological status of children with Tourette's syndrome with and without attention deficit hyperactivity disorder. *Neurology, 46*, 958–965.

Singer, H. S., & Walkup, J. T. (1991). Tourette syndrome and other tic disorders: Diagnosis, pathophysiology, and treatment. *Medicine, 70*, 15.

Sverd, J., Gadow, K. D., & Paolicelli, L. (1989). Methylphenidate treatment of ADHD in boys with Tourette syndrome. *Journal of the American Academy of Child and Adolescent Psychiatry, 28*, 574–579.

Swanson, J. M., Cantwell, D., Lerner, M., McBurnett, K., & Hanna, G. (1991). Effects of stimulant medication on learning in children with ADHD. *Journal of Learning Disabilities, 24*(4), 219–230.

Swanson, J., & Castellanos, F. (1998). Cognitive neuroscience of attention deficit hyperactivity disorder and hyperkinetic disorder. *Current Opinion in Neurobiology, 8*(2), 243–271.

Tallal, P., & Piercy, M. (1973). Defects of nonverbal auditory perception in children with developmental aphasia. *Nature, 241*, 468–469.

Tomblin, B. J., Zhang, X., Buckwalter, P., & Carts, H. (2000). The association of reading disability, behavioral disorders, and language impairment among second-grade children. *Journal of Child Psychology and Psychiatry, 41*, 473–482.

Urbain, E. S., & Kendall, P. C. (1980). Review of social-cognitive problem-solving interactions with children. *Psychology Bulletin, 88*, 109–143.

Vygotsky, L. (1962). *Thought and language.* New York: Wiley.

Walker, H. M. (1979). *The acting out child: Coping with classroom disruption.* Boston: Allyn & Bacon.

Walkup, J. T., Leckman, J. F., Price, R. A., Hardin, M., Ort, S. I., & Cohen, D. J. (1988). The relationship between obsessive-compulsive disorder and Tourette's syndrome: A twin study. *Psychopharmacology Bulletin, 24*, 375–379.

Whalen, C. K., & Henker, B. (1991). Social impact of stimulant treatment for hyperactive children. *Journal of Learning Disabilities, 24*(4), 231–241.

Wodrich, D. L., Banjamin, E., & Lachar, D. (1997). Tourette's syndrome and psychopathology in a child psychiatry setting. *Journal of the American Academy of Child and Adolescent Psychiatry, 36*(11), 1618–1625.

Chapter 4

Language Learning Disabilities

Lisa Schoenbrodt, Ed.D., CCC-SLP

CHAPTER OBJECTIVES

Upon completion of this chapter, the reader should be able to:

1. Have a clear concept of the exclusive nature of learning disabilities (LD) and how this term came to acquire its various definitions
2. Understand the environmental and genetic factors linked to LD
3. Be aware of the variety of characteristics that can signal an LD
4. Have a clear concept of what constitutes an LLD and understand the difference between isolated LD and LLD
5. Understand the connections between spoken and written language, as well as the evolutionary stages for both, especially in regard to the needs of a student with an LD or LLD
6. Understand the nature of and need for norm-referenced and naturalistic assessments and techniques for both
7. Have a grasp of the range of techniques available for intervention

INTRODUCTION

For many years, researchers in the area of learning disabilities have debated numerous definitions. Even at the time of this writing, while there is a generally accepted definition, many others still exist depending on the web site, support group, or literature you may consult. The definitions all support the fact that language (reading, writing, speaking, and listening) coexists frequently as part of the learning disability spectrum. Language disorders are frequently diagnosed during the preschool years and change to learning disabilities as children engage in more academic tasks when entering grade school. **Speech-language pathologists** (SLPs) and those in training need to be aware of the organic bases, historical context, characteristics, and definitions of the disorder. This chapter provides that information as well as methods for successful assessment and intervention with this population.

Research documents that the field of learning disabilities (LD) constitutes one of the newest, largest, and most hotly contested categories of disabilities at this time. Simply defining LD alone proves a difficult and controversial task; experts in all areas offer a variety of explanations as to the true nature of an LD. LD did not achieve official recognition until the 1960s. Prior to this recognition, children with LD were diagnosed with minimal brain dysfunction (MBD). In 1963, Samuel Kirk suggested the term **learning disability** (LD) to describe those children with deficits in processes such as auditory, visual perception, symbol recognition, short- and long-term memory, concept formation, reasoning, and fine and/or gross motor functions, as well as those having problems with receptive and expressive language, reading, writing, and mathematics (Goldstein & Reynolds, 1999).

Smith, Dowdy, Polloway, and Blalock (1997) identified several phases in the LD movement, including the foundations phase, the early years of the LD movement, and the modern phase. During the foundations phase a variety of theories regarding LD abounded. Gall's early investigations in the 1800s led him to propose the existence of specific localization of brain function. Following Gall, Broca described motor aphasia in an individual and identified the defect's location in the brain. Broca's research resulted in the discovery that alterations in the left side of the brain could result in speech and language problems. Another researcher, Wernicke, made further contributions to the field of LD, leading to the location of the auditory speech area in the left side of the brain. A lesion in or damage to this area leads to difficulties in comprehending speech, reading, and writing. Disorders in reading and writing began to be linked to the same problems that were associated with aphasia. In 1887, an ophthalmologist named Berlin used the term **dyslexia** to describe persons who have difficulty reading in the absence of visual problems. While Berlin made early discoveries in the area of dyslexia, Hinshelwood is credited for the idea of word blindness and its relationship to injury or underdevelopment in the parietal lobe on the left side of the brain, which may be due to "disease, birth injury, or abnormal development" (Richardson, 1992, as cited in Smith, Dowdy, Polloway, & Blalock, 1999). In the early 1900s, a neuropathologist named Orton asserted that listening, speaking, reading, and writing are all related functions. He stated that problems with any of these functions could be related to deficits in neurological functioning and identified several syndromes, including developmental aphasia, auditory aphasia, agraphia, motor speech deficits, and stuttering (Smith et al., 1999).

Smith et al.'s second proposed phase covers the early years of the LD movement, beginning with Samuel D. Kirk's use of the term *LD*. This period also witnessed the birth and growth of many professional and advocacy organizations, including the Council for LD and the LD Association of America (LDA). These associations gave way to the development of the Division for LD and the National Joint Committee on LD (NJCLD), whose membership includes the American Speech Language Hearing Association (ASHA), the Association of Higher Education and Disability, the Council for LD, the Division for Children with Communication Disorders, the Division for LD, the International Reading Association, the LD Association of America, the National Association of School Psychologists, and the Orton Dyslexia Society (Hammill, 1993).

Many legislative changes and changes in educational services provided to children with LD also occurred during this phase. Major legislative changes included PL 89-10, the Elementary and Secondary Education Act of 1965; the Rehabilitation Act of 1973, specifically Section 504; PL 94-142, the Education for All Handicapped Children Act of 1974; the Individuals with Disabilities Education Act (**IDEA**) in 1990; and PL 101-336, the Americans with Disabilities Act (ADA). Due to these legislative changes, children with LD can now receive better educational and support services.

The final phase discussed by Smith et al. (1999) is the modern phase. From the 1990s to the present, service delivery models have continued to evolve. In the past, services were more categorical in nature, in that children with LD were educated in self-contained classrooms with other children with LD. During the 1990s a shift occurred in favor of the **inclusion** model, which calls for more fully incorporating children with disabilities in general education classrooms. This movement, which Madeline Will termed the Regular Education Initiative, called for a blending of special and general education services for children with disabilities. Children with LD would therefore be educated in the least restrictive environment (LRE) possible through methods such as mainstreaming. Other issues that continue to emerge during this phase include (a) resolution of the definition of LD; (b) more efficient methods of identifying individuals with LD; (c) new methods for intervention, including more effective early intervention techniques; and (d) better teacher training in the areas of mild to moderate disabilities as well as research into outcomes of these training techniques.

ETIOLOGY

Defining LD continues to be a difficult task given the fact that these disorders do not share a common cause. LD falls into several categories based on the associated etiological factors. These categories include both environmental and genetic factors.

Environmental Factors

There are many prenatal, perinatal, and postnatal environmental factors that may be related to brain development and that could be considered causes of LD. These factors may directly produce the overall LD or may contribute to the disorder.

During prenatal development, deficits in maternal nutrition may affect brain development (Pirozzolo & Bonnefil, 1996; Pollitt, Golub, Gorman, Grantham-McGregor, Levitsky, Schürch, et al., 1996). Various organs and systems go through critical developmental stages during this period and are sensitive to teratogens. The central nervous system (CNS) is most sensitive during the third and sixth weeks of embryonic development, when the brain begins to develop. Substance abuse during the prenatal period is particularly detrimental. Fetal alcohol syndrome (FAS), fetal cocaine exposure (FCE), and maternal smoking are three major causes of deficits in fetal development.

Fetal Alcohol Syndrome

The effects of alcohol abuse during pregnancy were first documented as a specific syndrome in the 1970s. During this decade, researchers began to note a pattern of congenital malformations and developmental disabilities in children of alcoholic mothers (**fetal alcohol syndrome** [FAS]) that includes central nervous system (CNS) dysfunction, cognitive impairments, growth retardation, facial malformations, learning problems, behavioral problems, and symptoms of attention deficit disorder (distractibility, short attention span, hyperactivity). **Fetal alcohol effect** (FAE) is a less severe form of FAS and is similar to FAS except that the child may display some but not all of the clinical features associated with FAS (Schoenbrodt & Smith, 1995).

Fetal Cocaine Exposure

Prenatal exposure to cocaine may lead to several complications, including **intrauterine growth retardation** (IUGR, which occurs when an unborn baby is at or below the 10th weight percentile for his or her age [in weeks]), premature birth, and low birth weight. In addition, a pattern of intellectual and cognitive deficits exists as do sensory deficits in hearing and sight, a compromised nervous system, and difficulties in school performance.

Maternal Smoking

In 1993, the National Institute of Mental Health (NIMH) documented that maternal smoking during pregnancy produces infants who have a lower birth weight, which may increase the risk of developmental disabilities such as LD. In addition, studies show that there is an increased risk for hyperactivity, impulsivity, and reduced attention span (Nichols & Chen, 1981; Streissguth, Martin, Barr, Sandman, Kirchner, & Darby, 1984).

Perinatal Factors

Perinatal factors are those that occur during the time of birth. Several studies showed that birth histories that include hard labor, prolonged labor, or a combination of the two, fetal distress, and/or anoxia may lead to problems in neurobehavioral development. In addition, Goldstein and Reynolds (1999) reported a higher rate of birth complications among children with LD in comparison with "normal" children.

Postnatal Factors

Postnatal factors include any events that occur after birth that may cause injury to the brain. Postnatal causes of LD include head injuries, lead exposure, and diet. Head injuries, or traumatic brain injury, as discussed in Chapter 1, produce deficits in learning that parallel the profile of an individual who has an LD. There are differences between the two disabilities, but certainly the trauma to the brain causes changes that affect learning, emotional, and behavioral characteristics and outcomes.

Children who are exposed to significant levels of lead may display a variety of clinical signs, including retardation, seizures, irritability, hyperactivity, LD, and gastrointestinal problems. Lead poisoning is caused by the ingestion of lead-based paint, which is generally found in older homes (1950 and older). Studies evaluated the deciduous teeth shed by children exposed to lead, finding that higher levels of lead concentration in children produced clinical signs. More research is under way in order to document the effects of low-level lead exposure in children.

Other environmental factors that may contribute to impaired neurological development generally involve the home environment and childrearing practices, such as authoritarian parenting styles, a lack of structure and/or organization at home, a lack of parenting preparation or readiness (as is the case in teen pregnancy), cognitive limitations of parents, and lack of stimulation (Smith et al., 1997). It is difficult to isolate the effects of these factors, which can work in combination with a biological predisposition to LD. Nevertheless, these factors are critical to development and should not be ignored.

Genetic Factors

Currently there are many research studies that strongly support the basis for genetic factors in some forms of LD (e.g., deficits in reading, spelling, and writing), including family studies, twin studies, and multiple regression studies using twins. Each investigation showed that reading disabilities run in families and are inherited at a rate of 50 percent.

Severe reading disability, or dyslexia, is characterized by difficulty in learning to read in individuals who have no clear neurological, emotional, or intellectual problems. In 1990, Pennington showed that dyslexia has no one cause, but is instead associated with a number of genes. Smith, Kimberling, Pennington, and Lubs (1983) found evidence that in some families there are links between reading disability and a marker on chromosome 15p. Cardon, Smith, Fulker, Kimberling, Pennington, and De-Fries (1994) linked phonological segmentation with chromosome 6, a finding later supported by Pauls's

1996 study. More research continues to be conducted in order to isolate the component processes of reading.

In addition to a genetic predisposition to LD, many chromosomal disorders are associated with learning deficits, including Turner syndrome, Klinefelter syndrome, and fragile X syndrome (particularly in females, who carry the gene for this condition). Single-gene disorders associated with LD include neurofibromatosis, achondroplasia, and phenylketonuria (PKU).

DEFINITION

Practitioners in the field of LD have struggled to identify a common definition for the disorder, due perhaps to the field's youth. This difficulty in pinning down a definition may also be related to the fact that LD theories have arisen from a wide range of individuals of various backgrounds and representing different organizations. This continual struggle has led to the development of many different definitions, some of which are presented herein.

According to Kirk (1962), a learning disability "refers to a retardation, disorder, or delayed development in one or more of the processes of speech, language, reading, writing, arithmetic, or other school subjects resulting from psychological handicap caused by a possible cerebral dysfunction and/or emotional or behavioral disturbances. It is not the result of mental retardation, sensory deprivation, or cultural and instructional factors" (p. 263). This 1962 definition was the first to indicate that LD involves psychological process disorders. Kirk also noted the influence of processing problems on academic performance, and the existence of central nervous system dysfunction. Kirk's definition served as the foundation for the development of later definitions.

Barbara Bateman offered another early definition in 1965: "Children who have learning disorders are those who manifest an educationally significant discrepancy between their estimated intellectual potential and actual level of performance related to basic disorders in the learning process, which may or may not be accompanied by demonstrable central nervous system dysfunction, and which are not secondary to generalized mental retardation, educational or cultural deprivation, severe emotional disturbance, or sensory loss" (p. 200). Bateman's definition was the first to cite underachievement as a necessary component of LD, identifying its relationship to learning. While her definition is also the first to discuss discrepancy, Bateman does not indicate the level of discrepancy required or the best way to measure intellectual potential. While her definition was not widely accepted, the idea of significant discrepancy has been utilized in many of the criteria for identifying LD (Kavale & Forness, 2000; Smith et al., 1997).

Moving forward into the 1970s, regulatory and legislative definitions began to appear. The first such definition emerged from the United States Office of Education (USOE, 1976): "A specific LD may be found if a child has a severe discrepancy between achievement and intellectual ability in one or more of several areas: oral expression, written expression, listening comprehension or reading comprehension, basic reading skills, mathematics calculation, mathematics reasoning, or spelling. A 'severe discrepancy' is defined to exist when achievement in one or more areas falls at or below 50 percent of the child's expected achievement level, when age and previous educational experiences are taken into consideration" (p. 52405).

A large debate ensued following this publication over the idea of employing a mathematical formula to identify children with LD. Due to the high volume of criticism received, the USOE published another definition in 1977, which reads as follows: "The term 'specific LD' means a disorder in one or more of the basic psychological processes involved in understanding or in using language, spoken or written, which may manifest itself in an imperfect ability to listen, speak, read, write, spell, or to do mathematical calculations. The term includes such conditions as perceptual handicaps, brain injury, minimal brain dysfunction, dyslexia, and developmental apraxia. The term does not include children who have LD which are primarily the result of visual, hearing, or motor handicaps, or mental retardation, or emotional disturbance or of environmental, cultural, or economic disadvantage" (IDEA amendments of 1997, PL 105-17, June 4, 1997, 11 stat 37 [20 USC 1401 (26)]).

This definition continues to be the most widely used across the United States. Kavale and Forness (2000) report problems with this definition, however. While it does indicate that process disorders (in the language area) interfere with basic academic achievement, it contains no explicit conceptualization about the descriptions and relationships to LD. In addition, the USOE 1997 definition provides information about the similarities between LD and other conditions, but lacks explicit language describing what does *not* constitute an LD.

Several other definitions need to be introduced. The first of these comes from the National Joint Committee on Learning Disabilities (NJCLD) and is accepted by all the organizations except for the Learning Disability Association of America (LDA), which formulated its own definition. "LD is a generic term that refers to a heterogeneous group of disorders manifested by significant difficulties in the acquisition and use of listening, speaking, reading, writing, reasoning, or mathematical abilities. These disorders are intrinsic to the individual and presumed to be due to central nervous system dysfunction. Even though a LD may occur concomitantly with other handicapping conditions (e.g., sensory impairment, mental retardation, social and emotional disturbance) or environmental influences (e.g., cultural differences, insufficient/inappropriate instruction, psychogenic factors), it is not the direct result of those conditions or influences" (NCJLD, 1981, as cited in Smith et al., 1997, p. 39).

In 1986, the Learning Disabilities Association of America (LDA) developed the following definitions, after disagreeing with the NJCLD definition. "Specific learning disability is a chronic condition of presumed neurologic origin, which selectively interferes with the development, integration, and/or demonstration of verbal or nonverbal abilities. Specific learning disability exists as a distinct handicapping condition and varies in its manifestation and in degree of severity. Throughout life, the condition can affect self-esteem, education, vocation, socialization, and/or daily activities" (LDA, 1986, p. 15).

While the two definitions appear similar, the LDA definition excludes the reading, writing, and listening qualifications. In addition, some practitioners argue that the language of the LDA is vague and employs ambiguous vocabulary (Hammill, 1993; Kavale & Forness, 2000). In 1987, the Interagency Committee on Learning Disability (ICLD) similarly proposed its own definition, also in response to the earlier NJCLD definition. The ICLD's 12 member agencies (all in the U.S. Department of Health and Human Services and the U.S. Department of Education) developed the following definition: "LD is a generic term that refers to a heterogeneous group of disorders manifested by significant difficulties in the acquisition and use of listening, speaking, reading, writing, reasoning, or mathematical abilities, or of social skills. These disorders are intrinsic to the individual and presumed to be due to central nervous system dysfunction. Even though a LD may occur concomitantly with other handicapping conditions (e.g., sensory impairment, mental retardation, social and emotional disturbance), with socio-environmental influences (e.g., cultural differences, insufficient or inappropriate instruction, psychogenic factors), and especially attention deficit disorder, all of which may cause learning problems, a LD is not the direct result of those conditions or influences" (Interagency Committee on LD, 1987, p. 222).

This definition evoked a public outcry over the inclusion of social skills in the list of primary LD manifestations. In addition, the U.S. Department of Education (USDOE) refused to endorse this definition on the grounds that (a) it would require a change in the law (IDEA), (b) it would increase confusion regarding the criteria for eligibility, and (c) it would increase the number of students identified as learning disabled (Kavale & Forness, 2000; Hammill, 1993). The NJCLD modified its earlier definition twice in response to changes in knowledge, as well as in response to the ICLD definition, resulting in the following 1990 definition: "LD is a general term that refers to a heterogeneous group of disorders manifested by significant difficulties in the acquisition and use of listening, speaking, reading, writing, reasoning, or mathematical abilities. These disorders are intrinsic to the individual, presumed to be due to central nervous system dysfunction, and may occur across the life span. Problems in self-regulatory behavior, social perception, and social interactions may exist with LD but do not by themselves constitute a LD. Though LD may occur concomitantly with other handicapping conditions (for example, sensory impairment, mental retardation, serious emotional disturbance) or with extrinsic influences (such as cultural differences, insufficient or inappropriate instruction), they are not the result of those conditions or influences" (NJCLD, 1994).

In 1993, Hammill reviewed the various definitions published in many LD textbooks and found they generally shared several important elements. First the definitions referred to the notion that underachievement is necessary for identification of an LD. Second, the definitions described underachievement using the concepts of discrepancy of ability or achievement (Gregg & Scott, 2000).

Hammill (1993) and Kavale and Forness (2000) both reported that the current NJCLD definition and the IDEA definition appear to reach consensus on the following concepts: (a) LD appears to be the result of central nervous system dysfunction; (b) LD is a condition involving psychological process disorders; (c) LD can occur across the life span; (d) LD involves underachievement; and (e) while LD can be manifested in spoken and written language disorders as well as academic disorders, it is not a result of other conditions. Kavale and Forness (2000) warn that this consensus should not be misconstrued as "closure for the problem of definition" (p. 245), arguing that while the definitions are increasingly similar, both still identify the exact characteristics of a LD. Instead they propose the construction of an operational definition that employs a hierarchical perspective to identify LD.

Kavale and Forness's (2000) model uses a five-level hierarchy that begins with documentation of the presence or absence of underachievement (level I) and then moves through the identification and elimination of various underlying deficits (levels II through IV), concluding with a clear definition of what constitutes an LD for that student (level V). In this model, the identification of LD ceases if a student does not meet the criteria at any level. While the authors' model is very different from the other definitions presented thus far, it does provide a more concise way of identifying LD. Having identified the characteristics to be associated with LD, the next section focuses upon specific academic and speech and language characteristics of students with LD.

CHARACTERISTICS OF LD

Numerous problems can be related to the lack of basic skills necessary for successful academic achievement in students with LD, including:

1. Phonological awareness of sounds
2. Memorization of sound-symbol association
3. Speed of pronouncing words for reading
4. Comprehension of sentences and paragraphs

5. Memory for reading
6. Summarization of information that was read
7. Spelling difficulties related to remembering letters and sounds
8. Visualization of words for spelling
9. Application of spelling rules consistently for words and in written narratives
10. Fine motor coordination for handwriting
11. Writing mechanics (punctuation, spelling, grammar)
12. Organization of written narratives
13. Conceptual knowledge of math
14. Memory for operations and order of operations for math
15. Comprehension of the "language" of mathematics
16. Utilization of problem-solving skills
17. Translation of mathematical concepts into word problems
18. Practical application of mathematical knowledge to the real world

The psychological processes involved in LD can be auditory-verbal, visual-motor, and/or perceptual. Auditory-verbal process deficits result in reading disorders and other language-based LD. Visual-motor and perceptual process deficits may result in reading problems, but more than likely will affect handwriting and mathematics (Goldstein & Reynolds, 1999).

Children whose difficulties relate primarily to visual-motor skills but which are independent of a reading disability (e.g., a non-language-based LD) are identified in neuropsychology as having a "non-verbal LD" (Pennington, 1991; Rourke, 1989, as cited in Goldstein & Reynolds, 1999). These children have problems with spatial organization, mathematics, handwriting, memory for facts, attention to detail, and judgment and reasoning. In addition, these students are more likely to have problems related to depression and anxiety.

Children who have difficulty in a variety of language areas, including reading, have a language-based LD. While the term **language learning disability** is not universally accepted, the number of students demonstrating an LD concomitantly with communication disorders is on the rise.

LANGUAGE LEARNING DISABILITY

The boundaries of communication disorders and LD often overlap, making it difficult to determine the individual effects of each disorder versus their combined impact. Many researchers report that language impairments and LD are one and the same problem observed at different times throughout the life cycle. Haynes, Moran, and Pindzola (1990) found that students with a language impairment may be "rediagnosed" at different points throughout their school experience. Younger children may be identified as language impaired prior to entering school whereas older, school-age children are identified as learning disabled.

In younger children, parents or family members quickly realize if there are language-based problems when children have difficulty expressing their wants and needs. As the children age and go to school, academic needs become the main issue. According to some researchers (Carrow-Woolfolk & Lynch, 1982; Cornett & Chabon, 1986), once the child enters school, language-based problems will affect performance in the school setting and will consequently be recognized as an LD. The use of terminology such as "language learning disability" and "language-based learning disability" often suggests the existence of one specific disability rather than two distinctly different disorders that coexist. This confusion in terminology reflects the earlier difficulty in defining LD and language disorders. Nevertheless, the "accepted" definitions for both terms clearly reflect the similarities and differences between the two.

The 1987 NJCLD definition stated that LD is manifested by significant difficulties in listening, speaking, reading, writing, reasoning, mathematics, or social skills. There is obvious overlap in the area of language, as listening, speaking, reading, and writing comprise language as a whole. In addition, social skills fall under the realm of pragmatic language. Language also has a role to play in mathematics.

In 1990, the American Speech-Language Hearing Association (ASHA) published the following definition: "Specific LD means a disorder in one or more of the basic psychological processes involved in understanding or in using language, spoken or written, which may manifest itself in an imperfect ability to listen, think, speak, read, write, spell, or to do mathematical calculations. The term includes such conditions as perceptual handicaps, brain injury, minimal brain dysfunction, dyslexia, and developmental aphasia. The term does not include children who have learning problems which are primarily the result of visual, hearing or motor handicaps, of mental retardation, or emotional disturbance, or of environmental, cultural or economic disadvantage" (ASHA, 1990, pp. 55–56).

In addition to this definition, which strongly parallels that of the NJCLD, ASHA stated that "a language disorder is the impairment or deviant development of comprehension and/or spoken, written and/or other symbol system" (1982, p. 938). In 1993, Gerber reported that neuropsychological research supports the subtyping of groups of individuals with LD. The child with a concomitant language disorder and LD may at some point be recognized as a specific subtype group within the larger disabilities of language disorders or LD.

A review of individual state definitions of LD revealed that 48 of the states incorporate language disorders into their definitions of learning disabilities and into their criteria for service delivery (Mercer, King-Sears, & Mercer, 1990). Estimates of co-occurrence between the two disorders range from 35 to 60 percent, with language disorder syndrome as the primary presenting syndrome among children and adolescents with LD (Cantwell & Baker, 1992; Denckla, 1981; Satz & Morris, 1981; Wiig & Semel, 1984).

Wallach and Butler (1994) offer additional research to support the overlap. The authors undertook a study of adolescents with LD and identified three major patterns in language and learning disorders: (a) significant language disorders exist at an early age; (b) the teen has a history of academic difficulty; and (c) language-related academic problems did not appear until adolescence. In 1984, Wiig and Semel concluded that language disorders change over time and during the school years frequently manifest as learning problems in reading, writing, and spelling. Despite all the reported overlap, not all students with LD have language disorders because this group is highly heterogeneous (Schoenbrodt, Kumin & Sloan, 1997).

Characteristics

In 1978, Bloom and Lahey described language as a code whereby ideas about the world are represented through a conventional system of arbitrary symbols used for communication. This model included three major components: (a) form, which includes phonology, morphology, and syntax; (b) content, also known as **semantics**; and (c) use, also known as **pragmatics.**

In 1988, Lahey applied an earlier model of language to demonstrate an overlap between LD and language impairments in five areas. According to Lahey, both groups demonstrated the following:

(1) difficulty with language form; (2) disruption of content; (3) impairment to use; (4) distortions in interactions among form, content, and use; and (5) separation of form, content, and use. The difficulties exhibited by children with language and LD may appear clearly early on in life or may develop later and present somewhat more subtly in any one or all five components of this model.

Many researchers have described numerous characteristics of this population. In general, investigators note difficulties in basic vocabulary and information processing, as well as problems in cognition, comprehension and production of linguistic features, narrative and conversational discourse, nonverbal communication, and survival language (Chappel, 1985; Larson & McKinley, 1987, as cited in Schoenbrodt, Kumin, & Sloan, 1997). In addition, Gerber (1993) characterized the language and learning disabled (LLD) population as having delayed phonological acquisition, difficulty with perception and production of complex phonemic configurations, and difficulty in phonological awareness.

Studies documenting the characteristics of younger children with language disorders found that they typically (a) have more difficulty with sentence repetition and completion; (b) have more difficulty with auxiliaries, modals, prepositions, conjunctions, and other grammatical markers; (c) use a small number of verb types; (d) have difficulty with pronoun case marking; (e) produce their first words later and acquire words more slowly; (f) produce fewer lexical categories per sentence; and (g) have problems processing rapidly presented acoustic signals (Ingram, 1975; Rescoria, 1989; Rice & Bode, 1993, Snyder & Downey, 1991; Tallal, 1976; Watkins, Rice, & Moltz, 1993; Wiig, 1990).

Sawyer (1985) reported the following characteristics in school-age children with LLD: word-finding difficulties, limited spontaneous speech, use of immature grammatical forms, difficulty untangling relationships in complex sentences, and trouble remembering and repeating information presented orally. In academic tasks, children demonstrated difficulty with spelling and decoding as well as comprehension in reading in the early grades. Both the younger child and the school-age child with LLD demonstrate greater difficulty with communication tasks associated with daily living activities. These children frequently have problems with pragmatic and social skills, which may become more apparent during school years (Osman, 1982).

Gerber and Bryan (1981) reported on the characteristics of adolescents with LLD completing both basic and higher-level tasks. These adolescents had trouble following oral directions, processing and recalling critical information, retrieving words, making inferences, and comprehending basic classroom vocabulary and concepts. In addition, they demonstrated a reduced ability to organize their thoughts prior to oral output and to engage in flexible thinking. The researchers also reported impairments in auditory memory, comprehension, and attention.

Teachers report that, in the classroom, students with LLD have more difficulty interacting appropriately with their peers, particularly with comprehending and participating in adolescent banter (Gerber & Bryan, 1981; Mathinos, 1988; Rice, Sell, & Hadley, 1990). Rice went on to conclude that when students with LLD are less adept at conversational skills, opportunities for social communicative interaction are lessened, which decreases the opportunity for practice (1993). Conderman (1995) further stated that students who violate the classroom communication rules have more difficulty being accepted by their peers, creating problems with fitting in and acceptance, the quest for which is the hallmark of the adolescent years.

The connections between spoken and written language are clear. The 2001 Position Statement from the American Speech Language Hearing Association, regarding the roles and responsibilities of speech-language pathologists with respect to reading and writing in children and adolescents, supports this connection. According to the Position Statement, "the connections between spoken and written language are well established in that a) spoken language provides the foundation for the development of reading and writing; b) spoken and written language have a reciprocal relationship, such that each builds on the other to result in general language and literacy competence, starting early and continuing through childhood into adulthood; c) children with spoken language problems frequently have difficulty learning to read and write, and children with reading and writing problems frequently have difficulty with spoken language; and d) instruction in spoken language can result in growth in written language, and instruction in written language can result in growth in spoken language" (Position Statement, Guidelines, p. 17).

Four conclusions emerge from the literature on literacy in nondisabled children: (a) the process of learning to read and write is a continuum that begins at birth; (b) reading, writing, speaking, and listening develop concurrently and interrelatedly and not sequentially; (c) the functions of literacy are as integral to literacy learning as the forms; and (d) children learn written language through active engagement in their world.

The above statement defines reading as the processes one uses to construct meaning from printed symbols. Reading can be divided into two areas: decoding and comprehension. Decoding incorporates word recognition processes that transform print into words. Comprehension involves the processes for understanding and interpreting language, where the development of meaning can occur at the word, sentence, and discourse levels. According to Kamhi (1989), a reciprocal relationship exists between decoding and comprehension. In other words, decoding without comprehension is not reading, and comprehension without decoding is not reading. In order for the reader to recognize written words, the reader uses lexical knowledge acquired during early language development. Difficulty learning to read and write may involve many of the components of language, including phonology, morphology, syntax, semantics, and pragmatics. In fact, the comprehension of spoken language provides the core for the development of reading comprehension. According to Juel (1988), the effects of literacy learning problems are negative and long-lasting. Children who experience problems in literacy in early years may remain poor readers and writers throughout their school years. In addition, these children are less likely to be accepted by their peers in school, and may be limited in vocational options as they get older.

Children learn to read by progressing through a series of developmental stages. According to Frith (1985), the first stage is referred to as the logographic stage, in which children associate spoken words with visual stimuli such as the first letter of each word. In the second stage, known as the transition stage, children use some letter-sound cues in order to recognize words. It is during this stage that children begin to develop sight-word vocabulary for frequently used words. During the alphabetic stage, children learn to use letter-sound relationships in order to decode words. Children next begin to analyze words into units without phonological conversion, known as the orthographic stage. By the final stage, automatic word recognition, children have mastered the earlier stages in order to read words. Children who have difficulty in acquiring accurate and fluent word-identification skills may have the central deficit in a specific reading disability known as dyslexia.

Reading comprehension also involves a developmental process that begins in preschool and progresses throughout the life span. As preschoolers, children are exposed to narrative and expository texts and learn to identify relevant and irrelevant information. They also learn to question and respond to information that is read to them at home and at school.

During the elementary school grades, children refine their self-monitoring skills as they expand their knowledge for different types of text structures. They begin to develop skills for reading higher-level texts in a variety of styles and genres that are more linguistically complex. From the upper elementary grades through to adolescence and into early adulthood, students are expected to read lengthy material as part of the curriculum. Much of this material contains abstract and unfamiliar language.

The skilled reader needs to self-monitor comprehension and rely on metacognitive skills in order to develop strategies to facilitate comprehension.

Like reading, writing is a developmental process, which starts when children realize that they are "drawing" speech when representing objects, places, and ideas. In the early elementary years, children write sentences that mimic the length of their own utterances. Early writing is ungrammatical and contains numerous spelling errors. By the time children reach the later elementary grades, their sentences exceed their spoken utterances and have become more grammatically correct. The process of revising drafts and proofreading the product continues to develop and is further refined during the secondary and postsecondary years.

In order to be a good writer, the child needs to be fluent in spelling. Read (1971, 1975, 1986) found that young spellers used an inventive system of grouping sounds together according to some "shared phonetic features." Bissex (1980) and Gentry (1978, 1982) identified five stages through which children progress in developing their spelling: (a) the precommunicative stage, in which spellings are randomly selected letter strings that represent words; (b) the semi-phonetic stage, in which children begin to understand that letters have sounds that are used to represent the sounds in words and that the letters are only a partial "mapping" of the word that is being spelled; (c) the phonetic stage, in which children phonetically segment words and the spellings therefore contain a description of the sequence of the sounds in the pronunciation of the word; (d) the transitional stage, in which children begin to conform to the rules of spelling and vowels appear in every syllable; and (e) the correct spelling stage, in which children have mastered many of the rules, including those of silent consonants.

Given the information concerning literacy, it is evident that spelling problems in this area are related to spoken-language difficulties. Therefore, young children who demonstrate specific language impairments may encounter difficulties in the development of literacy as well. Many longitudinal studies support this notion. Kamhi and Catts (1989) and Wagner and Torgesen (1987) reported that reading disabilities are language-based disorders that can be identified long before children begin reading. Several symptomatic problems may appear, including expressive morphology, syntax, understanding words and sentences, and understanding what is read. In addition, written language is "highly decontextualized and its comprehension relies heavily on a well-developed vocabulary and clear understanding of the structural components and rules of language" (Kamhi & Catts, 1989, p. 86).

While some LD children may not exhibit the above difficulties, they may have trouble with phonological processing, such as a lack of awareness of speech sounds in words, difficulty with word retrieval, verbal short-term memory, and speech production (Badian, McAnulty, Duffy, & Als, 1990; Bradley & Bryant, 1983; Torgesen, 1986). Research has documented a relationship between phonological awareness and reading: phonological awareness develops prior to and influences reading acquisition. Other studies indicate that reading acquisition influences phonological awareness in children.

Though literature regarding children with developmental disabilities is limited, researchers have drawn some conclusions. Children with developmental disabilities experience "literacy" in a much different manner than do their nondisabled peers. Children with severe physical problems, for instance, may not have access to writing implements or have the opportunity to use them; for example, children with Down syndrome may not come in contact with books until later, perhaps age 8 or 9. The reasons for this delay in exposure range from physical, sensory, communicative, and cognitive deficits that limit opportunities for interaction with materials to problems in making modifications in the environment so the child can participate. In addition, the developmental delay label may influence caregivers' perceptions of the child. The caregiver may negatively underestimate the child's abilities based upon the child's behaviors or lack of engagement. In 1999, Katims demonstrated the opposite in a study with young children with disabilities. The study used children with a variety of disabilities, including mild to moderate mental retardation. The results found that these children demonstrated many emergent literacy behaviors when they were exposed to the material and received instructions in modeling the use of the materials.

Based on the definitions and characteristics presented, there is an obvious overlap between language disorders and LD. This is not to say that all children with LD will evidence language disorders, or that all students with language disorders will eventually be defined as learning disabled. The child diagnosed with LD alone is likely to encounter difficulty in academic settings, whereas the child with both a language disorder and LD will struggle in social situations as well. A practical way to think about the two groups is to remember that the child with LD will struggle from 9 to 5, whereas the child with LLD will struggle around the clock (Schoenbrodt, Kumin, & Sloan, 1997). Because both disabilities can be present in the same individual, assessment and intervention must imperatively surpass the traditional boundaries. Documenting both disorders requires multiple models for assessment and intervention.

ASSESSMENT

Norm-Referenced Assessments

Discrepancy scores are frequently used to determine eligibility for services for the student with both a language disorder and an LD, and generally use three common eligibility criteria: cutoff scores; a discrepancy criterion; and a clinical diagnostic model (Gregg & Scott, 2000). Gerber (1993) reported that the use of discrepancy scores does account for the cognitive, pragmatic, or social deficits present in such students. Additional support for that premise exists in other literature: Berninger, Hart, Abbott, and Karovsky (1992) found that intelligence did not consistently match the upper limit on achievement. In addition, Aram, Morris, and Hall (1992) questioned the clinical validity of definitions of developmental language disorders based upon the IQ-language discrepancy criteria. The sole use of discrepancy criteria to identify students with language disabilities and LD excludes many students who have difficulty with pragmatics, auditory processing, and **executive function** (problem-solving/organizational abilities) (Gerber, 1993).

In order to identify cognitive strengths and weaknesses and establish baseline behavior, the student with a language disorder and LD should undergo an in-depth multidisciplinary evaluation. The assessment team should consist of individuals with the skills, training, and qualifications to use the diagnostic tools. At the minimum, the speech-language pathologist (SLP), special and general education teachers, and the psychologist should be involved as part of the diagnostic team. Other specialists, such as the occupational therapist, may be called in for evaluation if the child demonstrates a specific problem in a particular area (e.g., speed and formation of letters for handwriting). Parents also play an important role on the assessment team, as they can provide critical information regarding the student's functioning in the home and community environments. Eligibility for educational services depends on the outcome of norm-referenced assessments and naturalistic assessments and on the student's ability to use language function appropriately in the academic setting (Schoenbrodt, Kumin, & Sloan, 1997).

Standardized or formal evaluation is necessary to document comparable scores and eligibility for educational and support services for the student with language and LD. In addition to having good reliability and validity, a formal assessment battery should evaluate functioning in the following areas: intelligence, problem solving, attention, concentration, memory, receptive and expressive vocabulary, listening comprehension, auditory processing, and academic ability, including performance using language (speaking, listening, reading, and writing).

Equally as important as choosing the assessment tool is determining the appropriate derived score to be reported. The most frequently reported derived scores are age-equivalent scores, percentile ranks, and standard scores. Standard scores are considered the most accurate of the three (Anastasiow, 1986) as well as the most meaningful way to compare the score of the test taker to that obtained by a normative sample. The best method of reporting performance uses the standard error of measurement, which provides a confidence range of performance within which the true score falls, instead of assigning one specific value to test performance. Unfortunately, not all assessment manuals report the standard error of measurement.

In terms of assessment, the examiner should be evaluating the student not only for his or her best performance, but also for performance as compared to peers when placed under the pressure of environmental constraints, such as a timed test (Lahey & Bloom, 1994). In any event, some modifications to the testing may be necessary in order to obtain important information about the student's level of language functioning. While the examiner must adhere to the instructions and time constraints outlined in the standardized assessment to ensure reliability, validity, and performance under stress, information obtained with modifications is invaluable. The student's abilities may be misinterpreted or, worse, missed altogether, if some modifications cannot be made.

Naturalistic Assessment

Norm-referenced tests are often necessary in order to determine eligibility for services and often provide important data regarding overall language performance. However, there are many reasons for not relying completely on this type of assessment alone. According to Launer (1994), norm-referenced tests (a) do not reflect actual communicative abilities, including pragmatics or language usage; (b) tap very specific skills with very specific methods; (c) produce anxiety and do not elicit realistic or optimal performance; (d) are not interactive, in that the student is in a position only to respond and not to initiate; (e) do not usually allow for creativity of response or flexibility in scoring and interpretation; (f) do not reflect language and communication in the classroom; and (g) are frequently culturally biased and do not reflect the diversity of cultures in the clinical population.

In order to counter these deficiencies, an in-depth assessment, which should also include an informal or naturalistic assessment, can provide important information regarding the language functioning of a student with language learning disability—information that may not be tapped by the norm-referenced assessment. Naturalistic assessments can take many forms, such as observation of performance through interviews, questionnaires, performance rating scales, behavioral observations, task analyses (in the form of narrative analysis or language samples), curriculum-based assessment (CBA), and ethnographic assessment (Damico, 1990). The student should be observed in a variety of settings and contexts that sample the type of environmental factors that exist in the natural setting, including the gymnasium, cafeteria, playground, classroom, and home. An observation of the student in the cafeteria, for example, may yield information regarding his or her ability to process information in a noisy environment, communicative competence with peers, ability to communicate under time constraints, word-finding difficulties, problem-solving abilities, and so forth. This type of invaluable information is not captured by a norm-referenced assessment. An informal evaluation can be descriptive, as it allows for a description of the student's communication patterns. Some informal assessment tools include:

1. Task analysis: According to Sohlberg and Mateer (1989), task analysis relies on four basic principles: (a) identification of the task parameters before the student completes the task; (b) evaluation of environmental factors, including the actual environment, and people, including teachers, peers, parents, and so on; (c) identification of the measurement criteria in a qualitative and quantitative manner; and (d) identification of the levels of cueing and compensatory strategies needed to complete the task.

2. Narrative assessment: A minimum of four samples should be collected from the student in the following areas: a personal-experience narrative, a television or movie program narrative, a book summary narrative, and a fictional story narrative. The samples should then be analyzed for style and story grammar development. Story grammar analysis determines if the narrative is a focused chain or a true narrative and answers questions such as: Is a setting given? Are the characters described? Is a goal presented? Narrative assessment evaluates true narrative by answering questions such as: Is the narrative grammatical? Is one topic presented? Is the vocabulary precise? and so forth (Hutson-Nechkash, 1990; Westby, 1984).

3. Curriculum-based language assessment (CBLA): CBLA starts with the identification of curricular contexts in which language-related problems exist, and uses those contexts to develop assessments and interventions. CBLA assesses the types of language skills and strategies the student with an LD employs to process the language of the curriculum, the types of resources he or she uses to meet the demands of the curriculum, the additional abilities and strategies the student might need to make processing more effective and efficient, and the changes that could be made in the curriculum or its presentation to make it more accessible to the student (Nelson, 1994). In the CBLA process, the following should occur: (a) schoolwork should be reviewed as a final product; (b) the student should be observed over several contexts or situations at various times of the day; and (c) once problem areas are identified, the student should be interviewed to obtain samples of expository and narrative discourse.

4. Portfolio assessment: This assessment approach involves collecting and retaining nonrandom samples of information over a period of time. The content of these samples should be identified so as to provide assessment data related to the goals of intervention. Examples of items to include are: narrative discourse samples, writing samples, student comments regarding assignments, samples of tests (essay writing), and observations of student behavior in terms of processing information (Scott, 1994).

Naturalistic assessments provide the most functional information and depict the student's communicative abilities in the school environment. In terms of intervention, it makes sense to assess the areas in the school setting that are the most troublesome to the student with language LD. The information obtained from the entire assessment should be used not only to determine eligibility of services, but also to provide a basis for the formulation of functional and meaningful goals and objectives for the student (Schoenbrodt, Kumin, & Sloan, 1997).

INTERVENTION

Once the student with a language learning disability has been evaluated, a profile of his or her strengths and weaknesses is developed. Students with language learning disability exhibit oral language deficits that affect both language comprehension and production. The type of intervention strategies provided to the student with language learning disability depends upon the results of the comprehensive assessment. In addition, there are many types of intervention strategies reported in the literature—far too many to outline here. The remainder of this chapter presents some intervention strategies that are particularly effective for students with language impairments and LD. For any intervention to be effective, however, it is important to present methods for enhancing these students' language environments. Additionally, collaboration between general and special education teachers, as well as specialists, is necessary for defining the problem, planning and providing services, and evaluating the outcomes of interventions. Critical elements in this process include interaction, communication skills, and assessment of consultation outcomes (Coufal, 1993; West & Cannon, 1988).

Enhancing the Language Environment

It is imperative that the education of students with LLD combine collaborative planning, problem solving, effective teaching methods, and learning strategies. The most effective language learning environments provide opportunities for frequent interaction: students encounter many opportunities to talk and hear talk used for various purposes and in a variety of settings. Dudley-Marling and Searle (1988) identified several principles for creating a language environment favorable for language learning. The first of these involves providing a physical setting that promotes talking. Rather than structuring the classroom in rows of desks, the instructor could provide larger tables for seating, or set aside an area in the classroom for students to gather for short periods, or provide time for students to collaborate on schoolwork, which encourages students to use language. In addition, teachers can facilitate talk in the classroom by providing students with ideas that elicit talk. For example, teachers can provide concrete materials, such as pet animals, photographs, objects related to class projects, and so forth, which promote opportunities to explain, share information, and ask questions. These materials and displays should be changed frequently to stimulate continued opportunity for talk.

The second principle requires that the teacher provide opportunities for students to interact and use language while they learn. Meaningful discussions about learning activities in the classroom enable students to use discourse for the purpose of learning. The teacher's key task for the student is providing opportunities for discussion related to the classroom learning activity. For example, a story about animals that live in the zoo might promote student discussion regarding their personal experiences with these animals. Most students will have visited a zoo while others will have seen pictures or toy versions of these animals. Discussions about personal experiences can enhance students' background knowledge as they continue to read the story. This type of sharing can also improve students' understanding of someone else's perspective in relation to their own.

The third principle specifies that the teacher should provide opportunities for using language for a variety of purposes and with different audiences, so that students learn to shift their language to accommodate the change. Opportunities to interact with younger or older students by sharing ideas, explaining the rules of a game, acting out a play, or collaborating on school projects are just a few examples of ways to interact with different audiences.

The final principle documents the need for teachers to respond effectively to student discourse. According to Dudley-Marling and Searle (1988), "children learn language best when they are directing the conversation to their own ends" (p. 141). To accomplish this, teachers should facilitate conversation by following students' initiations and keeping conversation flowing. Teacher responses should be positive in nature and indicate to the student that the listener is interested. Evaluative comments regarding the student's use of vocabulary or structure should be limited. Teachers should also be aware of the types of experiences upon which students have to draw: students with limited experiences may have difficulty contributing to the conversation if the underlying knowledge is not there. Similarly, students from various cultural backgrounds will have experiences to share that may be unfamiliar to the teacher. In such cases, teachers should be careful to encourage conversation and not highlight differences in the content. These four principles facilitate effective intervention in a naturalistic setting. After establishing an effective language environment, various techniques can be used to stimulate language production.

Targeting Classroom Vocabulary

Within the classroom environment, teachers need to target their instructional language, in addition to textbook language, identifying (Bashir & Scavuzzo, 1992) vocabulary words that are relevant, functional, and individualized for each student. According to Hamersky (1993), the choice of vocabulary must take into consideration the nature and severity of the student's communication deficit, that student's particular interests and needs, and the language needed for the home and school environments. Words can be chosen from the academic curriculum, various literature forms, classroom units, or functional "survival" words.

For older students who are taking vocational courses or working, teachers should target vocabulary that is meaningful, functional, and appropriate for the student's level of functioning in that environment. This type of approach integrates language instruction across the curriculum, providing a more naturalistic and unified approach to intervention.

Content Enhancement Strategies

Content enhancement strategies involve the use of semantic information and discussion for organizing information in class, a technique more commonly known as a semantic organizer. These strategies are excellent in that they not only extend oral language production but also facilitate reading comprehension and writing production for students with LLD.

Visual format strategies are types of semantic organizers that help students to learn the meanings of and relationships among new words, recognize words they already know, and identify relationships among new and familiar words (Hamersky, 1993, 2000). There are five visual format strategies:

1. Attribute webs: In this format, the key word is written in the center of the web. The students generate different attributes of the word, which are then written on extensions of the web. These characteristics are generated in a brainstorming session in which all responses are recorded on the web. A second web is then generated after students discuss similarities among the recorded characteristics.
2. Venn diagram: This strategy is used to help students visualize, understand, compare, and contrast the meanings and characteristics of two concepts. The ideas are written on an appropriate circle and similarities between concepts are written in the overlapping portion of the circle.
3. Multiple-meaning trees: A multiple-meaning tree can be used to help students visualize various meanings for content words. The concept is written in a rectangle (depicting the center of the

tree) with various meanings of the word then written on branches that extend from the tree. Once the tree is completed, students should generate sentences for each meaning.

4. Semantic continuum: This strategy can be used to help students understand that groups of related words can be ranked according to changes in their meaning. Students must have an understanding of the specific attribute that is changing between the words. A key word or concept is identified, and students then generate words that relate to the key word. The concept and related words are then placed on a continuum.

5. Associated words format: This format targets the interrelationships among word meanings. Students apply the target concept to each of nine categories: (a) similar meaning, (b) part/whole relationships, (c) class name, (d) class member, (e) opposite meaning, (f) where something exists, (g) when something occurs, (h) function, and (i) rhyming (Hamersky, 1993, 2000).

Narrative Discourse

Another type of intervention strategy that concentrates on the development of **syntax** (structure) and semantics (content) involves narration. According to Feagans and Appelbaum (1986), the discourse, or narrative, level requires the use of both syntax and semantics that exceed use at the sentence level. This type of language is what is used in the school environment and text information. Specifically, in **narrative discourse** teachers present information by lecturing and reading stories aloud. In response, students present reports or related events. Given the fact that narrative discourse is used extensively in the school environment, students need to understand and use this form of discourse (Kaderavek & Sulzby, 2000; Roth, Spekman, & Fye, 1995).

Discourse can take the form of conversational skills (to be discussed in the following section) or narrative skills, which are similar in that they require a sense of purpose, the selection of relevant information, a method for exchanging the information, the ability to assume the listener's perspective, and the ability to make any needed repairs. Differences in these forms are apparent, however. According to Roth and Spekman (1985), the generation of narratives requires the production of extended units of text. In addition, narratives should contain an introduction and a series of organized events that lead to a logical conclusion. Narratives also require that the speaker produce a monologue, during which the listener maintains a passive role and is responsible for obtaining clarification if something is unclear. In narrative discourse, words take primary responsibility for carrying the overall meaning. In dialogue, meaning is carried by words, the physical environment, intonation, and prosody (Westby, 1984).

Many intervention programs and literature focus on narrative language intervention. One program, developed by Hutson-Nechkash (1990), centers on the remediation of oral narrative skills. The goals of this intervention include exposure to literature, development of the oral narrative, and use of scaffolding techniques to aid in narrative construction.

Conversational Discourse

Conversational discourse involves an interaction between two individuals in which the speaker/listener roles and topics change frequently (Westby, 1984). Conversation is a complex event that is governed by certain rules regarding negotiation in turn-taking, the ability to maintain a discourse topic, and the ability to use repair techniques to recover from breakdowns in conversation (Brinton & Fujiki, 1989). These rules are further complicated by the influence of context, which provides the background for the way in which language is to be used. Context is determined by the number of participants in the conversation, the nature of their relationship, their shared experiences, the subject matter discussed, and the physical surroundings. In addition, speakers must be able to make assumptions about what their listeners know, otherwise known as presuppositional skills (Brinton & Fujiki, 1989; Roth & Spekman, 1989).

Some students with language impairments may have difficulty with the use of language because they demonstrate poor syntactic and semantic skills (Leonard, 1986). Others may have specific difficulty understanding the social uses of language (McTear, 1985). These deficits may change in nature as the student gets older. Evidence suggests that students with LLD do not grow out of their deficits in comprehending and using syntactic and semantic structures. As the student gets older, these deficits may impair the learning of slang and idiomatic expressions, which in turn may interfere with the interpretation of jokes and sarcastic remarks (Donahue & Bryan, 1984; Hall & Tomblin, 1978).

Students with LLD also have difficulty perceiving and interpreting social cues and frequently violate classroom rules by talking out and being off-task. These deficits may further inhibit the student's ability to gain social acceptance into the peer group (Conderman, 1995). For intervention to be effective, strategies such as those listed below, including direct and indirect instruction in social and communicative skills, must take place and the environment should be enhanced to provide increased opportunities for learning to take place (Duchan, Hewitt, & Sonenmeier, 1994).

- Direct pragmatic intervention: The primary goal of this approach is not just to teach behaviors such as turn taking, topic manipulation, and repair strategies, but also to facilitate these skills so that communication is enhanced in a variety of settings. This instruction is accomplished through the use of scaffolding techniques and representational play and story enactments, which include a theme of the script that is individualized for each student.
- Indirect instruction: This strategy structures the environment so that communication can occur in a naturalistic way. It is important that the student's peers be included in social interactions. Group activities in both academic and social settings, for example, offer a context for communication. This type of interaction provides a more natural way for students to gain information about slang terms and other expressions common to the peer group. Indirect instruction should also enhance the generalization of these skills across people and across settings.

The interventions presented thus far are just a few of many that are used in the remediation of language problems in students with LLD. While each intervention can be used to facilitate the development of form, content, and use, they are also complementary, sharing similar principles and based on the premise that intervention must be functional and meaningful to the student with LLD.

CONCLUSION

An LD can be a disorder either in isolation or in coexistence with other disorders, such as a language disability. A great deal of controversy surrounds the definition of an LD and this chapter presented an overview of the many methods of assessment and intervention for students with language LD. Research in assessment and intervention will continue to identify methods for the identification and remediation of language learning disability.

Case Study 1: Elena's Case History

Elena was diagnosed with a language disability at age 4 when her preschool teacher noticed that she consistently had difficulty following directions that were presented orally. She also noticed that Elena had some difficulty interacting with her peers appropriately. Her teacher commented that Elena tends to "stand on the outside and wait for her peers to ask her to join." Once she does join the activity, she either makes comments that are off-topic or delayed in response to the question. Elena was evaluated for speech and language difficulties by an SLP at the local school system. The SLP ruled out hearing loss, but noted that receptive and expressive vocabulary skills were delayed and suspected a central auditory processing disorder, though Elena was too young to test. Speech-language therapy was recommended and continued while Elena entered kindergarten and first grade.

Once Elena entered public school, her teachers continued to note the same language issues but began to notice that Elena's academics were beginning to slip. Elena had a great deal of difficulty with sight word recognition for reading and seemed frustrated and distracted with activities related to reading. By the end of first grade, the school assessment team recommended a complete multidisciplinary evaluation. Elena's parents were supportive of the team and were eager to help in any way possible. Following assessment, the team documented that an LD did exist and support services for reading and continued speech language therapy were recommended. It was also recommended that Elena participate in social skills groups and support groups to build self-esteem with the guidance counselor. She currently is excelling in these programs and her parents are pleased with the services offered by the school.

Case Study 2: John's Case History

John is currently attending middle school and is in the eighth grade. John is the product of a full-term pregnancy with no reported exposure to known gestational risk factors. The delivery was complicated by the umbilical cord being wrapped around his neck during labor. Apgar scores were remembered to be normal and birth weight was reported at 7.5 pounds. John experienced chronic ear infections. Developmental milestones were within normal limits with the exception of speech, which was delayed. John began talking at 1 year of age but it was difficult for others to understand him. The family history is significant for speech problems in the father and paternal uncle and depression in the maternal aunt.

John was cooperative during all three evaluation sessions. He was observed to be very aware of as well as frustrated by his speech difficulties. He displayed very slow processing and verbal formulation. Formal and informal evaluations revealed a severe speech disorder consistent with apraxia of speech. Oral peripheral examination revealed structures adequate for speech production. Dental crowding was observed. John was able to imitate isolated and motor movements, but had difficulty imitating alternating speech movements. Diadochokinetic rate was slow and imprecise. He displayed significant phonologically processing error patterns and significant motor planning and sequencing difficulties. Spontaneous connected speech was unintelligible at times to both familiar and unfamiliar listeners.

Overall language skills were in the below average to the average range. Receptive language skills ranged from slightly below average to average range, whereas expressive language skills were significantly below average. Weakness was indicated in auditory memory for sentences, following oral directions containing linguistic concepts, expression of word definitions, sentence formulation, sentence assembly, and word retrieval. Motor planning and speech difficulties also negatively impacted communicative performance.

John's communicative skills significantly impact his performance in academic and nonacademic tasks. Poor oral motor and sequencing for speech movements impact even the word choices he makes. In addition, he simplifies his vocabulary and sentence length due to difficulties with sequencing of sounds, syllables, and words. Reading and written language performance is significantly impacted. His written language reflects his speech and language patterns and contains poor spelling and grammar. John's impairment impacts his ability to listen to instructions, follow directions, complete reading and written language tasks, answer questions, participate in classroom discussions, and interact with peers and adults within the school environment. Direct and indirect intervention is recommended. In addition, a home program is recommended to involve the family in the remediation process.

REVIEW QUESTIONS

1. What characteristics/potential outcomes of students with LD make it particularly important for teachers to provide an effective language environment?

2. Kavales and Forness noted deficiencies in the widely used 1977 U.S. Department of Education definition of LD. Why are these problematic for the speech-language pathologist, the teacher, and others (e.g., legislators, administrators)?

3. What are the advantages and disadvantages of using a more operational definition of LD (à la Kavale and Forness, 2000) versus some of the more formal definitions?

4. Given the varieties of interventions discussed, what suggestions for modifications could you make to a math teacher dealing with a student with an LLD?

5. You are a speech-language pathologist in a middle school with a student recently diagnosed with an LD/LLD. How can you help facilitate his fitting in?

6. Suppose you are responsible for assembling Elena's assessment team. Whom would you include? What techniques would you use? What modifications might you make and why? What red flags would you be looking for?

7. Why do you think age-equivalent percentage ranks and standard scores are considered the most accurate of the derived scores? Why is it important that a student's scores be examined in comparison to those of his or her peers and while in a pressure-intensive situation?

8. How can cultural bias create problems during assessment and intervention? Give examples.

REFERENCES

American Speech-Language-Hearing Association. (1990). A model for collaboration service delivery for students with language learning disorders in public schools. *ASHA, 33,* 44–50.

Anastasiow, M. (1986). *Development of disability: A psychobiological analysis to special education.* Baltimore, MD: Paul H. Brookes.

Aram, D., Morris, R., & Hall, N. (1992). The validity of discrepancy criteria for identifying children with developmental language disorders. *Journal of Learning Disabilities, 25,* 53–65.

Badian, N. A., McAnulty, G. B., Duffy, F. H., & Als, H. (1990). Prediction of dyslexia in kindergarten boys. *Annals of Dyslexia, 40,* 152–169.

Bashir, A., & Scavuzzo, A. (1992). Children with language disorders: Natural history and academic success. *Journal of Learning Disabilities, 25,* 53–65.

Bateman, B. (1965). *The Illinois Test of Psycholinguistic Abilities in Current Research: Summaries of studies* (ERIC Document Reproduction Service No. ED011417).

Berninger, V. W., Hart, T., Abbott, R., & Karovsky, P. (1992). Defining reading and writing disabilities with and without IQ: A flexible, developmental perspective. *Learning Disabilities Quarterly, 15*(2), 103–118.

Bissex, G. (1980). Patterns of development in writing: A case study. *Theory Into Practice, 19*(3), 197–201.

Bloom, L., & Lahey, M. (1978). *Language development and language disorders.* New York: Wiley.

Brinton, B., & Fujiki, M. (1989). *Conversational management with language-impaired children.* Rockville, MD: Aspen.

Cantwell, D., & Baker, L. (1992). Association between attention-deficit hyperactivity disorder and learning disorder. *Journal of Learning Disabilities, 24,* 88–95.

Cardon, L. R., Smith, S. D., Fulker, D. W., Kimberling, W. J., Pennington, B. F., & DeFries, J. C. (1994). Quantitative trait locus for reading disability on chromosome 6. *Science, 266,* 276–279.

Carrow-Woolfolk, E., & Lynch, J. (1982). *An integrative approach to language disorders in children.* New York: Grune & Stratton.

Chappel, G. (1985). Description and assessment of language disabilities of junior high school students. In C. Simon (Ed.), *Communication skills and classroom success* (pp. 207–242). Eau Claire, WI: Thinking Publications.

Conderman, G. (1995). Social status of sixth- and seventh-grade students with learning disabilities. *Learning Disability Quarterly, 18*(1), 13–24.

Cornett, B. S., & Chabon, S. S. (1986). Speech-language pathologists as language-LD specialists; Rules of passage. *ASHA, 28,* 29–31.

Coufal, K. (1993). Collaborative consultation: An alternative to traditional treatment for children with communicative disorders. *Dissertation Abstracts International, 51*(2), 694.

Damico, J. S. (1990). Descriptive assessment of communicative ability in limited English proficient students. In E. V. Hanayn & J. S. Damico (Eds.), *Limiting bias in the assessment of bilingual students* (pp. 157–218). Austin, TX: PRO-ED.

Denckla, M. (1981). Minimal brain dysfunction and dyslexia: Beyond diagnosis by exclusion. In M. Blau, I. Rapin, & M. Kinsbourne (Eds.), *Child neurology* (pp. 471–479). New York: Spectrum.

Donahue, M., & Bryan, T. (1984). Communicative skills and peer relations of learning disabled adolescents. *Topics in Language Disorders, 4*(2), 10–21.

Duchan, J. F., Hewitt, L. E., & Sonenmeier, R. M. (1994). Three themes: Stage two pragmatics, combating marginalization, and the relation of theory and practice. In J. F. Duchan, L. E. Hewitt, & R. M. Sonnemeier (Eds.), *Pragmatics: From theory to practice* (pp. 1–9). Englewood Cliffs, NJ: Prentice-Hall.

Dudley-Marling, C., & Searle, D. (1988). Enriching language learning environment for students with learning disabilities. *Journal of Learning Disabilities, 21*(3), 140–143.

Feagans, L., & Appelbaum, M. I. (1986). Validity of language subtests in learning disabled children. *Journal of Educational Psychology, 78*, 358–364.

Frith, U. (1985). The usefulness of the concept of unexpected reading failure: Comments on "reading retardation revisited." *British Journal of Developmental Psychology, 3*(1), 15–17.

Gentry, J. R. (1978). Early spelling strategies. *Elementary Schools Journal, 79*(2), 88–92.

Gentry, J. R. (1982). Developmental spelling assessment. *Diagostique, 8*(1), 52–61.

Gerber, A. (1993). *Language-related learning disability.* Baltimore: Paul H. Brookes.

Gerber, A., & Bryan, D. (1981). *Language and learning disability.* Baltimore: University Park Press.

Goldstein, S., & Reynolds, C. R. (1999). *Handbook of neurodevelopmental and genetic disorders in children.* New York: Guilford Press.

Gregg, N., & Scott, S. S. (2000). Definition and documentation: Theory, measurement, and the courts. *Journal of Learning Disabilities, 33*(1), 5–13.

Hall, P., & Tomblin, J. (1978). A follow-up study of children with articulation and language disorders. *Journal of Speech and Hearing Disorders, 43*, 227–241.

Hamersky, J. (1993). *Vocabulary maps: Strategies for developing word meanings.* Eau Claire, WI: Thinking Publications.

Hamersky, J. (2000). *Vocabulary maps: Strategies for developing word meanings.* Eau Claire, WI: Thinking Publications.

Hammill, D. (1993). A brief look at the learning disabilities movement in the United States. *Journal of Learning Disabilities, 26*, 295–310.

Haynes, W., Moran, J., & Pindzola, R. (1990). *Communication disorders in the classroom.* Dubuque, IA: Kendall/Hunt.

Hutson-Nechkash, P. (1990). *Storybuilding: A guide to structuring oral narratives.* Eau Claire, WI: Thinking Publications.

IDEA amendments of 1997, PL 105–17, June 4, 1997, 11 stat 37 [20 USC 1401 (26)]

Ingram, D. (1975). If and when transformations are required by children. In D. Dato (Ed.), *Developmental psycholinguistics* (pp. 225–291). Washington, DC: Georgetown University Press.

Interagency Committee on LD, 1987, p. 22.

Juel, C. (1988). Learning to read and write: A longitudinal study of 54 children from first through fourth grades. *Journal of Educational Psychology, 80*(4), 437–447.

Kaderavek, J., & Sulzby, E. (2000). Narrative production by children with and without specific language impairment: Oral narratives and emergent readings. *Journal of Speech, Language, and Hearing Research, 43*, 34–48.

Kamhi, A. G., & Catts, H. W. (1989). *Reading disabilities: A developmental language perspective.* Boston: College-Hill Press.

Katims, D. S. (1999). Emergence of literacy in preschool children with disabilities. *Language Disorders Quarterly, 17*(1), 58–69.

Kavale, K. A., & Forness, S. R. (2000). What definitions of language disorders say and don't say: A critical analysis. *Journal of Learning Disabilities, 33*(3), 239–256.

Kirk, S. (1962). *Educating exceptional children*. Boston: Houghton Mifflin, 415.

Kirk, S. (1963). *Behavior research on exceptional children* (ERIC Document Reproduction Service No. ED017084).

Lahey, M. (1988). *Language disorders and language development*. New York: Macmillan.

Lahey, M., & Bloom, L. (1994). Variability and language learning disability. In G. Wallach & K. Butler (Eds.), *Language Learning Disability in school-aged children and adolescents*. New York: Macmillan.

Larson, V., & McKinley, N. (1987). *Communication assessment and intervention strategies for adolescents*. Eau Claire, WI: Thinking Publications.

Launer, P. (1994). Keeping on track to the twenty-first century. In G. Wallach & K. Butler (Eds.), *Language learning disability in school-aged children and adolescents*. New York: Macmillan.

Leonard, L. (1986). Conversational replies of children with specific language impairment. *Journal of Speech and Hearing Research, 29*, 114–119.

Mathinos, D. A. (1988). Communicative competence of children with learning disabilities. *Journal of Learning Disabilities, 21*, 437–443.

McTear, M. F. (1985). *Children's conversations*. Oxford, UK: Blackwood.

Mercer, C. D., King-Sears, P., & Mercer, A. R. (1990). Learning Disability definitions and criteria used by state education departments. *Learning Disability Quarterly, 20*, 43–60.

Nelson, N. W. (1994). Curriculum based language assessment and intervention across the grades. In G. Wallach & K. Butler (Eds.), *Language learning disabilities in school-aged children* (pp. 104–131). New York: Macmillan.

Nichols, P. L., & Chen, T. C. (1981). *Minimal brain dysfunction: A prospective study*. Hillside, NJ: Lawrence Erlbaum Associates.

Osman, B. (1982). *No one to play with: The social side of learning disabilities*. New York: Random House.

Pauls, D. L. (1996, March). Genetic linkage studies. In G.R. Lyon (Chair), *Critical discoveries in LD: A summary of findings by NIH research disabilities*. Workshop conducted at the International Conference of the LD Association, Dallas, TX.

Pennington, B. F. (1990). Annotations: The genetics of dyslexia. *Journal of Child Psychology and Psychiatry, 31*, 193–201.

Pennington, B. F. (1991). *Diagnosing learning disorders: A neuropsychological framework*. New York: Guilford Press.

Pirozzolo, F. J., & Bonnefil, V. (1996). Disorders appearing in the prenatal and neonatal period. In E. S. Batchelor, Jr. & R. S. Dean (Eds.), *Pediatric neuropsychology: Interfacing assessment and treatment for rehabilitation* (pp. 55–84). Needham Heights, MA: Allyn & Bacon.

Pollitt, E., Golub, M., Gorman, K., Grantham-McGregor, S., Levitsky, D., Schürch, B., et al. (1996). A reconceptualization of the effects of undernutrition on children's biological, psychological, and behavioral development. In S. Goldstein & C. R. Reynolds (1999) (Eds.), *Handbook of neurodevelopmental and genetic disorders in children* (pp. 108–144). New York: Guilford Press.

Read, C. (1971). Pre-school children's knowledge of English phonology. *Harvard Educational Research, 41*(1), 1–34.

Read, C. (1975). *Children's categorization of speech sounds in English* (NCTE Committee on Research Report No.17–200). (ERIC Document Reproduction Service No. ED112426).

Read, C. (1986). *Children's creative spelling.* London, UK: Routledge and Kegan Paul.

Rescoria, L. (1989). The language development survey: A screening tool for delayed language in toddlers. *Journal of Speech and Hearing Disorders, 54,* 587–599.

Rice, M. (1993). Don't talk to him; he's weird: A social consequences account of language and social interaction. In A. Kaiser & D. Gray (Eds.), *Enhancing children's communication: Research foundations for intervention.* Baltimore: Brookes.

Rice, M., & Bode, J. (1993). General all-purpose verbs. *First Language, 13,* 132–133.

Rice, M., Sell, M. A., & Hadley, P. A. (1990). The social interactive coding system: An on-line clinically relevant descriptive tool. *Language, Speech, and Hearing Services in Schools, 21,* 2–14.

Richardson, S. D. (1992). Historical perspectives on dyslexia. *Journal of Learning Disabilities, 25,* 40–47.

Roth, F., & Speckman, M. (1985). *Story grammar analysis of narratives produced by learning disabled and normally achieving students.* Paper presented at the Symposium on Research in Child Language Disorders, Madison, WI.

Roth, F. P., & Speckman, N. J. (1989). The oral syntactic proficiency of learning disabled students: A spontaneous story sampling analysis. *Journal of Speech and Hearing Research, 32,* 67–77.

Roth, F. P., Speckman, N. J., & Fye, E. C. (1995). Reference cohesion in the oral narratives of students with learning disabilities and normally achieving students. *Language Disabilities Quarterly, 18*(1), 25–40.

Rourke, B. P. (1989). *Nonverbal learning disability: The syndrome and the model.* New York: Guilford Press.

Satz, P., & Morris, R. (1981). Learning disability subtypes: A review. In F. J. Prizollo & M. C. Wittrock (Eds.), *Neuropsychological and cognitive processes in reading.* New York: Academic Press.

Sawyer, D. (1985). Language problems observed in poor readers. In C. Simon (Ed.), *Communication skills and classroom success.* Eau Claire, WI: Thinking Publications.

Schoenbrodt, L., Kumin, L., & Sloan, J. (1997). Learning disability existing concomitantly with communication disorder. *Journal of Learning Disability, 30*(3), 264–281.

Schoenbrodt, L., & Smith, R. (1995). *Communication disorders and interventions in low incidence pediatric populations.* Clifton Park, NY: Delmar Learning.

Scott, S. S. (1994). Determining reasonable academic adjustments for college students with learning disabilities. *Journal of Learning Disabilities, 27,* 403–412.

Smith, S. D., Kimberling, W. J., Pennington, B. F., & Lubs, H. A. (1983). Specific reading disability: Identification of an inherited form through linkage analysis. *Science, 219,* 1345–1347.

Smith, T. E., Dowdy, C. A., Polloway, E. A., & Blalock, G. B. (1999). *Children and adults with learning disabilities.* Boston: Allyn & Bacon.

Snyder, L. S., & Downey, D. M. (1991). The language-reading relationship in normal and reading-disabled children. *Journal of Speech and Hearing Research, 34,* 129–140.

Sohlberg, M., & Mateer, C. (1989). The assessment of cognitive-communication features and head injury. *Topics in Language Disorders, 9(2),* 15–33.

Streissguth, A. P., Martin, D. C., Barr, H. M., Sandman, B. M., Kirchner, G. L., & Darby, B. L. (1984). Intrauterine alcohol and nicotine exposure: Attention and reaction time in four-year-old children. *Developmental Psychology, 20,* 533–541.

Tallal, P. (1976). Rapid auditory processing in normal and disordered language development. *Journal of Speech and Hearing Research, 19,* 561–571.

Torgesen, J. K. (1986). Learning disabilities theory: Its current state and future prospects. *Journal of Learning Disabilities, 19(7),* 399–407.

U.S. Office of Education. (1976). Proposed rulemaking. Federal rulemaking, 41(230), 52407.

Wagner, R. K., & Torgesen, J. K. (1987). The nature of phonological processing and its causal role in the acquisition of reading skills. *Psychological Bulletin, 101(2),* 192–212.

Wallach, G. P., & Butler, K. G. (1994). *Language learning disabilities in school-age children and adolescents.* New York: Macmillan.

Watkins, R., Rice, M., & Moltz, C. (1993). Verb use in language-impaired and normally developing children. *First Language, 13,* 133–144.

West, J. F., & Cannon, G. S. (1988). Essential collaborative consultation competencies for regular and special educators. *Journal of Learning Disabilities, 21,* 56–63.

Westby, C. (1984). Development of narrative language abilities. In G. Wallach & K. Butler (Eds.). *Language learning disabilities in school-age children* (pp. 103–127). Baltimore: Williams & Wilkins.

Wiig, E. (1990). Linguistic transitions and learning disabilities: A strategic learning perspective. *Learning Disabilities Quarterly, 13,* 128–140.

Wiig, E., & Semel, E. (1984). *Language assessment and intervention for the learning disabled* (2nd ed.). New York: Merrill.

Chapter 5
Autism Spectrum Disorders

Janet Preis, Ed.D., CCC-SLP

CHAPTER OBJECTIVES

Upon completing this chapter, the reader will be able to:

1. Define an autistic disorder as including qualitative impairments in social interaction and communication, with restricted and stereotypic patterns of behavior occurring before a child's third birthday
2. Identify the five conditions included in autism spectrum disorders
3. Identify social impairments as one of the defining characteristics of autism
4. List communication impairments, including delays or lack of spoken language, marked impairment in initiating and sustaining conversations with others, stereotypical use of language, and poor social and imaginative play
5. Describe Asperger's syndrome as contrasted with autism in its absence of delay or deviance in language acquisition, and as defined by the presence of severe impairments in social interaction and the presence of restricted and repetitive patterns of behavior
6. Describe Rett's disorder as a progressive developmental disorder affecting only girls and differing from autism in its severe deterioration of skills during the first through third year, resulting in profound mental retardation, loss of hand use and expressive language, and the development of chronic stereotypic hand movements
7. Define childhood disintegrative disorder as a low-incidence disorder that differs from autism in age of onset and pattern of development
8. List adequate and appropriate means of assessment of students with autism
9. Describe goals of intervention and modifications needed for students with autism
10. Describe types of communication interventions, including discrete trial teaching, incidental teaching, and an ecological communication model

INTRODUCTION

Autism (autistic disorder) is one of a spectrum of disorders characterized by a severe and pervasive impairment in communication and socialization. These hallmark characteristics negatively impact the success of daily interactions for the children, adolescents, and adults affected by the disorder. **Speech-language pathologists** (SLPs) are critical members of a professional team trained to provide intervention to these students. This chapter examines the diagnostic criteria, characteristics of communication and socialization, and issues related to assessment and service provision specific to autism spectrum disorders.

In 1943, Leo Kanner first proposed the diagnosis of infantile autism. Based on the observation of 11 children, Kanner outlined both social and communicative deficits, which are remarkably consistent with the definition currently in use more than 50 years later. Kanner's term *autistic* used to describe these "disturbances of affective contact" was borrowed from the field of schizophrenia, though there are distinct and remarkable differences between the two disorders. The most prominent distinction of autism from schizophrenia is its lack of development, rather than regression, and the absence of a private fantasy world necessary for the diagnosis of schizophrenia. Presently, autistic disorder is one of five conditions currently classified as a pervasive developmental disorder in the *Diagnostic and Statistical Manual of Mental Disorders* (DSM-IV) (APA, 1994) and one of eight conditions in the *International Classification of Diseases* (ICD-10) (WHO, 1993), the two major diagnostic systems. This chapter examines the diagnostic criteria, characteristics, and assessment and service provision issues for disorders.

The DSM-IV (APA, 1994) describes autism as a lifelong, early-onset disorder characterized by marked impairments in socialization and communication, in the presence of restricted, repetitive, and stereotypic behavior. Specifically, the DSM-IV definition includes the following criteria for the diagnosis of autistic disorder: "(a) qualitative impairment in social interaction, (b) qualitative impairments in communication, and (c) restricted repetitive and stereotyped patterns of behavior, interests, and activities" (p. 70). These delays must occur before age 3, affect the areas of social interaction, social language, and imaginative play, and may not be accounted for by Rett's syndrome or childhood disintegrative disorder. Current prevalence estimates yield rates of one per 1000 children with autism (Wing, 1993) with as many as two to five per 1000 children exhibiting some form of the disorder. The male to female ratio is 4:1 and is not related to any racial, social, or ethnic boundaries, nor does a family's income, lifestyle, or educational level affect the occurrence of autism spectrum disorders (Wing, 1993; Wing & Gould, 1979).

EPIDEMIOLOGY

In the 50 years since Kanner's original description, research has produced a myriad of products reflecting a constant search for cause, cure, and treatment. Autism is not considered to be curable, though significant progress has been made in recent years regarding potential factors influencing its presence. Knowledge of the neurological, neurochemical, and genetic influences is crucial, as researchers trace this developmental disorder to its underlying dysfunction leading to a more complete clinical profile. Recently it is recognized that seizure disorders occur in about 25 percent of the cases of reported autism (Minshew, Sweeney, & Bauman, 1997), and a significant association exists with both fragile X and tuberous sclerosis (Dykens & Volkmar, 1997).

DIFFERENTIATION BETWEEN THE PERVASIVE DEVELOPMENTAL DISORDERS

Diagnostically, **pervasive developmental disorders** (PDDs) are a group of disorders characterized by severe impairment in reciprocal social interaction and communication, with the possible presence of stereotyped behavior, interests, and activities (APA, 1994). This triad of deficits can occur at different levels of severity in affected individuals. All of the disorders in the PDDs category impact many areas of an individual's life, resulting in qualitative impairments relative to chronological age and level of development. The DSM-IV currently breaks down PDDs into five conditions: autistic disorder, pervasive developmental disorder not otherwise specified (PDD-NOS), Rett disorder (a.k.a. Rett's syndrome), childhood disintegrative disorder, and Asperger's disorder (a.k.a., Asperger's syndrome).

Though confusion does exist within and between the varying conditions, the purpose of these distinctions is to "organize professional experience and data, promote communication, and facilitate the provision of suitable treatments and interventions" (Cohen & Volkmar, 1997, p. 9). Cohen and Volkmar (1997), however, warn professionals (and students) of a number of common mistakes and trends noted in the field of autism. First, these researchers remind us that the classification into the general category of PDD does not require identification of etiologies and causes. Second, these classification systems can be abused, primarily by defining the person in terms of a diagnostic label (remember: person first, disability second). Third, the classification is not an explanation, nor should it be the primary basis of therapeutic intervention. Finally, a diagnosis of a PDD can potentially stigmatize both the family and the person educationally and medically, even affecting insurance coverage. It is important to recognize and understand that diagnostic criteria represent a current agreement among researchers, and that ongoing research and experience will lead to change in these agreements.

Presently, the term *PDD* can be used interchangeably with autism spectrum disorders (ASDs). Lord and Risi (2001) maintain that the term *ASD* most adequately describes the relationship between the varying PDDs. Specifically, autism is considered the prototype, that is, the disability most clearly defined by the threefold deficits in social reciprocity, communication, and repetitive behaviors or interests with onset occurring before age 3. Asperger syndrome, childhood disintegrative disorder, and Rett's syndrome overlap in symptoms with autism, though the disorders are distinct in onset, course, delay, severity, and the domains affected. Atypical autism, or PDD-NOS, extends from the prototype with a decrease in both the severity and number of specific domains affected.

Regardless of the terminology, it is important to recognize both the overlap and distinction between each of the diagnostic categories. Even within the same diagnosis, a great range of functioning can occur, all causing lifelong impairment. These factors are critical in the provision of appropriate, ongoing therapeutic intervention. As stated earlier, a diagnosis is not synonymous with an intervention plan, allowing therapeutic approaches to both differ and overlap within the spectrum of autism. In order to understand how each of the PDDs relate, an explanation and differentiation of each of the five subtypes of PDDs will be presented, including the definition, incidence, onset and course, and factors affecting communication.

Autistic Disorder

When examining the spectrum of autistic disorders, researchers consider autism the prototype or model on which the other PDDs are based. The critical features of autism are significant qualitative impairment in social interaction and communication, in the presence of restricted and stereotyped interests and behaviors. These impairments as well as delays in social interaction, communication, and imaginative play must be present prior to age 3. Autism, unlike other psychiatric disorders, does not "level off" into normalcy, nor does it reveal itself only under specific circumstances. Unfortunately, however, the significant range of severity and the specific manifestations of the disorder between individuals, especially in the area of cognitive functioning, can complicate the diagnosis of autism. Children of varying ages and developmental levels may exhibit the disorder in a variety of ways and levels of severity. Additionally, the symptoms of autism change with age and developmental level. It is important to examine each of the entities of the definition, while remembering that each of the three areas (social interaction, communication, and stereotypic behavior) must be affected simultaneously.

Social Impairment

As noted in the DSM-IV (APA, 1994) definition, social development in children and adults with autism is impaired. Specific areas of impairment are gaze, joint attention, imitation, play, attachment, and pragmatic skills (Volkmar, Carter, Grossman, & Klin, 1997). More specifically, the DSM-IV requires at least two of the following characteristics to be present: (a) marked impairment in the use of multiple nonverbal behaviors (e.g., eye gaze, facial expression, body posture, use of gestures to regulate social interaction); (b) failure to develop peer relationships appropriate to developmental level; (c) marked impairment in the expression of pleasure in other people's happiness; and (d) lack of social or emotional reciprocity. Descriptively these delays remain throughout development, though changes typically occur over time. In infancy the symptoms of social delay may include the failure to develop eye contact or a social smile along with disinterest in the human face and social interactions. Children are often described as aloof as they enter childhood, with significant delays noted in joint attention and affective responses (Mundy & Crowson, 1997). School-age children may make some gains, but typically remain passive or odd (Wing & Gould, 1979), choosing adults rather than peers to be the source of their relationships (Volkmar et al., 1997). Adolescence is occasionally marked by improved social skills, though problems continue to exist. Social interactions, exchanges, and social "rule following" are areas of difficulty. These needs continue into adulthood, and even if persons with autism desire social contact, the strategies to carry out such a plan are lacking.

Pattern of Social Behavior in Young Children. Developmentally, impairment in social interaction occurs before the acquisition of language. The primary features in very young children with autism that differentiate them from children without disabilities are the lack of reciprocal eye contact and a social smile. Human faces and social interaction are not of great interest, though minor environmental changes may be easily detected. Also, young children with autism do not seek as much physical comfort from their parents, share interesting or pleasing events, or appear to take pleasure in interacting with their caregivers, in sharp contrast to their nondisabled peers.

Similar to the pattern of normal development of speech with a (seemingly) abrupt loss, 25 percent of cases report normal early social development from 18 to 36 months of age. One study, performed by Osterling and Dawson (1994), specifically revealed that at the age of 12 months children with autism could be differentiated from nondisabled peers by their reduced incidence of pointing, showing, responding to their name, and orienting as a response. Other studies have reported similar results with additional differences in imitation and attentional skills. Generally, young children with autism are described as "socially aloof" with affective responses minimally related to ongoing events. Additionally, they may be easily disrupted by changes in routines.

For young children with autism four social processes are the primary arenas of impairment: social orientation, imitation and play, attachment, and pragmatic language skills. Social orientation includes gaze and joint attention, both apparent precursors to later developing social and language skills. As noted earlier, the human face holds little interest for young children with autism, resulting in significantly reduced eye contact. The absence of reciprocal gaze between child and caregiver severely interrupts early interpersonal patterns central to communication (e.g., turn taking, sharing of affective states) as well as intersubjectivity (i.e., co-construction of shared emotional meaning). Along with gaze, joint attention is a component of social orientation. Joint attention typically emerges at 8 to 12 months of age, and manifests itself as a communicative skill that occurs before the development of speech and allows a child to share objects and events with another person (e.g., pointing, point and look at a toy). Even if joint attention does exist in children with autism it is typically qualitatively impaired with a reduced positive affect. Specifically, these children typically use gaze and/or gesture to obtain an object or event (protoimperative function). Gaze and gesture intended to comment or show (**protodeclarative function**), however, are notably absent.

Imitation and play are the second social process observed to be impaired in young children with autism. Deficits in imitation are reported for gross motor movements, actions involving objects, actions of adults within routines, and reciprocal play (e.g., "peek-a-boo"). Imitation skills are impaired at both spontaneous and elicited levels. The impact of a deficit in imitation appears to negatively affect symbolic activities of language and play. Play styles for children with autism are described as repetitive and stereotypical, as well as being nonfunctional in the uses of play objects. Even when compared to children of the same cognitive level, much less symbolic play exists in children with autism.

Attachment and affective development comprise the third social process that is significantly impaired in young children with autism. Attachment may be absent or at least atypical, with connection to people notably impaired in the presence of attachments to objects. The belief that children with autism do not form attachments to their parents, however, is no longer supported. The difference is primarily in the form of attachment, rather than a total absence. For example, children with autism are reported to seek physical proximity to a parent more than to a stranger, and show increased attachment at the departure and return of a parent. The use of transition objects is atypical, as normal developing children also are noted to form attachments to objects. However, instead of choosing soft and cuddly objects (e.g., blankets, bears) children with autism typically choose odd objects such as cereal boxes, magazines, and strings.

Affective development follows the patterns of attachment—present but odd. Specific characteristics noted in young children with autism are the absence of seeking physical comfort, lack of desire to be held or cuddled, minimal to no response to speech of parents, and little response to the emotional state of another. Specifically, children with autism are typically unable to recognize the emotional state of others as well as produce, in imitation or spontaneously, emotional facial displays. The greatest area of difficulty in affective development is the ability to produce and respond in an ongoing social interaction.

Pragmatic language skills, or the use of language in social contexts, are the final social skills affected in young children with autism. Many of the previously noted areas, such as gaze, joint attention, play, and affect, appear as pragmatic social skills when used as expressive means of communication. In typically developing children pragmatic language skills begin to emerge by 3 months of age, primarily in the form of joint attention, reciprocal gaze, and turn taking. Each of these skills is typically absent or at least atypical in their development in young children with autism. These deficits continue for some children even in the presence of expressive language. Related deficits in pragmatic language skills for a young verbal child include difficulty talking about what someone else is looking at (**joint attention**), taking turns in conversation (turn taking), following the topic of another (joint attention), and discerning a conversational partner's facial expressions (**reciprocal gaze**).

Pattern of Social Behavior in School-Age Children. Though improvement may be noted in the area of social skill development during the school years due to intervention, the core deficits in this area persist. The specific form of the social need may change, however, as the child changes due to maturation, development, and experience. Researchers found that enough similarities do exist to classify the social skills of school-age children with autism into three groups: the aloof group, the passive group, and the active but odd group (Wing & Attwood, 1987). It is important to keep in mind that these categories are descriptive, not diagnostic, and are presented to assist in the identification and ultimately the intervention for children as they move through their school experience.

Children in the aloof group (the first of the three social descriptors) are often described as classically autistic. Contact with people in the environment is avoided, and distress may result if that contact is forced. Communication and other interaction is seldom, if ever, initiated regardless of the level of expressive language, with a general lack of responsiveness in interactions initiated by either peers or adults. Poor eye contact, apparent minimal attention to presenting events, and a lack of gaze and gesture is common. Children in the aloof group appear so removed from the impact of social and conversational events they often appear as if they are deaf. Adjustments to new situations are difficult, as are transitions between events. Frustration, even tantrums, may result when a routine is interrupted or control over events is reduced. Though these patterns are most typical in the preschool and early school years, persistence of the behavior into adolescence and adulthood may occur, especially in children with more severe mental retardation (Loveland & Tunali-Kotoski, 1997).

The second group is labeled passive, primarily due to their passive approach to social interactions. This group tends to be at a higher level of developmental functioning than the aloof group, and possesses more language and fewer stereotypic behaviors. As a group, these children tend to accept the social initiations of peers and adults, or at the very least do not avoid them, but are unable to respond to or initiate an exchange spontaneously.

The third social group of children with autism is the active-but-odd group. These children are typically categorized as having high-functioning autism (i.e., autism in the absence of cognitive impairment) or **Asperger's syndrome.** Socialization with others in the environment is actively sought, but the interactions are odd due to reduced social skills. These students typically have strong language skills as well as a desire to communicate. However, a narrow focus of topics, incessant questioning, poor response to a partner's interests or comprehension, and unusual facial expressions significantly interfere with successful exchanges. Predictable social routines are typically easier for children in this group to handle, as learned responses can be effectively implemented, rather than more fluid situations, where intent, topic, and audience can change. Because these are students with at least age-appropriate language and cognitive skills, they are often placed in situations where they are expected to interact socially. Their lack of social skills may be interpreted as a behavior or psychiatric disorder by unfamiliar adults and peers, or conversely lead others to assume that they have no feelings about people in their lives. Many of the children in this group are aware of their deficits, and depression and frustration over their inability to establish and maintain relationships are not uncommon.

Pattern of Social Behavior in Adolescents and Adults. Research on the impact of autism in later life is limited, as the emphasis has historically been on childhood. Research is promising, however, in that adolescents and adults with autism have repeatedly been found to continue in the development and expansion of their social interests (Mesibov & Handlan, 1997). But even in the face of such improvements, deficits remain in the establishment and maintenance of relationships. Rutter, in 1983, found that three specific areas affected most adolescents and adults with autism: lack of reciprocity in social exchanges, failure to seek physical contact, and an inability to understand what others are thinking or feeling. Additionally, significant difficulty is noted for the "extraction of rules" from social interactions. A deficit in any or all of these areas leads to confusion, a lack of success, and frustration in seemingly simple (and in the not so simple) daily social interactions.

Communication

A deficit in communication is often one of the first warning signs that a child with autism has a disability. According to the DSM-IV (APA, 1994), a "qualitative impairment in communication" is central to a diagnosis of autism. The DSM-IV definition specifies that in order for the diagnosis of autism to be made, a child must manifest the communication impairment in at least one of the following four areas: (a) delay or lack of spoken language; (b) if speech is present, a marked impairment in the ability to initiate or sustain a conversation with others; (c) stereotyped or repetitive use of language; and/or (d) lack of varied spontaneous make-believe play or social imitative play appropriate to level of development.

Understanding the patterns of communication impairment present in children with autism is important in both assessment and intervention. Language skills are often the predictor of later outcomes, specifically the presence of expressive language by age 5 (Rutter, 1970). High- and low-functioning autism are differentiated primarily by markers of language, specifically the use and flexibility of expression. Early development of social skills is often correlated with a child's use of non-verbal modes of communication (e.g., gestures, gaze), and atypical or deviant language patterns are often central to an appropriate differential diagnosis of autism versus other disabilities. The following section describes the language characteristics of children with autism in the areas of speech development, grammatical complexity, semantics, and pragmatic language use.

Speech. Generally children with autism speak at a later age and develop speech at a slower rate than children without autism (Lecouter et al., 1989). Approximately 25 percent of children with autism have been described as having words (at around 12 to 18 months) and losing them. Research (Kurita, 1985) has indicated that this typically occurs in children who have 10 or fewer words, and takes place over a period of time, placing the pattern in contrast to childhood disintegrative disorder, where loss of speech is sudden and dramatic. Some research indicates that 50 percent of children with autism are without "useful speech." The term *useful speech*, however, is often widely defined, placing these statistics in question. Regardless of a definitional controversy, verbal expression for many children with autism is (and will continue to be) an area of significant need.

In the area of expressive phonology, children who are verbal are unremarkable when compared to other disabled populations, with a similar pattern of the less frequently a phoneme occurs in language the greater the incidence of error. The presence of verbal apraxia appears, however, to impact children with autism, though little research has correlated the two disorders. For children considered to be non-verbal, motor planning deficits appear to interfere with the complex productions required for articulation of speech, with imitation of specific oral movements difficult. These difficulties are consistent with deficits in imitation for other motor movements typically found in children with autism.

Impairments in the paralinguistic features of voice quality, intonation, and stress patterns can also exist in subjects with autism. Tone of voice is frequently monotonous, but may have a singsong quality. Atypical prosodic features are noted as well, including reduced or unusual pauses and phrasing of words. Variations in voice quality, including hoarseness and hypernasality, as well as fluctuating and inappropriate voice volume, have also been reported.

Grammar. In the expressive arenas, sentence length and complexity, both functions of syntax and morphology, can be variable in children with autism. One study (Bartolucci, Pierce, & Streiner, 1980) found that children with autism produced the 14 grammatical morphemes (e.g., articles, present progressive -*ing*, plural *s*) less frequently than their cognitively matched, nondisabled peers, with most errors noted for the use of articles (i.e., a, the, an) and verb tenses. Development of syntax and the use of varying sentence forms appear to be similar to that of peers of equal cognition, with a relation to a developmental rather than age level. Some children with autism treat language as gestalt chunks and expressively produce phrases and sentences in such a manner. In these instances sentence length and grammatical complexity are not indicators of language development and increased complexity, but of an atypical style in language production. Pronoun reversal is also a commonly discussed error of expressive morphology noted in children with autism. Though this is an error in grammatical form, some researchers believe it is born of the deficits in joint attention and understanding another's perspective.

Receptively, less is known about the processing skills of children with autism in the areas of morphology and syntax. As noted previously, difficulty with pronouns is often reported both expressively and receptively. Syntactically, errors appeared to be related to associating sentences to the probability of real-life events, as children with autism had more errors in this arena than cognitively matched peers. Little research has been done, however, to analyze general patterns in receptive language for children with autism.

Semantics. **Semantics,** otherwise known as language content, is the area of language and communication involving the comprehension and use of vocabulary and concepts. Expressive development of vocabulary, including the loss of previously acquired words, is found in some cases of young children with autism to cease. It is significant, however, that this loss occurs before children have a vocabulary burst, a time when vocabulary is acquired quickly and widely generalized. Children with autism often remain in the first phase of lexical development, where words are learned slowly and only for significant people and events. Generalization of these words to other uses is reduced, and the method for learning is not systematic. The second phase of "normal" vocabulary development follows a vocabulary spurt in which words are learned rapidly, often with little exposure, and are generalized to new situations. Researchers believe that language learning in this phase is due to the underlying process of mapping words onto meanings that does not solely rely on associative learning. Children with autism may fail to reach the level of language learning that is not strictly associative, resulting in a limited repertoire of words and phrases. Semantically, children with autism appear to demonstrate a separation of language function and language form. Though they may possess the labels for objects and events, the appropriate use of these words in multiple and varied communicative situations is impaired.

Beyond this difference in development, children with autism differ in their use of words. Some words take on unusual meanings, associated with events or intents unfamiliar to most listeners. Some words may be modifications of the intended one, resulting in odd but understandable language (e.g., "cuts and blusers" for cuts and bruises). Other modifications include the use of **neologisms** in which the source of the word or phrase was not easily evident (e.g., "poomba" for hairdryer).

Previously, researchers believed that children with autism who acquire language did not follow the same stages or pattern as other children. This, however, is found to not be the case (Tager-Flusberg, 1997), as children with autism are more like other children with disabilities as well as children without impairments than they are different, particularly in the area of semantic development. Receptively and expressively it is often found that vocabulary and concepts depicting tangible, concrete events are more easily understood and used than abstract concepts and descriptors. Abstract linguistic concepts are often found to be difficult to understand (e.g., not, after, or, but) as are temporal concepts (e.g., later, yesterday), but these patterns are similar to typical language acquisition.

Pragmatics. The area of language found to be the most significantly impaired in children with autism is **pragmatics,** or the social use of language. For young children, or children at the emerging stage of language development, acquisition of "communicative intentionality" (Prizant, Schuler, Wetherby, & Rydell, 1997) is the major task. Once children use language, the challenge is to expand the range of communicative functions. Expressing these communicative functions in comprehensible and appropriate ways as well as across differing contexts becomes the primary pragmatic goal.

Children with autism may be slow to shift from preverbal communication to symbolic language, with patterns that are "idiosyncratic, less readable, and more context-bound than linguistic communication" (Prizant et al., 1997, p. 573). Additionally, children with autism may engage in **unconventional verbal behaviors** (UVBs), including echolalia, perseverative speech, and language with private meaning, making communication with a less familiar partner difficult or impossible. Though these forms of verbal expression are aberrant, they are not meaningless. Research (McEvoy, Loveland, & Landry, 1988; Prizant & Duchan, 1981) has found that both immediate and delayed echolalia may serve a purpose in the conversation of a child with autism. Some of the functions of echolalia may be turn taking, rehearsal, affirmative answers (i.e., "yes"), declaration of information, and making a request. **Echolalia** is generally viewed as a communicative strategy in the absence of consistent, spontaneous verbal expression, which typically reduces as more language is acquired (Loveland & Tunali-Kotoski, 1997).

Communicative intent is typically very restricted, with regulation of another's behavior, as demonstrated through requests and protests, noted to exist more frequently than socially driven communication (e.g., sharing feelings, commenting, requesting permission). Even in the presence of symbolic language, use is typically much less flexible across multiple environments. Typically, language forms and usage are context-driven, concrete, and cue-dependent. Communicative abilities can also be greatly influenced by a child's emotional state as well as variables in communicative environments, resulting again in great variability in skills dependent on setting. Additionally, children with autism have difficulties understanding verbal information as well as nonverbal signals. This difficulty will limit the reciprocity of a conversational exchange, as a child with autism is often unaware of what a listener is expecting of him or her. As children develop in their language skills, these needs translate into difficulties making conversational repairs and reading the emotional state of others.

Overall, children with autism differ from children without autism in their rate of communicative initiation, with most attempts directed at regulation rather than social interaction. The presence of perseverative comments or questions is reported, as well as reduced incidence of appropriate responses to a partner's comment in conversation. This deficit, as well as previously noted difficulties regarding taking the perspective of a listener, contributes to poor conversational skills. From reduced use of communicative intents at the prelinguistic level to breakdowns in conversational interactions at a more advanced social language level, children with autism manifest significant needs in the area of pragmatic language use.

Cognition

The cognitive, social, and linguistic development of children with autism, though often examined as separate entities, are interrelated, with each area affecting the other (Wetherby & Prutting, 1984). Kanner originally maintained that persons with autism had normal intellectual functioning. This fact, however, was disproven (Lockyer & Rutter, 1969; Volkmar, Hoder, & Cohen, 1985), with research finding that 70 to 80 percent of people with autism obtain IQ scores in the range of mental retardation, primarily falling into the moderate to severe categories (DeMeyer et al., 1972; Wing & Gould, 1979). Though the majority of individuals with autism are mentally retarded, a substantial minority demonstrate average to above-average cognitive skills (Volkmar, Klin, & Cohen, 1997). Therefore, assessment of individual cognitive performance is critical to the design of any treatment plan, considering intellectual functioning as well as adaptive skills.

According to Sigman, Dissanayake, Arbelle, and Ruskin (1997), autistic children are not delayed or deviant in spatial knowledge, perceptual organization, or short-term memory skills. Rather, primary difficulties are noted for the derivation of abstract information "necessary for sequencing material and in transforming this information into symbolic representations" (p. 259). These deficits in turn significantly impact both social and communicative functioning, as representational thinking is necessary to extract knowledge of other people, their language, and the environment.

Asperger's Syndrome

Asperger's syndrome (AS) is a developmental disorder with two critical features: severe and sustained impairments in social interaction; and the development of restricted, repetitive patterns of behavior, interests, and activities that severely impact social, occupational, or other important areas of functioning (APA, 1994). Asperger's syndrome is contrasted with autism in its absence of delay or deviance in language acquisition. The DSM-IV defines this as "single non-echoed words by age 2, and spontaneous communicative phrases by age 3" (p. 80). Additionally, children with AS do not manifest delays in cognition, demonstrating appropriate curiosity in the environment and the appropriate acquisition of learning skills and adaptive behavior with the exception of interactive social development.

The hallmark of this disorder is the severe and sustained impairment in social interaction and emotional relatedness. These impairments may be in one of four areas (manifestation of at least two is required for the diagnosis): nonverbal behavior, peer relationships, spontaneous sharing of interests, and emotional reciprocity. Mental retardation is not usually observed, but a pattern of strengths and weaknesses may be noted with typical strengths in verbal ability (e.g., vocabulary) and weaknesses in nonverbal areas (e.g., visual-spatial skills). Physically, clumsiness and poor body awareness may be present but are usually mild, with an odd posture or gait, possibly leading to further social awkwardness. Additionally, overactivity and inattention are often noted, sometimes yielding an initial diagnosis of attention deficit/hyperactivity disorder (ADHD).

According to the definition, a diagnosis of AS mandates an absence of a speech delay. It does not mean, however, that communication is not impaired. Typically individuals with AS demonstrate poor **prosody** of speech with intonation patterns not necessarily associative with their intent (e.g., humor, anger). Additionally, speech may be noticeably different from that of nondisabled peers in its rate (often too fast), fluency (often jerky), and appropriate modulation of volume (often too loud in close proximity) (Klin & Volkmar, 1997). Beyond noticeable differences in speech, expressive language is also impaired in the areas of both content and use (i.e., semantics and pragmatics). Individuals with AS are typically verbose, engaging in incessant talking (not necessarily conversation) about a favorite topic, regardless of a listener's level of interest or comprehension. Conversations are typically monologues that often appear to exist without a clear point or conclusion. Their expressive language may be confusing to a listener, as individuals with AS often fail to provide appropriate background information on a subject or clearly mark a change in topic. Conversation may also include internal thoughts seemingly inappropriate in an exchange, making a two-way conversation difficult to impossible.

Asperger's syndrome has mistakenly been labeled *high-functioning autism*, a term used to describe children with autism in the absence of mental retardation. "In contrast to the social presentation in autism, AS usually involves fewer symptoms and has a different presentation" (Klin & Volkmar, 1997, p. 102). Though social isolation and impaired interaction are critical to the diagnosis, individuals with

AS are aware of people in their environment. The social awkwardness is not because of a lack of desire for friendship necessarily, but rather the continued frustration that they experience when relating to others. Inappropriate responses are often noted for people with AS, especially regarding emotional interactions. They may be able cognitively to explain a situation and describe the emotions involved, even the unspoken intent of a conversational partner, but are unable to translate this knowledge into spontaneous affect. This "deficient intuition and lack of spontaneous adaptation" (Klin & Volkmar, 1997, p. 102) results in a social style that is rigid, formal, and seemingly unaffected. Individuals with autism are typically unaware of and disinterested in communication partners, whereas those with AS possess the interest, cognitive knowledge, and awareness but not the immediate skills to interact socially.

Onset and Course

Different than children with autism, children with AS do not present with early developmental delays. Language acquisition, cognitive development, and self-help skills are typically within normal limits, contrasted to children with autism who display needs in all three areas prior to age 3. According to Klin and Volkmar (1997), however, two characteristics of early development are strikingly noticeable. Children with AS are often precocious in their ability to speak, and have an unusual attraction to and recognition of numbers and letters. Young children with AS are often deemed to be "hyperlexic," indicative of an ability to decode letters and (occasionally) words with little to no comprehension of their meaning. The second notable feature of young children with AS is a pattern of attachment to members of their family that is generally appropriate. This distinctive feature separates AS from autism, as young children with autism often engage in withdrawal or aloofness, with limited family attachments.

Asperger's syndrome is a lifelong disorder, though differences are noted with age. Young children through school age may be misdiagnosed due to the strengths in verbal language and cognition. Children with AS demonstrate difficulty in social functioning in the early school years, but the inability to establish and maintain relationships may not be noticeable due to academic success. Often, social difficulties are attributed to behavior difficulties, stubbornness, or "adjustment" issues, again due to strong verbal skills. Adolescence presents additional difficulties as a desire for peer relationships usually increases. "Older individuals may have an interest in friendship but lack understanding of the conventions of social interaction and may more likely make relationships with individuals much older or younger than themselves" (APA, 1994, p. 82). Though outcome studies are few, the prognosis for adults with AS is better than for those with autism in terms of employment, independence, and creation of a family (Klin & Volkmar, 1997).

Rett's Syndrome

Rett's syndrome is a progressive developmental disorder affecting only females, characterized by initial normal development followed by a deterioration of skills. Rett's syndrome (termed *Rett's disorder* in the DSM-IV) is not a degenerative disease but a disorder characterized by arrested neurological development of unknown cause (VanAcker, 1997). Rett's syndrome is a subcategory of the PDDs in the DSM-IV, but differs significantly from autism. Though the etiology of Rett's syndrome is not yet established, a genetic origin is strongly suggested (VanAcker, 1997). Presently, as many as 10,000 girls in the United States are estimated to have Rett's syndrome, though only a small percentage have been accurately diagnosed (Moser, 1986). The various presentations of the disability contribute to misdiagnosis, as its appearance is different depending on the age of the child at diagnosis. Tracking back and following the disorder from birth is critical with Rett's syndrome to most accurately differentiate it from autism and other disabilities (e.g., cerebral palsy, hearing loss, psychosis).

Up to the age of 6 to 18 months, children with Rett's syndrome have normal development. At this time developmental stagnation occurs, with a deceleration of head and brain growth, resulting in profound mental retardation across all areas. From age 1 to 3 there is a progressive loss of hand use and expressive language/speech, with the development of chronic stereotypic hand movements. These hand movements include wringing, clapping, tapping, and mouthing, and occur simultaneously with little interest in manipulating objects. Seizures are present in at least 70 percent of the children in early childhood, with self-abusive behaviors also a common symptom. Motor skills become impaired as walking becomes progressively more difficult due to issues in gait, with the presence of both **ataxia** (muscle incoordination) and **apraxia** (inability to perform purposeful movements and motor planning difficulties).

Rett's syndrome differs from autism in a number of ways. The simultaneous regression of both language and motor skills in Rett's syndrome is a key element in a differential diagnosis from autism. Additionally, children with autism have a greater scatter of intellectual skills, often yielding stronger visual skills than verbal skills. Eye contact, often very intense, is usually present in Rett's syndrome, a characteristic typically absent in children with autism. Children with autism do engage in stereotypic, repetitive behaviors, but the repertoire is greater and more complex in autism, and rarely does it remain at midline (hands together at the center) as noted for Rett's syndrome.

Very little research has been conducted on the communication skills of persons with Rett's syndrome. Prior to regression, both language expression and comprehension are reported to be intact, with the rapid loss of skills appearing similar to that associated with a sudden hearing loss. Generally, girls with Rett's are nonverbal with extremely limited to absent verbalizations, restricted to consonant-vowel combinations (Woodyatt & Ozanne, 1993). Improvements are reported as the girls reach adolescence in the areas of eye contact, social interaction, and communicative intent. Communicative intent is manifested through vocalization, facial expressions, gestures, looking, and walking toward a desired object or event. Receptive language skills in girls with Rett's disorder may be stronger than their expressive skills, but the severe impairments in cognition and motor skills impede accurate assessment of language comprehension (i.e., difficulty pointing and/or verbally responding).

Childhood Disintegrative Disorder

Childhood disintegrative disorder (CDD) is an infrequently reported and uncommonly studied disorder that falls under the category of PDDs in the DSM-IV. CDD is a regressive developmental disorder marked by a prolonged period of normal development. The age of onset and pattern of development in CDD are the critical factors differentiating it from autism. Both disorders are characterized by qualitative impairments in social interaction and communication, and the presence of restricted, repetitive, and stereotyped patterns of behavior. Prior to the time of regression, individuals with CDD have a prolonged period (i.e., years) of normal development, with age 3 to 4 being the typical age of onset. This distinguishes CDD from autism in that autism must be present by age 3 (and is often suspected before age 2). Though "deterioration" is reported on occasion in autism, it is typically restricted to a loss or continued use of words. In CDD, deterioration occurs across domains, including speech, with a higher level of language initially acquired. Specifically, a definite loss in at least two of the following areas is necessary for diagnosis: expressive or receptive language, play, social skills, bowel/bladder control, and/or motor skills (WHO, 1993).

Once CDD is established, it resembles autism both clinically and behaviorally. Social skills may be slightly less impaired than those seen with autism (Volkmar, Klin, Marans, & Cohen, 1997), but the loss is still considered significant. A loss of self-care skills, especially toileting, is specific to CDD. Along with losses in social and self-care skills, language is notably affected. Children with CDD regress from using full sentences to possible complete mutism. The loss in language is striking and generally not regainable, as skills do not typically return intact. Language skills in CDD are similar to those seen in autism, with depleted communicative intents and marked impairments in semantic and pragmatic functions.

Pervasive Development Disorder-Not Otherwise Specified

The final category of the PDDs, **pervasive developmental disorder-not otherwise specified** (PDD-NOS), is the broadest. A diagnosis of PDD-NOS can be made when a child does not meet the criteria for a specific diagnosis, but demonstrates a severe impairment in reciprocal social interactions in the presence of impaired communication skills or restricted repetitive and stereotyped patterns of behavior. A diagnosis of PDD-NOS is only used when the criteria are not met for any of the PDDs (i.e., autism, Rett's syndrome, childhood disintegrative disorder, Asperger's syndrome), schizophrenia, schizotypal personality disorder, or avoidant personality disorder (APA, 1994).

PDD-NOS is a disorder in need of further research, as subjects diagnosed with it do not share a specific etiology (e.g., Rett's syndrome) or specific behavioral patterns (e.g., autism, CDD). The term *PDD-NOS* is literally defined as "not anything else in PDD." As a group, individuals with PDD-NOS are heterogeneous, with common core features of "delays in social relatedness and/or deficits in the capacity to reciprocate and understand social interactions, but these can be much milder than those seen in autism" (Towbin, 1997, p. 124). A diagnosis of PDD-NOS is, according to Towbin, used in the following circumstances: (a) as a default diagnosis when information is unreliable, inadequate, or otherwise unfavorable; used as a temporary diagnosis; (b) when the impairment in one of the three core features is too "light" for a diagnosis in another area of PDD, and too severe to qualify for a less severe disorder; considered as "mild" autism; (c) when the age of onset is later than 30 months; and (d) as a temporary category for children when the critical features of early onset and deficits in social relatedness may be accounted for by another disability (e.g., schizoid disorder, semantic-pragmatic disorder, reactive attachment disorder).

ASSESSMENT

Adequate and ongoing assessment of individuals with autism spectrum disorder is the foundation of any intervention program, yet its significance is often downplayed in clinical and educational settings. For an assessment to be adequate it must be comprehensive and, according to researchers, involve "evaluating multiple areas of functioning that are relevant to the child's adaptation, taking the developmental aspects of each of these areas into consideration, and analyzing interrelationships between domains" (Klin et al., 1997, p. 412). Klin et al. (1997) describe six principles that should drive the assessment of children with autism: (a) assess multiple areas of functioning; (b) adopt a developmental perspective; (c) profile any variability in skills; (d) analyze variability in performance across settings; (e) evaluate the impact on everyday life and functional adjustment; and (f) document both delays and deviancies. Assessment methods must consider the quality of measures used and the information obtained, with specific consideration given to a child's variability in performance over time and across settings, as well as any possible impacting environmental factors.

Assessment also requires continuous contact, tracking progress from the diagnostic phase to the phase of intervention to ensure the information obtained is adequately and appropriately translated into functional goals. To most adequately achieve this end, assessment should focus on multiple areas of functioning, including current level of functioning, behavioral components, and functional abilities. A developmental perspective allows students with ASD to be considered in relation to their developmental level, especially as mental retardation is prevalent in many children in this population. Delineation of strengths and needs is also critical, as variability across differing skills is common and a general "score" or single result gives little information regarding such variability. Variability across settings, including people and structure, is also common. Information regarding optimal environments and less optimal settings is valuable. Relating and interpreting assessment information into everyday settings has a multilayered benefit; that is, it considers what a child does in "real life," relates the assessment immediately to intervention, and correlates social/emotional functioning to both assessment and intervention.

Lastly, both delays and deviancies need to be considered. Though a standardized instrument can often easily measure delays, deviance from the norm cannot be as easily measured. This does not mean, however, that the deviancies are irrelevant, but that alternative methods must be employed to obtain the information. Parents and service providers from multiple disciplines need to be involved to create a cohesive picture of strengths and needs in academic as well as social, communicative, and behavioral performance.

Regardless of the area assessed (e.g., communication, cognition, motor function) some guidelines need to be followed. First, the testing environment should be considered in terms of simplicity, use of effective reinforcers, pacing of tasks, and structure. The level and intensity of the social demands involved in the testing should also be monitored. Typically as the level of social demands increases, the performance level on a task decreases for children with ASD. The component of impaired social interaction impedes the assessment process as issues of motivation are often questioned in relation to a child's test performance. Second, parents/caregivers should be involved to the maximum extent possible. Parent input is crucial regarding the testing environment and its impact on their child and the "typicalness" of the child's performance, and as a source of information about specific strengths and needs. An even more critical reason for parent involvement may be a family's ability to associate assessment results and intervention recommendations immediately to specific observable behaviors during testing. Third, multiple examiners should combine their results into a single report, one that is cohesive rather than solely chronological. Discussion of findings should be integrated with each other; for example the communication results should be interpreted in light of the psychological and education findings and vice versa. Finally, assessments, by nature, should be ongoing and geared toward the development of goals and objectives.

Educational and speech/language assessments for young children with autism should follow in this form. As the two primary disabling components of a child with autism are communicative functioning and social interactions, these should be of key interest. Additionally, information regarding level of cognitive functioning should be obtained, using measures that rely less on language. Educational and communication assessments should focus on a child's adaptive functioning, or skills in real-life situations, as well as the performance in a clinical setting.

Communication Assessment

Marked impairment in communication skills is a central characteristic in the diagnosis of autism spectrum disorders. Given the impact an individual's communication skills have on the ability to function in a primarily language-based society, thorough understanding of what a child can and cannot do is crucial. Comprehensive and ongoing assessment is key to designing appropriate interventions to address the individual needs in the domain of communication. Typically, a communication evaluation addresses speech production as well as receptive and expressive functioning in the areas of form (**morphology, syntax**), content (semantics), and use (pragmatics). Information about a student's communicative functioning, as mentioned previously, must be considered in light of the whole student functioning in multiple environments. Standardized tests are one part of an assessment, but it is necessary to understand that the results of formal testing often do not capture all of a child's strengths and needs. Typically, pragmatic and social functioning cannot be assessed through formal testing, particularly in the area of communicative intent. According to Prizant et al. (1997) it is especially important when working with children with ASD to determine the communicative intent of prelinguistic, preverbal, and verbal behavior, as well as unconventional verbal output. A functional communication assessment, including interview, direct observation, and experiment, is also suggested to determine the purpose of an atypical or unusual behavior and its correlation to communicative intent (Carr, Levin, McConnachie, Carlson, Kemp, & Smith, 1994).

Speech

Though many students with autism do not differ from nondisabled peers in articulatory development (Lord & Paul, 1997), 50 percent of the population are nonverbal. The presence of limb and/or verbal dyspraxia has significant implications for the protocol of treatment. The inability to motor-plan limb and oral movements will negatively affect a child's ability to gesture, imitate sounds, and use phonemes in connected speech. These motor-planning and praxis issues need to be considered when evaluating nonverbal motor movements and oral functioning. Along with the specific motor functions associated with speech, precursors for the development of language, such as joint attention, turn taking, and imitation, must be assessed. Some researchers believe these are the building blocks for learning as they are certainly prerequisites for successful communicative interaction.

Due to the variation in speech production among children with ASD, the terminology of language as "expressive" must be considered beyond the scope of speech. Comprehension and use of augmentative and alternative communication systems should be evaluated as well as the role and impact of visual stimulus (e.g., pictures, words, photographs). For subjects who are verbal, assessment of their phonemic repertoire is beneficial to determine the ability to form and produce sounds in the language. Oral motor issues, especially dyspraxia of speech, should be considered, as intervention may vary greatly depending on the type of speech disorder present.

Language

The remaining two areas of language form, morphology and syntax, can be assessed both through standardized tests and the collection of a language sample. Language content or semantics can be evaluated again through standardized tests and informally with the focus on comprehension and use of vocabulary, including labels, descriptors, temporal language, and concepts. Additionally, comprehension and use of questions, negation, and simple and complex directives should be assessed, all of which require syntactic and semantic skills.

Pragmatics. Language use or pragmatic language is often the most overlooked area of a communication assessment, but could be the most informative for the creation of an intervention program. As more than 50 percent of individuals with autism are mute, communicative intent is a critical component of evaluation. Even subjects who are verbal may engage in unconventional verbal behavior (UVB) consisting of echolalia for almost 75 percent of their utterances (Prizant et al., 1997). Wetherby and Prizant (1993) developed the **Communication and Symbolic Behavior Scales** (CSBS) to assess the communicative, symbolic, and social-affective abilities of "developmentally young" children. The CSBS is exceptionally relevant for the assessment of young children with autism, as it evaluates areas of communication often overlooked in standardized tests, but critical to the development of intervention. Specifically it measures the communication parameters of (a) communicative functions (i.e., range of functions, behavioral regulation, joint attention); (b) gestural communicative means (i.e., conventional gestures, distal gestures, coordination of gesture and vocal acts); (c) vocal communicative means (i.e., isolated vocal acts, inventory of consonants, syllable shape, multisyllables); (d) reciprocity (i.e., discourse structure including respondent acts, rate, repair strategies); (e) social-affective signaling (i.e., gaze shifts, positive affect with eye gaze, episodes of negative behavior); (f) verbal symbolic behavior (i.e., expressive language, language comprehension); and (g) nonverbal symbolic behavior (i.e., symbolic play, combinatorial play). Results of such an assessment for young children with ASD should lead, according to Wetherby and Prizant (1997), to the development of specific intervention approaches.

Correlation of Assessment with Intervention

For students with ASD, as with all communicatively impaired children, functionality should drive intervention. Remembering this, goals for intervention at all stages of development should be able to answer the question of, "So what?" For example, when developing expressive and receptive vocabulary goals focus should be on "power words," or words that facilitate a response in the environment, rather than the presentation of predictable vocabulary units. Specifically, teaching the vocabulary for individual items and events with which a child comes in contact such as names of family and peers, labels for routine events, and language for desired items and routines is far more effective and meaningful than teaching standard vocabulary units of "farm animals, clothing, household items," and the like. Assessment results will be especially helpful in answering this question, as a student's inability to be successful in many domains is often correlated with a delay or deviance in communication. The goals for language intervention should, therefore, be presented similarly to any other functional goals, following the sequence of acquisition, demonstration across environments, and spontaneous initiation. Spontaneous communication is the desired outcome, in the absence of adult intervention to the greatest degree possible.

INTERVENTION

The goal of intervention for all students, including those with ASD, is the development of skills necessary to function as independently as possible within a community. Autism spectrum disorders are lifelong disorders that begin early in life, with changes occurring across the life span. ASD is by definition a descriptive disorder, with variations noted across subjects in cognition, language, level of socialization, and concomitant disorders. These individual differences make the goal of intervention a significant and often daunting challenge. Each student with autism has unique strengths and weaknesses that must be taken into account when designing a treatment plan. Along with variations in ability, chronological age and developmental functioning must be considered in designing an effective program. Development of skills is central, but adaptive functioning must be held to be equally important. The constant and critical focus of any intervention program, therefore, must be the development of skills that allow a person to participate ultimately at the highest level possible in his or her family, with peers, and in the community.

Academic Content and Environmental Modifications

Throughout the assessment process and into the development of goals for intervention, the emphasis should be on the criterion of ultimate functioning (Brown, Nietupski, & Hamre-Nietupski, 1976). This philosophy emphasizes "that assessment efforts and intervention objectives should specifically target behavior that will be functional in real environments for the individual with a disability" (Powers, 1997, p. 449). Educational programs for students with autism have been cited to have "little likelihood of positively impacting (on) their adult functioning" (Donnellan, Mesaros, & Anderson, 1985, p. 506). Keeping this in mind, specific academic content should therefore be geared toward independent functioning in the community.

Little empirical research currently exists on the specific content of an academic program. Research does exist, however, to support how to most effectively teach students with autism. The concept of structured teaching has received substantial support, and should be considered in the development of educational and academic programs. A review of the literature (Fischer & Glanville, 1970; Halpern, 1970; Graziano, 1970; Schopler, Brehm, Kinsbourne, & Reichler, 1971) indicates that intervention incorporating structured teaching yields greater success than that found in teaching environments with less structure. Overall, the goal of structured teaching is to promote independence and reduce interference from supervising adults (Schopler, 1997). According to Schopler, Mesibov, and Hearsey (1995), teaching within a structured framework serves to compensate for typical areas of need in students with autism, including impairment in receptive and expressive language, attention, abstractions, organization, auditory processing, generalization, and change in routine. Typical strengths in students with ASD are special interests, rote memory, and visual processing, all upon which structured teaching is based. Structured teaching is not a specific curriculum; rather, it is a framework in which vocational, social, and daily living skills are taught. Adaptations are made for each individual student, adjusting to chronological and developmental age, with ongoing assessment determining the needed levels of support. It encompasses modifications made to the physical environment, the use of schedules, individual and individualized work areas and systems, and specific organization of presented tasks.

The physical environment should also be modified to meet the needs of the student and the task at hand. Strategies successfully employed at **TEACCH (*Treatment and Education of Autistic and related Communication handicapped Ch*ildren)** in North Carolina have been the use of individual workstations and areas of the room specifically designated for academic and leisure activities. This visual structure, according to the founders of TEACCH (Schopler et al., 1995), allows a student to make associations between locations and events, as well as between work and leisure, and to understand the expectations of others for her or his performance. Separation of areas may or may not be necessary, depending on a student's individual ability to remain focused and his or her tolerance for separation. Initially it is advisable to reduce auditory and visual distraction when teaching a task (Duker & Rasing, 1989), with gradual reentry into an environment similar to that encountered in a community setting. The ability to tolerate noise, visual movement, and multiple distractors is a key component in ongoing assessment, in order to determine the appropriate level of support needed in this area.

Issues of sequencing tasks and requests, task size, and student preference and choice are factors that influence student performance. Specifically, the interspersement of acquired and novel tasks increases learning (Dunlap, 1984) and reduces inappropriate behavior (Charlop, Kurtz, & Milstein, 1992). Similarly, sequence of requests impacts success. In two separate studies (Davis, Brady, Williams, & Hamilton, 1992; Davis, Brady, Hamilton, McEvoy, & Williams, 1994) subjects with autism performed better when low-probability requests were preceded by high-probability ones; finding the "behavioral momentum" of the initial success affected the more difficult requests. Finally, consideration should be given to task size and the motivation of the student regarding the specific materials or activity. Logically, if a task is too large, success decreases (Sweeney & LeBlanc, 1995), and preferable activities increase attention, motivation, and appropriate behavior (Foster-Johnson, Ferro, & Dunlap, 1994).

Overall, academic content must be individually driven, with continued and vigilant focus on independent functioning in a community. Thorough and ongoing assessment is crucial to determine both strengths and needs in individual students. The presence of structure in the learning environment is suggested and can be achieved by organizing both the environment and the tasks into clear, predictable segments as needed. Within the content of the established curriculum, instructional variables of sequence of activities and requests, size of task, and student interest and choice should be strongly considered.

Communication Intervention

Early Intervention

Therapeutically, significant attention and time should be given to language intervention for young children with autism. Acquisition of expressive language by age 5 has been positively correlated with behavioral and vocational success (Rutter, 1970). Three factors found to predict later language development are social responsiveness, phoneme production, and skills in verbal imitation (Windsor, Doyle, & Siegel, 1994). Some research has found that children with autism appear to benefit most substantially when intervention is initiated between ages 2 and 4, with a minimum of 15 hours per week of "focused treatment" involving a very low student to teacher ratio (Rogers, 1996).

Some intensive behavioral treatment programs have been criticized, however, for their absence of natural communicative interactions. Specifically, limitations of a strict behavioral approach have been cited for their obsessive focus on form (i.e., how to talk) with little attention given to communicative function (i.e., why to communicate) (Carr, 1983). The adaptive skill of communication by definition requires the ability to understand and use symbolic and nonsymbolic behaviors, including those necessary to understand and convey requests, emotions, comments, protests, and rejection. Intervention must therefore be analyzed in terms of its ability to promote independent communication rather than isolated verbal behavior. As indicated by Wetherby, Schuler, and Prizant (1997), "the focus of communication enhancement efforts must be the development of functional communication abilities, rather than just the development of communicative means or behaviors" (p. 513). An integrated approach combining intensive treatment with functional communication intervention appears to be a logical marriage of current intervention practices.

Direct Communicative Instruction

Language curriculum, though used by many, does not fit all students. Yet once the goals have been specifically and individually matched to a student's strengths and needs, as well as to multiple communicative environments, methods of intervention can be similar. As mentioned previously, early intervention has proven to be a necessary component in successful instruction for children with autism. If a student is without the form of language, that is, she or he does not speak or possess communicative precursors, discrete-trial teaching may be suggested to address these needs. **Discrete-trial teaching** is considered to be a traditional method of language instruction incorporating drills, often with large numbers of trials until a child reaches a high level of performance (typically 90 to 100 percent). Discrete-trial teaching is an effective means to teach communicative skills that can be task-analyzed into component parts, or skills, considered to be prerequisite for further language development (Lovaas, 1977, 1981). Sitting in a chair or responding to simple commands (e.g., "give to me") may be considered prime examples of skills appropriate for discrete-trial intervention, especially if more naturalistic means of intervention are not successful. In a discrete-trial model the student is requested to respond to the discriminative stimulus (e.g., the verbal command, "give to me") in a massed trials format (possibly 10 to 15 consecutive trials). Reinforcement is provided for accurate responses, with inaccurate responses negated (i.e., student told "no") and subsequently prompted (e.g., provide an outstretched hand with the verbal command). This format is continued until the goal is achieved to a high accuracy level over multiple sessions.

Though historically discrete-trial teaching typically involved reinforcers unrelated to the goal of intervention (Matson, Benavidez, Compton, Paclawskyj, & Baglio, 1996), assimilation to a natural language paradigm is suggested for the promotion of more natural speaking situations. The natural language teaching paradigm incorporates the reinforcers into the teaching, thus associating communicative intent with communicative form in a discrete-trial format (Koegel, O'Dell, & Koegel, 1987). All skills taught in the structured format must be directly related to functional communication, and involve the domains of receptive language, expressive communication, and social interaction.

Incidental teaching is an intervention technique incorporating naturally occurring interactions designed to facilitate language use. The primary contrast between it and discrete-trial teaching is that incidental teaching allows the child to initiate the interaction, thus choosing the location and content of the teaching (Carr, 1983). Typically, a "teaching episode" consists of only a few trials and is followed by natural and meaningful reinforcement. Using the example involving the command "give to me," an incidental approach would focus on this goal within a natural routine and teacher-child interaction. For example, if the child was unable to open a container holding items he desired, the teacher could request that the child "give to me." The desired outcome of responding appropriately to the verbal request is the reinforcer, as the intervention follows the student rather than the student following the intervention. Combining the techniques of discrete-trial and incidental teaching could allow for the acquisition of language form as well as promote language use.

Parental and family involvement is critical on every level of intervention, regardless of the specific methodology chosen. A family's concerns and preferences for their child must be taken into account when developing goals, objectives, and intervention strategies. Some language intervention models take the family into consideration, with application to families in naturalistic settings. Specifically, the **ecological communication model (ECO)** focuses on both the child and the parent during play and addresses activity level, joint focus of attention, balance of turns, imitation, initiated communication, and topic selections (MacDonald & Carroll, 1992). Research has found that children with disabilities (including autism) communicate more frequently and with higher quality when the interactions are child-initiated (Norris & Hoffman, 1990). Specifically the ECO model includes a three-step process: the adults organize the environment with appropriate toys and activities; adults interpret the child's behavior and provide communication opportunities; and adults provide natural consequences to continue communication.

Generalization

Spontaneous use of established skills is the ultimate goal of communication intervention. Providing a child with strategies for self-initiation should accelerate progress for content and form as well as promote the goal of independence (Koegel & Koegel, 1995). Self-initiation can be fostered through antecedent interventions involving environmental modifications and the use of visual supports. Spoken language is a transient signal, with the phonemic form unrelated to its semantic content. Therefore, the use of pictures, symbols, and/or text allows a fleeting auditory message to become iconic and concrete, increasing the probability of comprehension. According to Quill (1995), "the simultaneous presentation of spoken and written language enhances the child's ability to focus attention on the message, organize and extract meaning from the language, and respond more efficiently" (p. 181). Providing visual supports throughout the environment as well as during the directive and incidental teaching phases of intervention could allow a child with autism to more efficiently generalize a skill into multiple environments with reduced adult interference. McClannahan and Krantz (1999) reported an increase in spontaneous verbalizations in children with both limited and extensive language repertoires in the presence of visual supports. The use of auditory or pictured scripts successfully prompted children with autism to expand on a topic spontaneously. Overall, the environment must be assessed to determine the role and level of prompts needed that can be accomplished in the absence of an adult.

In sum, all goals and objectives of intervention should be communicatively correlated across domains as often as possible, at all levels of language development. Intervention at an early age is critical, with specific attention and effort given to the expansion of a communicative repertoire, receptively and expressively. Focused, early communication intervention may prevent the development of aberrant behavior, often associated with the inability to communicate traditionally. The 1985 study conducted by Carr and Durand found that problem behaviors could be effectively reduced and ultimately replaced by strengthening relevant communication skills (Durand & Carr, 1991). It could then be assumed that communication training designed to enhance pragmatic aspects of language, specifically to satisfy the functions of attention, escape, request, comments, and sensory needs, would preclude some aberrant behaviors from developing. Clearly, communication training is not a "cure-all," but it is a wise investment in time and energy, as functional independence cannot occur in its absence.

Case Study 1: Child with Autism

Jessie is a 4-year-old girl presenting with limited to absent communication skills, occasional outbursts of hitting herself and others, and limited social skills. Her parents initially became concerned about her lack of expressive communication, believing that "she understood all of what others said to her." She appeared, according to parental report, to be very independent, easily entertained by certain toys (especially dolls), and to experience frustration primarily due to her inability to communicate with others. When questioned how Jessie had her needs met, her parents reported she usually obtained items on her own (e.g., pushing a chair to a counter to open a cabinet containing food; placing videos in the VCR independently), or led them by the hand to desired items and events. Both parents were anxious to rule out the diagnosis of autism based on the consistently "good eye contact" observed at home with members in and outside of the family as well as her demonstration of affection.

Diagnostic testing was conducted over a period of two weeks, consisting of a psychological evaluation to determine her level of cognitive functioning, a speech-language evaluation to determine her current level of communicative functioning, an educational evaluation to assess present levels of preacademic skills, and an occupational therapy evaluation to determine the level of self-help skills and sensory functioning. A combination of parent interview, direct observation, and standardized testing was conducted. The Psychoeducational Profile-Revised (PEP-R) was administered to identify characteristic uneven learning patterns exhibited by children with autism or related developmental disorders. The scores are distributed among seven Developmental Scales and four Behavioral Scales. The Developmental Scales are norm-referenced and indicate where a child is functioning relative to peers. Jessie.'s overall Developmental Score was 20 months, well below her chronological age. Her strengths were in the areas of fine and gross motor and eye hand coordination. Her weakest areas were cognitive performance and cognitive verbal, as she had not yet mastered some of the early skills necessary for preschool learning, such as matching pictures to objects, recognizing shapes and letters, and labeling colors. Limited attention to task also affected her performance. Encouragement to continue to work was met with resistance when the task was not preferred. Alternately, she had difficulty transitioning from preferred tasks and made attempts to escape from less desirable ones by whining and arching her back as a form of resistance.

The Vineland Social Maturity Scales, an instrument using parent report to measure functional skills and adaptive behaviors not readily observed in an assessment session, was administered. Jessie's overall Adaptive Behavior Composite score fell in the range of moderate deficit with all areas of adaptive behavior affected (i.e., communication, daily living skills, socialization, and motor). Her strength was in the motor domain, with overall functioning similar to that of a child 18 months old. However, when Jessie's skills were compared with the special population of children with autism under age 10 who are nonverbal, her adaptive behavior skills were considered to be average, with the exception of daily living skills.

The Childhood Autism Rating Scale (CARS) was also administered. This is an observational measure of behaviors characteristic of autism that was completed at the time of assessment. Behaviors are rated in terms of severity for the following areas: (a) relating to people, (b) imitation, (c) emotional response, (d) body use, (e) object use, (f) adaptation to change, (g) visual response, (h) listening response, (i) taste, smell, and touch response and use, (j) fear or nervousness, (k) verbal communication, (l) nonverbal communication, (m) activity level, (n) level and consistency of intellectual response, and (o) general impressions. Jessie's total score was indicative of "mildly to moderately autistic."

In the communicative assessment, Jessie was evaluated using the Communication and Symbolic Behavior Scales (CSBS) in the areas of (a) communicative functions, (b) gestural communicative means, (c) vocal communicative means, (d) reciprocity, (e) social-affective signaling, (f) verbal symbolic behavior, and (g) nonverbal symbolic play. Results of the assessment revealed the primary function of Jessie's communication to be requesting desired items or events, with occasional episodes of protesting. Jessie communicated for behavioral regulation but did not communicate for the purpose of calling, showing off, or commenting. The function of joint attention was limited, as she had difficulty attending to both objects and people, clearly focusing most frequently on only the objects. During the evaluation, J.P. communicated primarily through the conventional gesture of giving with no distal gestures observed. She often manipulated the hand of the examiner or her mother to request assistance or request items that were difficult to obtain independently. Occasionally, vocalizations were observed during these requests, primarily in the form of a single vowel sound with rising intonation. Repair strategies were attempted through the repetition of behaviors to request items or events, with few gaze shifts observed. Positive **affect** (i.e., facial expressions of pleasure or excitement with or without vocalization) was limited, with two instances of negative affect (i.e., vocal expressions of distress or frustration).

A limited number of vowels and consonants was observed in Jessie's spontaneous phonemic repertoire, including four vowels (i.e., *ah, ih, uh, eh*) and five consonants (i.e., *b, d, k, m, n*), primarily during solitary play. These sounds were observed in isolation and occasional consonant-vowel combinations (e.g., *buh, kuh, dih*). No expressive language forms were heard. Impaired language comprehension was illustrated through Jessie's inconsistent response to verbal requests when accompanied by gestural cues. She did, however, point to a variety of pictures on demand, given up to a field of three choices. Jessie engaged in play with dolls, appearing to have them kiss and walk. She did not respond to the play of the examiner and had difficulty relinquishing these items when presented with alternate toys. Other areas evaluated included imitation of gestures and oral movements. Jessie attempted to imitate a variety of gestural movements, including signs for "more, done, stop, go, and eat." Oral movements appeared more difficult, though she imitated mouth opening and closing, lip presses, and lip rounding when given assistance with oral positioning. Attempts to imitate the vowels within her repertoire were unsuccessful with the exception of *ah*. No consonants were imitated.

Based on the evaluation, communication intervention for Jessie will focus on: (a) the expansion of communicative functions (i.e., behavioral regulation, social interaction, joint attention); (b) imitation of gestural, vocal, and verbal behavior; (c) improved comprehension of gestural and verbal language; and (d) development of action play schemes used with familiar and novel objects. These goals will be addressed through the use of instructional routines to help develop anticipatory and intentional behaviors, replacing idiosyncratic communicative means (e.g., hitting, pushing away) with more conventional means (e.g., verbalizing "no"; head shake), and developing multiple means of communication. Jessie shows an interest in and a level of comprehension for pictures that will be used to establish a communication system for both receptive and expressive language development. Additionally, gestures and signs will be presented along with simple vocalizations for familiar and high-frequency intents. Oral motor functioning will be concurrently addressed through oral motor intervention specifically directed toward the imitation of sounds and the correlation of sounds to meaningful utterances. Finally, play and communication will be simultaneously addressed thorough imitation of novel play schemes with a peer and/or an adult, including turn taking, cooperative behavior, and tolerance of shared materials.

Case Study 2: Adolescent with PDD-NOS

Louis is a 16-year-old presenting with a long history of academic and social difficulties first evident in his early childhood. He initially received services at age 2 through the infants and toddlers program. He subsequently received special education services from age 3 until the present, including education services, occupational and physical therapies, speech and language therapy, and psychological services. Presently Louis receives instructional support in the areas of English, science, and social studies. Additionally, he receives speech and language services one hour a week, and participates in a social skills group co-led by the SLP and the school psychologist. Louis's current disabling condition is autism due to pervasive developmental disorder-not otherwise specified (PDD-NOS).

The diagnosis of PDD-NOS was determined in January 1997 by a psychiatrist not affiliated with the public school system. The medical report indicated uneven patterns of cognitive development and deficits in executive functioning leading to difficulties in attention, tendencies toward obsessiveness/perseveration, and poor impulse control. Additionally, Louis was diagnosed with severe anxiety with obsessive-compulsive disorder, separation anxiety, and poor self-esteem. A review of Louis's medical history revealed hypotonia and failure to thrive. Genetic testing was negative for fragile X and Langer Giedion. An audiological evaluation in 1996 revealed mild hearing loss in the right ear and hearing within normal limits in the left ear.

Louis received multiple psychological evaluations in his academic history. His most recent results (February 2002) indicate his overall cognitive abilities are in the borderline range of functioning. Strengths noted in testing, falling in the average range, were visual-spatial reasoning, short-term auditory memory, and fund of factual knowledge. Significant weakness was revealed in the areas of mental mathematical reasoning, social reasoning, and visual-motor speed.

The communication assessment, conducted across four sessions in May 2002, revealed significant needs in the areas of language content, auditory processing, and pragmatic language use. Articulation testing revealed no errors in single words or during a storytelling task. Informally, Louis's conversational speech is often less intelligible, with imprecise articulation and a rapid rate of speech. Oral motor functioning is borderline, with needs noted for tongue tip strength and difficulty with tongue and jaw stability and separation. Standardized testing was administered to assess receptive and expressive language form (morphology, syntax) and content (semantics). Specifically, the Peabody Picture Vocabulary Test-III (PPVT-III), the Clinical Evaluation of Language Fundamentals-3rd edition (CELF-3), and the Test of Adolescent/Adult Word Finding (TAWF) were administered. Louis revealed age-appropriate skills in his receptive vocabulary, with borderline below age level skills noted for both receptive and expressive language skills. Specific areas of need were identified for word retrieval, rapid naming, comprehension of idioms and figurative language, question comprehension related to verbal information, and recalling sentences. Significant needs also exist in the area of pragmatic use of language. Difficulties were noted and reported for staying on topic, continuing a topic not of his own initiation, social problem solving, eye contact, and appropriate use of facial expressions. Louis appeared to be impulsive regarding his verbalizations, often making negative comments about an activity and about himself. He often became frustrated when a task was difficult and adopted a depressed and negative affect, occasionally hitting himself on the head when he interpreted a response as incorrect. Louis was also impulsive behaviorally, often grabbing for materials that belonged to the examiner, getting out of his seat to look out the window, and rocking in his chair. He was generally responsive to a verbal cue and appeared to have little awareness of his behavior. Parent and teacher report that Louis continues to present with poor impulse control, poor social judgment, and obsessive/perservative thought patterns.

Based on the evaluations, communication intervention for Louis will focus on (a) increasing intelligibility of speech; (b) improving word retrieval and specific verbal expression; (c) expanding expressive vocabulary; (d) understanding and applying figurative language, including idioms; (e) social problem solving; and (f) identification and modification of physical aspects of social language (body posture, eye contact, movement, facial expressions, etc.). These goals will be addressed through direct instruction, clinician and student identification of areas of need, role-play, and "real-time" implementation of strategies. Specifically, word retrieval and specific verbal expression will be presented using a "visualize/verbalize" approach, addressing various strategies to retrieve information necessary across a variety of tasks and interactions. Expressive vocabulary and figurative language will also be addressed primarily through direct instruction, correlating the content to current academic topics across a variety of subjects. Pragmatic language skills will be addressed through self-identification of social skills critical for successful peer and adult interactions. Louis will identify the presence of social skills that both facilitate and inhibit successful interactions with others through the use of videotape and, eventually, in "real time." An ecological assessment will be conducted by Louis to determine specific factors or "triggers" for target behaviors, leading to role-play to practice more appropriate strategies. Finally, strategies will be implemented across a variety of settings with varying conversational partners, allowing Louis to self-evaluate and self-monitor his level of success and need.

REVIEW QUESTIONS

1. How does each of the five diagnostic categories of the autism spectrum disorders overlap? How are they distinguished from each other?

2. For young children with autism there are four social processes that are the primary areas of impairment. Name these and explain how they could interfere with subsequent development.

3. School-age children with autism can be described socially as "aloof, passive, or active-but-odd." How do these groups differ, and what are the implications for intervention?

4. What are the four diagnostic areas considered in the "qualitative impairment in communication"? How does each of these manifest itself in children with autism? Give examples.

5. In the areas of communication form, content, and use, what is a typical language scenario for a child with autism?

6. What are the six principles that should drive the assessment of children with autism? Why is each of these important to the development of an intervention program?

7. What are some specific areas that should be addressed during a communication evaluation for a child with autism?

8. What factors need to be considered when designing an intervention program for a child with autism? Why?

9. How could you present various goals under differing intervention models? For example, what would specific goals "look like" using a discrete-trial model, incidental teaching, and ECO? How would you determine which intervention is most appropriate?

REFERENCES

American Psychiatric Association. (1994). *Diagnostic and statistical manual* (4th ed.). Washington, DC: American Psychiatric Association.

Bartolucci, G., Pierce, S., & Streiner, D. (1980). Cross-sectional studies of grammatical morphemes in autistic and mentally retarded children. *Journal of Autism and Developmental Disorders, 10,* 39–50.

Brown, L., Nietupski, J., & Hamre-Nietupski, S. (1976). Criterion of ultimate functioning and public school services for severely handicapped students. As cited by Powers, M. D. (1997). Behavioral assessment of individuals with autism. In D. J. Cohen & F. R. Volkmar (Eds.), *Handbook of autism and pervasive developmental disorders* (2nd ed., pp. 448–459). New York: Wiley.

Carr, E. G. (1983). Behavioral approaches to language and communication. In E. Schopler & G. B. Mesibov (Eds.), *Communication problems in autism* (pp. 37–57). New York: Plenum.

Carr, E. G., & Durand, V. M. (1985). Reducing behavior problems through functional communication training. *Journal of Applied Behavior Analysis, 18,* 111–126.

Carr, E. G., Levin, L., McConnachie, G., Carlson, J. I., Kemp, D. C., & Smith, C. E. (1994). *Communication based intervention for problem behavior: A user's guide for producing positive behavior change.* Baltimore: Brookes.

Charlop, M. H., Kurtz, P. F., & Milstein, J. P. (1992). Too much reinforcement, too little behavior: Assessing task interspersal procedures in conjunction with different reinforcement schedules with autistic children. *Journal of Applied Behavior Analysis, 25,* 795–808.

Cohen, D. J., & Volkmar, F. R. (Eds.). (1997). *Handbook of autism and pervasive developmental disorders* (2nd ed.). New York: Wiley.

Davis, C. A., Brady, M. P., Hamilton, R., McEvoy, R., & Williams, R. E. (1994). Effects of high-probability requests on social interactions of young children with severe disabilities. *Journal of Applied Behavior Analysis, 27,* 619–637.

Davis, C. A., Brady, M. P., Williams, R. E., & Hamilton, R. (1992). Effects of high-probability requests on the acquisition and generalization of responses to requests in young children with behavior disorders. *Journal of Applied Behavior Analysis, 25,* 905–916.

DeMeyer, M. K., Alpern, G. D., Barton, S., DeMeyer, W. E., Churchill, D. W., Hingtgen, J. N., Bryson, C. Q., Pontius, W., & Kimberlin, C. (1972). Imitation in autistic, early schizophrenic and nonpsychotic subnormal children. *Journal of Autism and Childhood Schizophrenia, 2,* 264–287.

Donnellan, A. M., Mesaros, R. A., & Anderson, J. L. (1985). Teaching students with autism in natural environments: What educators need from researchers. *Journal of Special Education, 18*(4), 505–522.

Duker, P. C., & Rasing, E. (1989). The effects of redesigning the physical environment on self-stimulation and on task behavior in three autistic type developmentally disabled individuals. *Journal of Autism and Developmental Disorders, 25,* 449–460.

Dunlap, G. (1984). The influence of task variation and maintenance tasks on the learning and affect of autistic children. *Journal of Experimental Child Psychology, 37,* 41–64.

Durand, V. M., & Carr, E. G. (1991). Functional communication training to reduce challenging behaviors: Maintenance and application in new settings. *Journal of Applied Behavior Analysis, 24,* 251–264.

Dykens, E. M., & Volkmar, F. R. (1997). Medical conditions associated with autism. In D. J. Cohen & F. R. Volkmar (Eds.), *Handbook of autism and pervasive developmental disorders* (2nd ed., pp. 388–407). New York: Wiley.

Fischer, I., & Glanville, B. (1970). Programmed teaching of autistic children. *Archives of General Psychiatry, 23,* 90–94.

Foster-Johnson, L., Ferro, J., & Dunlap, G. (1994). Preferred curricular activities and reduced problem behaviors in students with intellectual disabilities. *Journal of Applied Behavior Analysis, 27,* 493–504.

Graziano, A. M. (1970). A group-treatment approach to multiple problem behaviors of autistic children. *Exceptional Children, 36,* 765–770.

Halpern, W. I. (1970). The schooling of autistic children: Preliminary findings. *American Journal of Orthopsychiatry, 40,* 665–671.

Klin, A., Carter, A., Volkmar, F., Cohen, D. J., Marans, W. D., & Sparrow, S. S. (1997). Assessment issues in children with autism. In D. J. Cohen & F. R. Volkmar (Eds.), *Handbook of autism and pervasive developmental disorders* (2nd ed., pp. 411–417). New York: Wiley.

Klin, A., & Volkmar, F. (1997). Asperger's syndrome. In D. J. Cohen & F. R. Volkmar (Eds.), *Handbook of autism and pervasive developmental disorders* (2nd ed., pp. 94–122). New York: Wiley.

Koegel, R. L., & Koegel, L. K. (1995). *Teaching children with autism: Strategies for initiating positive interactions and improving learning opportunities.* Baltimore: Brookes.

Koegel, R. L., O'Dell, M. C., & Koegel, L. K. (1987). A natural language teaching paradigm for teaching nonverbal autistic children. *Journal of Autism and Developmental Disorders, 17,* 187–200.

Kurita, H. (1985). Infantile autism with speech loss before the age of 30 months. *Journal of the American Academy of Child Psychiatry, 24,* 191–196.

Lecouter, A., Rutter, M., Lord, C., Rios, P., Robertson, S., Holdgrafer, M., & McLennan, J. D. (1989). Autism Diagnostic Interview: A semi-structured interview for parents and caregivers of autistic persons. *Journal of Autism and Developmental Disorders, 19,* 363–387.

Lockyer, L., & Rutter, M. (1969). A five- to fifteen-year follow-up study of infantile psychosis: III. Psychological aspects. *British Journal of Psychiatry, 115,* 865–882.

Lord, C., & Paul, R. (1997). Language and communication in autism. In D. J. Cohen & F. R. Volkmar (Eds.), *Handbook of autism and pervasive developmental disorders* (2nd ed., pp. 195–225). New York: Wiley.

Lord, C., & Risi, S. (2001). Diagnosis of autism spectrum disorders in young children. In A. Wetherby & B. Prizant (Eds.), *Autism spectrum disorders: A transactional developmental perspective* (pp. 11–30). Baltimore: Brookes.

Lovaas, O. I. (1977). *The autistic child: Language development through behavior modification.* New York: Irvington.

Lovaas, O. I. (1981). *Teaching developmentally disabled children.* Baltimore: University Park Press.

Loveland, K., & Tunali-Kotoski, B. (1997). The school-age child with autism. In D. J. Cohen & F. R. Volkmar (Eds.), *Handbook of autism and pervasive developmental disorders* (2nd ed., pp. 283–308). New York: Wiley.

MacDonald, J., & Carroll, J. (1992). A social partnership model for assessing early communication development: An intervention model for preconversational children. *Language, Speech, and Hearing Services in the Schools, 23,* 113–124.

Matson, J. L., Benavidez, D. A., Compton, L. S., Paclawskyj, T., & Baglio, C. (1996). Behavioral treatment of autistic persons: A review of research from 1980 to the present. *Research in Developmental Disabilities, 17,* 433–465.

McClannahan, L. E., & Krantz, P. J. (1999). *Activity schedules for children with autism.* Bethesda, MD: Woodbine House.

McEvoy, R., Loveland, K., & Landry, S. (1988). Functions of immediate echolalia in autistic children. *Journal of Autism and Developmental Disorders, 18,* 657–688.

Mesibov, G., & Handlan, S. (1997). Adolescents and adults with autism. In D. J. Cohen & F. R. Volkmar (Eds.), *Handbook of autism and pervasive developmental disorders* (2nd ed., pp. 309–322). New York: Wiley.

Minshew, N. J., Sweeney, J. A., & Bauman, M. L. (1997). Neurological aspects of autism. In D. J. Cohen & F. R. Volkmar (Eds.), *Handbook of autism and pervasive developmental disorders* (2nd ed., pp. 344–369). New York: Wiley.

Moser, H. (1986). Preamble to the workshop on Rett syndrome. As cited by VanAcker, R. (1997). Rett's syndrome : A pervasive developmental disorder. In D. J. Cohen & F. R. Volkmar (Eds.), *Handbook of autism and pervasive developmental disorders* (2nd ed., pp. 60–93). New York: Wiley.

Mundy, P., & Crowson, M. (1997). Joint attention and early social communication: Implications for research intervention with autism. *Journal of Autism and Developmental Disorders, 27*, 653–675.

Norris, J., & Hoffman, P. (1990). Comparison of adult-initiated vs. child-initiated interaction styles with handicapped prelanguage children. *Language Speech, and Hearing Services in the Schools, 21*, 28–36.

Osterling, J., & Dawson, G. (1994). Early recognition of children with autism: A study of first birthday home videotapes. *Journal of Autism and Developmental Disorders, 24*(3), 247–257.

Powers, M. (1997). Behavior assessment of individuals with autism. In D. J. Cohen & F. R. Volkmar (Eds.), *Handbook of autism and pervasive developmental disorders* (2nd ed., pp. 448–459). New York: Wiley.

Prizant, B., & Duchan, J. (1981). The functions of immediate echolalia in autistic children. *Journal of Speech and Hearing Disorders, 46*, 241–249.

Prizant, B., Schuler, A., Wetherby, A., & Rydell, P. (1997). Enhancing language and communication development: Language approaches. In D. J. Cohen & F. R. Volkmar (Eds.), *Handbook of autism and pervasive developmental disorders* (2nd ed., pp. 572–605). New York: Wiley.

Quill, K. A. (1995). Enhancing children's social-communicative interactions. In K. A. Quill (Ed.), *Teaching children with autism: Strategies to enhance communication and socialization* (pp. 163–189). Clifton Park, NY: Delmar Learning.

Rogers, S. J. (1996). Brief report: Early intervention in autism. *Journal of Autism and Developmental Disorders, 26*, 243–247.

Rutter, M. (1970). Autistic children: Infancy to adulthood. *Seminars in Psychiatry, 2*, 435–450.

Rutter, M. (1983). Cognitive deficits in the pathogenesis of autism. *Journal of Child Psychology and Psychiatry, 24*, 513–531.

Schopler, E. (1997). Implementation of TEACCH philosophy. In D. J. Cohen & F. R. Volkmar (Eds.), *Handbook of autism and pervasive developmental disorders* (2nd ed., pp. 767–795). New York: Wiley.

Schopler, E., Brehm, S., Kinsbourne, M., & Reichler, R. (1971). Effects of treatment structure on development in autistic children. *Archives of General Psychiatry, 24*, 415–421.

Schopler, E., Mesibov, G. B., & Hearsey, K. (1995). Structured teaching the TEACCH system. In E. Schopler & G. B. Mesibov (Eds.), *Learning and cognition in autism* (pp. 243–268). New York: Plenum Press.

Sigman, M., Dissanayake, C., Arbelle, S., & Ruskin, E. (1997). Cognition and emotion in children and adolescents with autism. In D. J. Cohen & F. R. Volkmar (Eds.), *Handbook of autism and pervasive developmental disorders* (2nd ed., pp. 248–265). New York: Wiley.

Sweeney, H. M., & LeBlanc, J. M. (1995). The effects of task size on work-related and aberrant behaviors of youths with autism and mental retardation. *Research in Developmental Disabilities, 16*, 97–115.

Tager-Flusberg, H. (1997). Perspectives on language and communication in autism. In D. J. Cohen & F. R. Volkmar (Eds.), *Handbook of autism and pervasive developmental disorders* (pp. 894–900). New York: Wiley.

Towbin, K. (1997). Pervasive developmental disorder not otherwise specified. In D. J. Cohen & F. R. Volkmar (Eds.), *Handbook of autism and pervasive developmental disorders* (2nd ed., pp. 123–147). New York: Wiley.

VanAcker, R. (1997). Rett's syndrome: A pervasive developmental disorder. In D. J. Cohen & F. R. Volkmar (Eds.), *Handbook of autism and pervasive developmental disorders* (2nd ed., pp. 60–93). New York: Wiley.

Volkmar, F., Carter, A., Grossman, J., & Klin, A. (1997). Social development in autism. In D. J. Cohen & F. R. Volkmar (Eds.), *Handbook of autism and pervasive developmental disorders* (2nd ed., pp. 173–194). New York: Wiley.

Volkmar, F., Hoder, L., & Cohen, D. (1985). Compliance, "negativism" and the effects of treatment and structure in autism: A naturalistic behavior study. *Journal of Child Psychology and Psychiatry, 26,* 865–877.

Volkmar, F., Klin, A., Marans, W., & Cohen, D. (1997). Childhood disintigrative disorder. In D. J. Cohen & F. R. Volkmar (Eds.), *Handbook of autism & pervasive developmental disorders* (2nd ed., pp. 47–59). New York: Wiley.

Volkmar, F., Klin, A., & Cohen, D. J. (1997). Diagnosis and classification of autism and related conditions: Consensus and issues. In D. J. Cohen & F. R. Volkmar (Eds.), *Handbook of autism and pervasive developmental disorders* (2nd ed., pp. 5–40). New York: Wiley.

Wetherby, A., & Prizant, B. (1993). *Communication and Symbolic Behavior Scales.* Baltimore: Brookes.

Wetherby, A., & Prutting, C. (1984). Profiles of communicative and cognitive-social abilities in autistic children. *Journal of Speech and Hearing Research, 27,* 364–377.

Wetherby, A., Schuler, A. L., & Prizant, B. M. (1997). Enhancing language and communication development: Theoretical foundations. In D. J. Cohen & F. R. Volkmar (Eds.), *Handbook of autism and pervasive developmental disorders* (2nd ed., pp. 513–538). New York: Wiley.

Windsor, J., Doyle, S. S., & Siegel, G. M. (1994). Language acquisition after autism: A longitudinal case study of autism. *Journal of Speech and Hearing Research, 37,* 96–105.

Wing, L. (1993). The definition and prevalence of autism: A review. *European Child and Adolescent Psychiatry, 2,* 61–74.

Wing, L., & Attwood, A. (1987). Syndromes of autism and atypical development. In D. J. Cohen, A. Donnellan, & R. Paul (Eds.), *Handbook of autism and pervasive developmental disorders* (pp. 3–19). New York: Wiley.

Wing, L., & Gould, J. (1979). Severe impairments of social interaction and associated abnormalities in children: Epidemiology and classification. *Journal of Autism and Developmental Disorders, 9,* 11–29.

Woodyatt, G., & Ozanne, A. (1993). A longitudinal study of cognitive skills and communication behaviors in children with Rett syndrome. *Journal of Intellectual Disability Research, 37,* 419–435.

World Health Organization. (1993). *The ICD-10 classification of mental and behavioral disorder: Diagnostic criteria for research.* Geneva: World Health Organization.

Chapter 6

Mental Retardation

Libby Kumin, Ph.D., CCC-SLP

CHAPTER OBJECTIVES

Upon completing this chapter, the reader should be able to:

1. Classify mental retardation according to IQ score or according to levels of support needed in daily life
2. Describe mental retardation as being caused by prenatal, birth, or postnatal complications
3. List major causes of mental retardation
4. List etiologies, characteristics, and associated medical conditions in Down syndrome and their impact on speech and language
5. List etiologies, characteristics, and associated conditions for fragile X syndrome
6. List evaluation and treatment protocols for children with Down syndrome, fragile X syndrome, and mental retardation

INTRODUCTION

Many people with disabilities have difficulties with the tasks of daily living. **Mental retardation** (MR) is the term used when people demonstrate substantial limitations in intellectual functioning and adaptive behavior that affect daily living. The limitations are observed in conceptual (e.g., receptive and expressive language), social (e.g., ability to follow rules, interpersonal skills), and practical adaptive (e.g., using the telephone, using transportation) skills. This disability originates before age 18. Mental retardation can be defined by evaluating intelligence. If a person earns an IQ score under 70 on a standardized intelligence test, the person can be classified as mentally retarded. It can also be defined by evaluating the person's intellectual limitations and difficulties in daily living, and defining the supports that the person will need to function. Usually, it is defined by a combination of test scores and consideration of the needs for supports in daily life. Mental retardation is characterized by significantly subaverage intellectual functioning, that is, an IQ score of 70–75 or below, existing concurrently with limitations in two or more adaptive skill areas, that is, communication, self-care, functional academics (reading, writing, basic math), self-direction, home living, social skills, community use, health and safety, leisure, and work. The population with mental retardation is generally divided into three levels based on the severity of the intellectual impairment. Mild mental retardation is most common, affecting over 85 percent of people diagnosed with MR. Mild mental retardation is defined as an IQ score 2 to 3 standard deviations below the mean IQ score of 100, that is, an IQ score of 75 or below. The levels that are used to differentiate the groups can be found in Table 6-1.

Sometimes the individuals with severe and profound retardation are grouped together as the severe and profound handicaps (SPH) population. But what do these levels mean? How do they help us understand how a child functions in daily life? These levels are not always meaningful or helpful when planning services for a child and his or her family. Many IQ tests are language based, so children with language and speech difficulties will often score at a lower level. For example, a child with Down syndrome who was enrolled in the speech and language center was tested by the school psychologist using the Wechsler Intelligence Test for Children (WISC). The result was an IQ score of 50. At the suggestion of the **speech-language pathologist** (SLP), the psychologist retested the child using a nonverbal IQ test, the Leiter International Scale, and the same child had an IQ of 79. A score of 79 would place that child in the low normal intelligence range, not in the range of mental retardation. Children whose native language is not English may also have scores that are not accurate representations of their overall level of function in daily life. Test results are usually reported as mental age scores or intelligent quotient scores. Mental age is a test construct which means that the individual answered the same number of items correctly on a standardized IQ test as the average for the test norms collected. But, it is not accurate to equate mental age with level of function. A 15-year-old who has 15 years of life experience but has test scores with a mental age of 10 does not function in daily life the same as a 10-year-old. So, the label of mental retardation, based on IQ test scores, is not always definitive. For these and other reasons, in 1992, the American Association on Mental Retardation (Schalock, Baker, & Croser, 2002) expanded the definition of mental retardation so that it would focus on assessing how the person functions in daily living, and the type and level of support that the person needs to function effectively, rather than relying on a test score to define the categories or levels of mental retardation. They also stated four important assumptions that are essential to ensure that the label of mental retardation is used appropriately. In 2002, a fifth assumption was added (Luckasson et al., 2002). The five assumptions are:

1. Limitations in present functioning must be considered within the context of community environments typical of the individual's age peers and culture.
2. Valid assessment considers cultural and linguistic diversity, as well as differences in communication, sensory, motor, and behavioral factors.
3. Within an individual, limitations often coexist with strengths.
4. An important purpose of describing limitations is to develop a profile of needed supports.

Table 6-1   Levels of Mental Retardation

Level	IQ score
Mild	50–75
Moderate	35–49
Severe	34 or below
Profound	need full assistance with self-help skills

5. With appropriate personalized supports over a sustained period, the life functioning of the person with mental retardation generally will improve.

The AAMR expanded diagnostic criteria, in addition to standardized test results of intelligence and adaptive skills, is a process of evaluating the individual's strengths and needs. The person's strengths and needs are described, in a variety of ways, across four dimensions:

1. Intellectual and adaptive behavior skills
2. Psychological/emotional considerations
3. Physical/health/etiological considerations
4. Environmental considerations

The descriptions may be based on observations, interviews with key people in the person's life, interviews with the person, interacting with the person in his or her daily life, and formal testing. Based on this analysis of strengths and needs, an interdisciplinary team determines the person's needs for support across the four dimensions. Supports are the resources and individual strategies and services that are needed to promote the development, education, interests, and well-being of an individual with mental retardation In 2002, an expanded system of supports was proposed that includes the need for support in the areas of human developmental, education and school learning, home living, community living, health and safety, behavior, social interaction, and protection and advocacy. Each support is classified as one of four levels of intensity:

- Intermittent: support on an "as needed basis." The person may need support to find a new job or new housing, but the support would be needed occasionally, not on a regular basis. The support may be needed in times of crisis.
- Limited: support may be needed for a limited time span. For example, during the transition from school to work, there will be a need for on-the-job training with a job coach. This level of support will be needed for a limited amount of time.
- Extensive: Support is needed on a daily basis for a specific area or for several areas of daily function. The person may have different levels of need for supports in different areas of daily function. For example, she or he may need assistance with transportation, but may not need assistance with bathing, dressing, and grooming.
- Pervasive: support that is needed on a constant basis across environments and all life areas.

So, there are different routes to the diagnostic label of mental retardation, based on testing and necessary supports for living.

ETIOLOGY

There are many causes of mental retardation, including prenatal trauma, infections and other problems during pregnancy, trauma at birth, and postnatal problems such as illness, injury, and environmental toxins. Biomedical, social, behavioral, and environmental risk factors can increase the chances that an individual will show mental retardation. Some problems are preventable, such as lead poisoning or alcohol or substance abuse by the mother. These conditions will be discussed in separate chapters.

Other problems, such as hypothyroidism and Rh-incompatibility, can be controlled through medical testing and treatment. Genetic causes account for approximately 45 percent of cases of mental retardation (Batshaw & Perret, 1992). Two common genetic syndromes that result in mental retardation are Down syndrome and fragile X syndrome. Since individuals with Down syndrome comprise the largest group with genetic etiology, the focus of this chapter will be on children with Down syndrome. The chapter will also include a discussion of fragile X syndrome, an inherited cause of mental retardation, with suggested readings and resources.

DOWN SYNDROME

Down syndrome is a genetically based syndrome that affects an individual's overall development, as well as speech and language development and function. Incidence is estimated at one in 1000 live births, with 3000 to 5000 infants born with Down syndrome every year. Though it was first described by Dr. John Langdon Down in 1866, it was not until 1959 that Dr. Jerome Lejeune identified the underlying chromosomal abnormality, an additional 21st chromosome. There are three different types of chromosomal abnormalities that may be the underlying cause of Down syndrome in an individual: trisomy 21, translocation, and mosaicism.

Approximately 95 percent of children with Down syndrome have an extra 21st chromosome in each cell, for example, each cell has 47 chromosomes instead of the usual 46 chromosomes. This is known as trisomy 21 or nondisjunction trisomy 21. It results from nondisjunction, or a failure of the 21st chromosome to separate correctly during cell division in the fertilized egg. Approximately 3 to 4 percent of children with Down syndrome have an extra chromosome 21 in which the long arm attaches or translocates onto another chromosome, usually chromosome 14, 21, or 22. This is known as translocation. Approximately 1 to 2 percent of children with Down syndrome have an extra chromosome in some cells, but not all cells, for example, some cells have 46 chromosomes, but other cells have 47 chromosomes. This type is known as mosaicism. This means that fewer cells are affected, as compared to trisomy 21.

Though the etiology of Down syndrome is known, the cause of the extra chromosome is not known. Older mothers have a higher risk of having a child with Down syndrome, but it is estimated that over 80 percent of babies born with Down syndrome have mothers under age 35 (NDSS, 2002). Paternal factors may play a role as well. Some researchers believe that environmental factors may have an influence. Others have theorized that hormonal problems, immunological problems, viral infections, and/or pollutants may result in the extra chromosome. Exactly how the extra chromosomal material affects development and function is not totally understood. Some researchers feel that there is a dosage effect of the extra material, for example, the extra chromosomal material affects the development of each organ system. Others feel that the extra chromosome results in incomplete development of the embryo. In the year 2000, as part of the human genome initiative, chromosome 21 was mapped. Research is now moving more quickly, and within the next decade we will probably have a better understanding of the genetic basis of Down syndrome.

Definition of the Disorder: Medical and Behavioral Definitions

How does the extra chromosome in Down syndrome affect development and function? How does the genotype affect the phenotype? There is a wide variety of physical and mental characteristics that may occur in individuals with Down syndrome, including physical signs, associated medical conditions, and behavioral and learning characteristics. Approximately 60 signs have been identified. Before there were tests to determine genetically that a child had Down syndrome, the diagnosis was made on the basis of the presence of seven or more of the clinical signs. An individual with Down syndrome may have few or many signs, and medical problems. Some of the more common signs include:

- Underdevelopment of the midface (midface hypoplasia)
- Flattening of the back of the head
- Slanting of the eyelids (palpebral fissures)
- Skin folds at the inner corner of the eyes (epicanthal folds)
- Small upper jaw (maxilla) relevant to the lower jaw (mandible)
- Depressed bridge of the nose
- Small outer ears (tops may fold over)
- Small ear canals
- Single line across the palm of the hand (simian crease)
- Low muscle tone (**hypotonia**)
- Loose ligaments (ligamentous laxity)
- Decreased muscle strength
- Short arms and legs
- Short stature
- Colored spots in the iris of the eye (Brushfield spots)

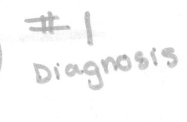

Associated Medical Conditions

There are many associated medical conditions seen in individuals with Down syndrome, which must be monitored and treated by the pediatrician. Hearing problems are very common in individuals with Down syndrome, and impact speech and language development. They will be discussed below. Other common medical and health concerns include:

- Congenital heart disease, including endocardial cushion defect, ventricular septal defect, and atrial septal defect
- Gastrointestinal abnormalities
- Metabolic difficulties
- Thyroid problems, especially hypothyroidism
- Celiac disease
- Enlarged tonsils and adenoids
- Skeletal difficulties, including atlantoaxial instability (neck alignment problem)
- Higher incidence of seizure disorders
- Higher incidence of leukemia
- Sleep apnea
- Hearing problems, including excess fluid, conductive and sensorineural hearing loss
- Visual problems, including congenital cataracts, strabismus, nystagmus, nearsightedness, and farsightedness
- Periodontal disease
- Skin conditions

The Down Syndrome Medical Interest Group has published guidelines for medical evaluation and treatment (Cohen, 1999), which are available and are used widely by physicians. See resources at the end of the chapter.

Communication Strengths and Challenges for Children with Down Syndrome

There is no single pattern of communication impairment in children with Down syndrome; however, there are areas of strength and weakness that occur in many children. But these difficulties may manifest in different symptoms. For example, most children with Down syndrome have difficulties with speech intelligibility, but for one child, this may manifest as articulation and fluency difficulty while for another child, resonance problems will be the major symptom. Speech and language development is greatly influenced by input from a child's environment. Children learn speech and language by watching and listening to the people in their environment, and then trying to make sense out of what they see and hear. Many children with Down syndrome have difficulty with sensory input and association systems, and this will impact on speech and language development. For example, hearing may be affected by fluid in the ears, or the child may be tactilely defensive and seek to avoid oral experiences; these factors will impact on speech and language development.

Early development is asynchronous in children with Down syndrome, for example, progress is not the same in all developmental areas. Children with Down syndrome may be more advanced in gross motor development than they are in speech. They usually learn better through the visual channel (reading and visual models) than they do through the auditory channel (verbal instructions). Speech and language development is usually more delayed than would be predicted by cognitive level. Language impairment may be linguistic-specific impairment, as children with Down syndrome are usually more advanced in vocabulary skills than they are in morphosyntactic skills. Receptive language skills are usually far more advanced than expressive language skills, so that children with Down syndrome understand more than they can say. Speech is usually the most difficult channel for communication for children with Down syndrome, far more difficult than sign language or picture communication systems.

The difficulties in expressive language and intelligibility often lead professionals to underestimate the intelligence and capabilities of children with Down syndrome. Even when children with Down syndrome increase their expressive language skills, their effectiveness in communicating with others depends, to a large extent, on whether their speech can be understood (Chapman, Seung, Schwartz, & Bird, 1998). When you cannot understand what someone is saying, it is very difficult to assess the person's abilities. Speech and language testing that uses expressive output as the measure may not be accurate in assessing the child's receptive language level and/or reading level. If we ask the child to give us a verbal answer, we cannot assume that he or she does not know the answer, only that he or she cannot tell us the answer. This impacts testing as well as educational opportunities. In the classroom, materials often need to be modified to accommodate the visual strengths and auditory and verbal difficulties of children with Down syndrome. Materials that use pictures or written instructions can enable the child to demonstrate knowledge and mastery of skills.

Communication difficulties may also relate to behavior difficulties. When children cannot express needs, they may use behavior such as screaming or running out of the room as a strategy to express frustration and make needs known. A functional behavioral assessment (FBA) can analyze the situations that come before and after the behavior and draw some conclusions regarding the function that the behaviors are serving for the child. Behavioral evaluations should always consider whether communication difficulties are affecting the behaviors exhibited. Behavioral treatment plans should provide augmented and assistive communication, when appropriate, to enable the child to communicate her or his needs.

Characteristics of Down Syndrome

The following are characteristics of Down syndrome as it affects language, speech development, hearing and auditory skills, voice, and fluency.

Language

Children with Down syndrome have more difficulty with expressive language than receptive language. Miller (1988) found that more than 75 percent of his subjects demonstrated deficits in language production when compared to language comprehension and cognitive skills, and that the expressive language difficulties increase over time (Miller, 1988, 1992; Miller, Leddy, Miolo, & Sedey, 1995). Studies comparing semantic and syntactic development in children with Down syndrome demonstrate that syntax is a far more difficult area for children with Down syndrome (Fowler, 1990, 1995; Miller, 1988) than semantics. The abstract nature of grammar and the sequencing skills required appear to be related to this difficulty.

Language level is often more impaired than would be expected by the child's cognitive level. Most testing involves language, both in making instructions and in making responses. Expressive language output is usually affected, resulting in shorter phrases and sentences. Bray and Woolnough (1988) reported that 11 children from ages 12 to 16 that they studied spoke primarily in single-word utterances. Rosin, Swift, Bless, and Vetter (1988) found that adolescents with Down syndrome use shorter phrases and sentences as evidenced by a significantly shorter mean length of utterance (MLU) than typically developing adolescents matched for mental age (MA) or adolescents with mental retardation due to other causes. The finding of shorter mean length of utterance is probably related to difficulties with syntax and with speech production, as well as difficulty encoding the language message. School involves language for learning, for following instructions, and for interacting with other children and teachers and school staff. Thus, having difficulty with language presents many problems for children with Down syndrome during the school years.

Semantics. Researchers find that vocabulary development and the words included in the early vocabularies of children with Down syndrome are similar to those of typically developing children (Cardoso-Martins, Mervis, & Mervis, 1985; Gilham, 1979; Kumin, Councill, & Goodman, 1998, 1999; Mervis, 1997), but that there is a slower rate of development (Cardoso-Martins et al., 1985; Kumin et al., 1999, 1998; Miller, 1995). There is also wide variability in vocabulary development in children with Down syndrome, ranging from rates of vocabulary growth consistent with mental age (Miller, 1995) to severe delays in vocabulary development.

When young children use their first spoken or signed word, they show that they can connect a symbol with an object, person, or event. The literature documents the first spoken word at an average age of 18 months in children with Down syndrome (Gilham, 1979), but children are often able to sign vocabulary words to identify toys or people, and to make requests before 12 months of age (Buckley, 2000; Buckley & Bird, 2001; Kumin, Goodman, & Councill, 1991). Studies of semantic development in children with Down syndrome match experimental and control groups by chronological age, mental age, linguistic age, or mean length of utterance (MLU). Chronological age (CA) and mental age (MA) matching both generally show delays in vocabulary development for children with Down syndrome, though MA is a better predictor of vocabulary development level. Studies that match by linguistic age or mean length of utterance (length of average output) generally get results that show vocabulary development level in children with Down syndrome closer to the matched group. Miller (1987) studied expressive vocabulary in children with Down syndrome 2 to 12.5 years (CA) and typically developing children matched by mental age or MLU using a 30-minute language sample taken while the children were conversing with a parent. Results showed that when children were matched by MA, children with Down syndrome produced fewer different words than children with typical development, but when children were matched by MLU, children with Down syndrome produced significantly more different words. This may be reflective of findings that suggest that syntactic development and MLU are areas of greater difficulty for children with Down syndrome than their cognitive level would suggest. Matching by MLU would therefore be sampling children who are at a more advanced language level than matching by mental age. A classic study by Rondal (1988), which matched children with Down syndrome and children with typical development by linguistic stage, found that children with Down syndrome had a broader vocabulary and used a greater number of different words than typically developing children who were at that same linguistic stage. Since children with Down syndrome were older at each linguistic stage, Rondal felt that the results reflected the influence of life experience.

When do children with Down syndrome shift from single-word to multiword utterance usage? Typically developing children combine words into two-word phrases when they have a 50-word vocabulary at an average age of 19 months to 2 years of age. In children with Down syndrome, multiword utterances usually occur later and when children have larger single-word vocabularies. Rondal (1988) documented the use of multiword utterances at ages 4 to 5, Buckley at 36 months (Buckley, 2000), and Kumin, Councill, and Goodman (1998) between ages 4 and 5. Though typically developing children combine words when they have a 50-word vocabulary, there is a wider range for children with Down syndrome. Buckley reported a range of 21 words to 109 words, with an average of approximately 100 words (Buckley, 1993). Kumin et al. (1998) found significant expressive vocabulary growth in children with Down syndrome from ages 1 to 8; however, there was a great deal of variability and a wide range of expressive vocabulary usage. Miller (1988) also noted variability and found that while some children with Down syndrome were delayed in lexical development, others were using the same average number of words as typically developing children.

Syntax. Morphosyntax, including word roots, prefixes, suffixes, word order, and sentence composition, are difficult areas for children with Down syndrome. They have greater difficulty in developing prepositions and connectives and other function words (Fowler, 1990; Miller, 1987, 1988). Fowler (1990, 1995) believes that a specific deficit in syntax learning based on underlying sequencing difficulties is a major language learning problem in children with Down syndrome. It is also possible that syntax presents more difficulty because it is more abstract, or because word endings such as suffixes and verb tense markers tend to be said with decreased volume, making it more difficult for children to hear these word endings. Grammatical markers and word order become a concern when children are using longer, more complex utterances, and more complex utterances are more difficult for children with Down syndrome, so, there may be multiple reasons why morphosyntax is a difficult area of language for individuals with Down syndrome. Researchers have not found definitive conclusions that can lead us to appropriate assessment and treatment strategies. There is a need for further research.

What has been identified as a vocabulary delay in children with Down syndrome may be affected by the specific difficulties in learning vocabulary words with grammatical meanings. Kumin et al. (1998) found a significant difference between the expressive vocabulary usage of referential vocabulary words (labels) and grammatical vocabulary words. Children with Down syndrome use significantly more labels than grammatical classification terms. Grammatical and morphosyntactic markers are not used by the majority of children with Down syndrome until at least age 5. Children appear to use plurals between ages 4 and 5, but even at age 5, they are not routinely using plurals. Since plural usage is documented through speech, this finding may also be related to phonological and articulatory development. Whether the child uses final consonant deletion and whether the child can produce the /s/ and /z/ sound in the final position in words can impact on whether the child is perceived to use plurals in speech. In analyzing expressive speech, we judge whether children are using plurals by whether they include a final /s/ (as in tops), final /z/ (as in cars), or final /ez/ (as in houses). Perhaps they are trying to use plurals, but because they leave out or cannot say certain final consonants, we assume that they are not using the plural marker. Though children can remember and talk about a past event between ages 3 and 4, 77 percent are still not using past-tense morphosyntactic markers (e.g., *ed*) by age 5 (Kumin et al., 1998). The concept of possession is mastered several years before children begin to use possessive markers (e.g., *'s*). Children with Down syndrome appear to understand concepts related to past, future, and possession, but do not use grammatical markers expressively to mark these concepts until much later. There is a need for further research in the area of syntax in children with Down syndrome.

Pragmatics. Pragmatics and social interactive language are strengths for children with Down syndrome. Though they may have difficulty with specific pragmatics skills, children with Down syndrome seek social interactions and use gestures (e.g., waving, high 5) and facial expressions (e.g., smiling and frowning) to enhance their verbal language (see Figure 6-1). In fact, most research on pragmatics in children with Down syndrome compares social interactive language in children with Down syndrome, autism spectrum disorders, and fragile X syndrome, and finds that individuals with Down syndrome are more advanced than the other populations. But, because the results are based on comparisons of the three groups, rather than separate analyses, they probably underestimate the pragmatic abilities of individuals with Down syndrome. Mundy, Sigman, Kasari, and Yirmiya (1988) found that young children with Down syndrome show strength in nonverbal social interactional skills. Thus, though we may need to

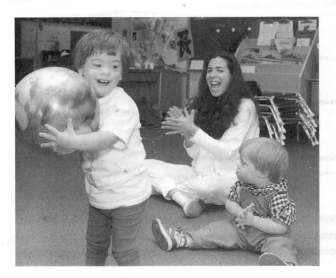

Figure 6-1
Children with Down syndrome typically seek social interaction and demonstrate strengths in nonverbal interaction skills.

teach "how to" use language in certain situations, children with Down syndrome "want to" interact and communicate with others. Children with Down syndrome generally use gestures appropriately. Attwood (1988) found that children with Down syndrome also respond appropriately to instrumental gestures (e.g., come here). Children with Down syndrome may need help in learning how to make requests (Attwood, 1988; Mundy et al., 1988). Though research demonstrates that children with Down syndrome acquire conversational skills at a later age, when young children with Down syndrome were matched with typically developing children by language level, instead of chronological age, children with Down syndrome demonstrate significantly greater conversational skills than the matched controls (Leifer & Lewis, 1984). Research shows that children with Down syndrome learn and respond well to social scripts (Loveland & Tunali, 1991). Since many conversational interactions are repeated over and over again in daily life (e.g., greetings, answering a telephone), children with Down syndrome can learn and practice these skills as social scripts. So, pragmatics is an area of strength for most children with Down syndrome. But children have more difficulty with advanced pragmatics skills that involve the use of figurative and abstract language. If children have great difficulty with social language interactions, further testing is indicated. Approximately 7 percent of children with Down syndrome have dual diagnoses of Down syndrome and autism spectrum disorders (Kent, Evans, Paul, & Sharp, 1999). This group may experience difficulty with pragmatic language and social interaction skills.

Speech Development

Research on early sound production demonstrates similar patterns of development for vowels and consonants during the first 15 months of age, and similar sounds in babbling and the occurrence of reduplicated canonical babbling for children with Down syndrome and typically developing children. Emergence of phonemes in children with Down syndrome in their early language productions follows a definite order, but there is a wide range of age of emergence, from 10 months to 8 years of age (Kumin, Councill, & Goodman, 1994).

There are many factors that influence speech production ability. Children with Down syndrome often have fluid in the ear, with fluctuating hearing loss that will affect speech sound development (Roizen, Wolters, Nicol, & Blondis, 1992; Shott, 2000). Difficulty with phonemic processing and sequencing will affect auditory discrimination and production of sounds (Fowler, 1990). Hypotonia (i.e., low muscle tone) will affect the precision and accuracy of speech sound production, as well as voice, resonance, and fluency (Leddy, 1999). Children with Down syndrome often have difficulty with planning and sequencing motor movements (i.e., developmental apraxia of speech) which affects consistency and accuracy of speech production, especially as words and phrases increase in length (Crary, 1993; Kumin & Adams, 2000). In almost all children with Down syndrome, speech is affected, and in many children, difficulty with speech intelligibility is a problem. The physical findings, anatomical and physiological, and the difficulty with neuromotor and neurosensory function result in secondary symptoms that directly affect speech. For example, enlarged tonsils and adenoids, with mild blockage of the nasal airways, in combination with low muscle tone of the palatal and pharyngeal muscles, result in **hyponasality,** that is, affected individuals sound as if they have a cold when they speak. Low muscle tone and mouth breathing result in open mouth posture, which will affect articulation (e.g., the child's ability to produce the /s/ and /z/ sounds correctly).

Articulation and Phonology. Producing correct sounds and sound combinations in speech is often difficult for children with Down syndrome, and they often continue to use phonological processes, the simplification rules that children use as they learn speech sounds, longer than other children. Dodd (1976) reported that children with Down syndrome show twice as many articulation errors and almost twice as many inconsistent substitutions as children with mental retardation matched for mental age. Rosin et al. (1988) found that consonant articulation at the word level shows significantly more errors for adolescents with Down syndrome than other adolescents with mental retardation. Stoel-Gammon (1980) noted more articulation errors in conversation than in isolated sound production.

The most frequent phonological process (i.e., simplification rule) used by individuals with Down syndrome from ages 13 to 22 is final consonant deletion, followed by consonant cluster reduction (Sommers, Patterson, & Wildgen, 1988). Initial cluster reduction and stopping are also used by younger children with Down syndrome, ages 3 to 4.6 (Bleile & Schwartz, 1984). More phonological processes are used as the length and complexity of the speech output increase, that is, as more phonological processes are used in connected language samples than in picture naming or imitative naming (Sommers et al., 1988). Phonological processes are used beyond the expected age by children with Down syndrome (Bleile, 1982). At ages 1.5 to 2, children with Down syndrome and typically developing children showed no significant qualitative or quantitative differences in phonological processes used, but by age 4, the children with Down syndrome showed quantitative differences, that is, they continued to use phonological processes at about the level of the typically developing child ages 2 to 2.5 (Smith & Stoel-Gammon, 1983). The most frequent phonological processes used by children with Down syndrome are:

- Final consonant deletion (saying "boo" for "boot")
- Consonant cluster reduction (saying "gas" for "glass")
- Stopping (saying "toup" for "soup")
- Fronting (saying "doe" for "go")
- Backing (saying "ko" for "toe")
- Weak syllable deletion (saying "nanas" for "bananas")

Speech Intelligibility. Intelligibility of speech is a major problem for children with Down syndrome. Rosin et al. (1988) found that adolescents with Down syndrome had more difficulty with intelligibility of speech than a matched group of adolescents with mental retardation due to other etiologies.

Speech intelligibility is defined as how clearly a person speaks so that his or her speech is comprehensible to a listener (Leddy, 1999). The presence of difficulties with speech intelligibility in children with Down syndrome is cited in the literature in clinical reports (Chapman et al., 1998, 1995; Horstmeier, 1988; Miller, Leddy, & Leavitt, 1999; Swift & Rosin, 1990; Rosin et al., 1988; Swift & Rosin, 1990) and in surveys of families (Kumin, 1994a). In a survey study of 937 families (Kumin, 1994a), over 95 percent of the respondents reported that their children had difficulty being understood by people outside of their immediate circle sometimes or frequently. When the age groups were examined individually, in every age group, over 50 percent of the parents indicated that the children had difficulty with intelligibility of speech frequently. Only approximately 5 percent of parents reported that their children rarely or never had difficulty in being understood. Speech intelligibility is a widespread problem in children with Down syndrome. Anatomical and physiological factors, neurofunctional patterns, and perceptual symptoms contribute to difficulty in speech intelligibility for individuals with Down syndrome (Kumin, 2001b).

Anatomical and Physiological Factors. Clinicians and researchers note anatomical and physiological differences in individuals with Down syndrome that make speech difficult (Miller & Leddy, 1999; Miller, Leddy, & Leavitt, 1999). Structural differences such as a high narrow palatal arch, irregular dentition and an open bite, or a relatively large tongue contribute to difficulties with speech. Physiological differences such as low tone in the oral facial muscles and lax ligaments in the temporomandibular joint play a role. Hypotonia (low muscle tone) contributes to difficulty in articulation. Bless, Swift, and Rosin (1985) report asynchrony of motor movements, which impacts the muscles of speech. Most children with Down syndrome also have a history of otitis media with effusion, which affects phonetic processing as the child is learning language.

Hearing and Auditory Skills

The incidence of both conductive and sensorineural hearing loss is increased in individuals with Down syndrome (Roizen et al., 1992; Shott, 2000). Children with Down syndrome have a history of persistent otitis media with effusion and fluctuating hearing loss (Shott, 2000). Hearing aids, assistive listening devices, and classroom amplification systems can help. Children with Down syndrome also have greater difficulties with auditory-motor and auditory-vocal processing than with visual-motor and visual-vocal processing (Hopmann & Wilen, 1993; Pueschel, Gallagher, Zastler, & Pezzulo, 1987). Their visual-motor skills are relatively strong and they learn best through the visual channel. These differences between auditory and visual skills should be considered when planning educational and treatment programs (Buckley, 1986).

Neurofunctional Patterns

Neurofunctional patterns will have an effect on production of the sounds of speech, as well as on respiration, voice, resonance, and fluency. Problems with any of these areas can impact on speech intelligibility. Oral motor problems, such as dysarthria, affect the strength and precision of muscle movement, resulting in speech that sounds thickened or imprecise. When muscle function is affected, the problem is consistent for all of the activities that would involve that muscle, so if lip muscles are affected, eating and keeping the lips closed would be affected as well as speech sound production.

Developmental apraxia of speech (DAS), or any other synonymous label, describes an inability of a child to voluntarily program, combine, organize, and sequence movements necessary for speech tasks (Kumin, 2001b). Historically, children with Down syndrome have been excluded from such studies. This is because the original researchers who defined developmental apraxia of speech included in their studies only subjects who met the following criteria: normal intelligence, absence of hearing loss, and absence of muscle weakness or paralysis. Their results and definitions of DAS were not generalized beyond the original subject groups. Children with Down syndrome frequently have hearing loss (Cohen, 1999; Roizen et al., 1992; Shott, 2000), mild to moderate retardation (Cohen, 1999), and low muscle tone (Cohen, 1999; Pueschel et al., 1987). Without the diagnosis being made, assessment and treatment programs have generally failed to address the motor-planning difficulties that are experienced by many children with Down syndrome (Kumin, 2001a). Rosin and Swift (1999), writing about planning treatment for Jay, a young man with Down syndrome, state: "There are aspects of Jay's speech that are consistent with characteristics reported for children with developmental apraxia of speech. . . . Regardless of whether the diagnosis of developmental apraxia of speech is appropriate for Jay, associated therapy techniques can be applied to his intervention" (Rosin & Swift, 1999, p. 144).

Some current definitions of motor-planning difficulties are beginning to include children with Down syndrome within the populations that experience motor-planning disorders. A study by Kumin and Adams (2000) documented that seven children with difficulties with speech intelligibility who were tested with the Apraxia Profile demonstrated test results indicative of DAS. There is a rich body of treatment literature for children with DAS that can and should be used to help children with Down syndrome who have difficulty with motor planning.

Voice

Voice production may be affected in several ways. Researchers report hoarse and breathy voice quality in some children with Down syndrome. The volume of the voice may be too loud, too soft, inconsistent and uncontrolled, or inappropriate to the occasion (e.g., screaming in school). Often this is not due to respiratory or voice production difficulties, but is related to the child's lack of awareness of volume. Some children shout and misuse their voice (vocal abuse). Resonance patterns vary. Some children are hyponasal. They sound as if they have a cold all of the time. This is often due to swollen tonsils and adenoids. Other children are hypernasal. This is often due to a high palatal vault, short palate, or weak muscles in the palate and pharyngeal wall (**velopharyngeal insufficiency**). A comprehensive medical ENT (ear, nose, and throat) evaluation to examine causes for some of these conditions is always needed before a speech assessment and before a treatment plan is developed.

Fluency

Stuttering or dysfluency is more prevalent in people with Down syndrome. Incidence of stuttering is estimated at 45 to 53 percent in individuals with Down syndrome (Devenny & Silverman, 1990). Results of parent surveys indicate that parents report that their children have difficulty with stuttering (Kumin, 1994b). Sometimes there is fluency difficulty as the child is developing language. But, more frequently, the fluency difficulty does not become evident until the child is using longer phrases and sentences and more complex language output. Devenny and Silverman (1990) suggest that there is a breakdown of the neural organization of speech at the consonant level, which results in verbal fluency difficulties. Elliott and colleagues hypothesize that there is a dissociation between right hemisphere speech perception and left hemisphere speech production in individuals with Down syndrome, which makes it difficult for them to complete any task that involves both speech perception and production (Elliott, Weeks, & Elliot, 1987; Heath & Elliott, 1999; Weeks, Chua, & Elliott, 2000), and affects the ability to produce fluent speech (Heath & Elliot, 1999). There is no general agreement among researchers and clinicians as to whether the fluency difficulty is based on motor performance difficulty or on language load and complexity. Clinically, we are able to document that the fluency patterns that we are seeing in children with Down syndrome (ages 7–15) present the same characteristics as stuttering seen in younger typically developing children. Stuttering is one condition that affects the smooth flow of speech. **Prosody** is the general term for the rhythm of speech output. Prosody includes pitch and inflection. It includes whether the voice goes up at the end of the sentence for a question or down for a statement. Children with Down syndrome may have a rapid rate, a slow rate, or an uneven and changing rate of speech. Prosody and rate patterns are not well documented in the literature.

Overview of Team Approaches to Assessment and Intervention

As previously discussed, speech is an output system, but, in order for speech to develop, there must be well-functioning sensory input systems, such as vision and hearing, and adequate sensory integration skills. Vision and hearing must be tested and monitored frequently. In infancy, difficulty with feeding is often noted. Since feeding uses the same structures and many of the same muscles as speech, early intervention for feeding can help develop the mechanism that will be used later in development for speech. The family provides speech and language stimulation at home, and can provide practice as well as feedback. There needs to be a close working relationship between families and SLPs (see Figure 6-2) (Kumin, 1994b). In infancy and toddlerhood, members of the team might include:

- Speech-language pathologist
- Occupational therapist
- Feeding specialist
- Audiologist
- Family
- Pediatrician
- ENT (otorhinolaryngologist)
- Audiologist

Most young children with Down syndrome will be ready to use language before they are able to speak. The SLP and family may want to consult with an augmentative communication or assistive technology specialist, in order to design an effective sign language, picture board, or high-technology communication system to help the child continue to communicate during the period when he or she is learning speech. During the school years, the regular education teacher, special education teacher, and school administrators would be part of the planning team. An individualized education plan (IEP) would be developed for the child, which would include school-based speech-language pathology treatment. According to IDEA, speech-language pathology services in the schools are designed to help children make progress in the regular educational curriculum. Criteria for eligibility for school services

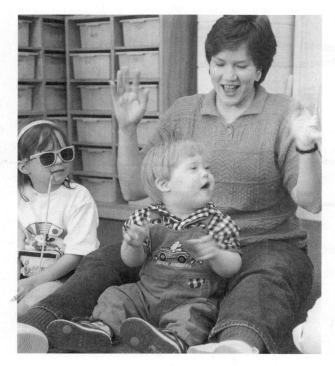

Figure 6-2
An SLP works closely with a toddler with Down syndrome to provide language stimulation and practice.

focus on providing access to the curriculum. Children with Down syndrome may need to continue to receive services outside the school environment through medical and rehabilitation centers, universities, and private practices, in addition to school services.

Psychosocial Issues—Functioning in the Home and Community Environments

There has been a revolution in the field of mental retardation in the past 25 years. Federal legislation in the United States now mandates that a free, appropriate public education be provided for every child, including children with special needs. More and more children with Down syndrome are being included in regular education classrooms during all or part of the school day. Children in special education are being integrated with other children for lunch, recess, music, art and other school activities. Children are being included in the community in scouting, religious activities, and other community events. These activities present many opportunities for speech and language practice and growth. In adulthood, individuals with Down syndrome are living with support or independently in community settings, and working within the community in supported or competitive employment settings. In adulthood, communication abilities, especially speech intelligibility, impact on employment opportunities and on the quality of life.

Speech and Language Skills: Evaluation and Treatment for Children with Down Syndrome

Children with Down syndrome have individual and complicated patterns of strengths and challenges related to communication, language, and speech. There are no evaluation methods or test instruments that are designed specifically for children with Down syndrome. The following discussion, while focusing on children with Down syndrome, could apply to children with mental retardation due to other causes. Evaluation and treatment are part of the same process leading to more effective functional speech and language skills. The speech and language evaluation should be the first step in the treatment planning process. The evaluation should clearly describe the child's communication and explore the best channels and approaches for that child, so that treatment can be planned to address any difficulties that a given child is experiencing. The purpose of a speech and language evaluation is to get an accurate picture of the child's present communication function in daily living activities, including those in the home, school, and community. The instruments that are chosen will vary depending on the cognitive level of the child, as well as whether the child is using speech, sign language, picture communication systems, or other forms of assistive technology. The evaluation should document the speech and language skills that the child has mastered and those that are difficult for her or him. This is difficult to accomplish when testing individuals with Down syndrome because:

- They may have difficulty following test instructions because of auditory or visual processing problems.
- They may have difficulty responding to questions if speech is the response mode.
- They may have difficulty generalizing their skills from a real-life situation to a testing situation.
- They may not perform well with an unfamiliar examiner in an unfamiliar situation.
- There is a wide range of communication abilities in children with Down syndrome. Some children may be speaking in sentences and participating in complex conversations, whereas other children will be at a one- or two-word level.

These factors make it very important to collaborate with families to get a more accurate picture of the child's functional communication abilities. The SLP can request that the family bring videotapes or audiotapes to the evaluation to assist in assessing the child's communication patterns at home. Checklists can be used to help the parents document the child's communication abilities in the home and community setting. Observations of parents and their child communicating may be part of the assessment. If possible, speech and language evaluation should be conducted over several sessions in a familiar environment with familiar people. Research has shown that the testing performance of a child with a language disorder is affected by whether the child knows the person doing the evaluation. Studies have shown that children with communication difficulties perform more poorly with unfamiliar examiners than with familiar examiners (Fuchs, Fuchs, Power, & Dailey, 1985).

In children with Down syndrome, there are usually difficulties in multiple systems that impact on speech and language. Children with Down syndrome may have difficulty with sensory reception (visual, auditory, tactile), processing, and memory, as well as oral motor, oral motor sequencing, encoding, and word retrieval (Kumin, 1996). They may also have difficulty with respiration, phonation, resonance, and articulation, which will affect speech. A comprehensive speech and language evaluation should include assessment of oral motor, speech, receptive and expressive language, and pragmatics skills (Kumin, 1999).

For infants and toddlers, feeding evaluation and sensory integration evaluation may be done by speech-language pathologists with advanced specialty training, or by occupational therapists, feeding therapists, neurodevelopmental specialists, or sensory integration specialists with advanced specialty training in these areas. For school-age children, evaluation should also include assessment of language and literacy skills, as well as curriculum-based language skills. Referrals should be made for audiological evaluation and otolaryngological evaluation (ENT). Referrals for neurological evaluation and evaluation of sensory integration skills should be made as needed.

An evaluation should include:

1. Case history
2. Observation of family and child
3. Family interview
4. Play or conversation (as appropriate for age and developmental level)
5. Formal testing
6. Informal testing
7. Consultation with family

The following speech and language skills should be evaluated through case history, observation, and/or testing, for all children with Down syndrome at that stage of development. Information on associated areas, such as audiological status and sensory integration skills, should be evaluated by specialists through referral, and considered when designing the speech and language treatment plan.

During the period from birth to when the child is able to use single words to communicate, evaluation should include assessment of:

- Prespeech skills
  1. Respiration
  2. Feeding
  3. Oral motor skills

- Pragmatics skills
- Prelanguage skills

The above areas can be assessed by the SLP using case history information, observation, and formal and informal testing. For example, it can be observed whether the infant makes requests, and how those requests are made. Does the infant point or look at the object, make grunting noises, say an approximation of the word, or actually say the word? Family reports can help to corroborate the observation. A battery such as the MacArthur Communicative Development Inventory (a parent survey) can be used to document the communication requesting behavior. A test such as the **Communication and Symbolic Behavior Scale,** which has items designed to elicit requesting behaviors can be used to assess the infant-toddler. Consultations with occupational therapists, audiologists, otolaryngologists, and pediatricians may be indicated to determine sensory skills and hearing status.

During the period when the child is using single words through the period when he or she is using multiword utterances, the child's skills in vocabulary, pragmatics, oral motor, and articulation/phonology should be determined. Mean length of utterance should be determined using a language sample. There is no formal test designed for children with Down syndrome so language tests developed for typically developing children will be used. There are currently no norms developed for children with Down syndrome. Tests used during this period may include Communication and Symbolic Behavior Scale, Clinical Evaluation of Language Function-Preschool (CELF-Preschool), Hawaii Early Learning Profile, Mac Arthur Communicative Development Inventory, Sequenced Inventory of Communication Development (Revised), Test of Early Language Development, Goldman-Fristoe Test of Articulation, Khan-Lewis Phonological Analysis, Peabody Picture Vocabulary Test, Receptive One-Word Picture Vocabulary Test, and the Expressive One-Word Picture Vocabulary Test. Hearing status and sensory integration skills should be monitored through consultation with specialists as during the earlier period.

During the preschool through kindergarten years, the child with Down syndrome is often speaking in multiword utterances, phrases, and short sentences. Morphosyntax and narrative discourse skills are usually not yet mastered and would be difficult to test at this stage. Areas assessed should include receptive language skills, expressive language skills, vocabulary, concept development (colors, shapes, and other early learning skills), pragmatics skills, and speech skills, including articulation, oral motor skills, and speech intelligibility. The tests cited above can also be used during the preschool and kindergarten years.

During the elementary and middle school years, there will be a wide range of functional communication abilities, as well as a variety of school experiences. Some children will be included in the regular education classroom, receiving any special education services within the classroom. Other children will be split between a regular classroom and a resource room for special help during the day. Others will be in a special education classroom with children who have a variety of disabilities. Still others will be in a special education classroom designed exclusively for children with mental retardation (see Figure 6-3). Other children will be in a special education school. Testing during the school years should include assessment of:

- Receptive language skills
  1. Comprehension
  2. Semantics
  3. Morphology/Syntax

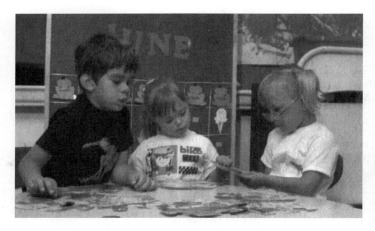

Figure 6-3
Children with mental retardation working together in a special education classroom to improve communication skills.

- Expressive language skills
  1. Semantics
  2. Morphology
  3. Syntax
  4. Mean length of utterance
- Pragmatics skills
  1. Social interactive skills
  2. Communication activities of daily living
  3. Narrative discourse skills
  4. Requests
  5. Clarification strategies/repairs
- Speech skills
  1. Articulation
  2. Intelligibility
  3. Oral motor skills
  4. Motor planning skills
  5. Voice
  6. Fluency

Treatment planning for children with Down syndrome and children with mental retardation due to other causes should focus on the child's short-term communication needs as well as long-term considerations for functional communication in school and later in the workplace and the community.

Communication needs and communication skills are different in infancy, toddlerhood, childhood, adolescence, and adulthood. This is true for everyone, including people with mental retardation. For people with Down syndrome who often experience difficulties with speech and language skills, it is essential to consider how to help them develop effective communication skills that will meet their needs at all ages and stages of life.

From what we know now, there is going to be a wide range of communication abilities in people with Down syndrome. We do not want to limit any child. There is no hard and fast rule as to how far any individual child will progress. We need to learn more so that we can maximize communication abilities and help each child reach her or his potential.

For some children and adults with Down syndrome, speech that can be easily understood is a reality by later childhood and adolescence. For some children and adults, complex language that is able to convey and support the rich experiences of daily living is a reality. For other children, their speech is difficult to understand and they need assistance in communication. For a small number of individuals, assistive communication systems and devices will be needed to be able to communicate effectively. But for most toddlers and young children, assistive communication systems (e.g., sign language) will be needed to support communication until and while the young children are learning to speak.

Treatment programs must therefore be based on ongoing evaluation of the communication needs and communication skills of the individual child (Kumin, 1999). Up until the past decade, treatment for children with Down syndrome involved general language stimulation. Behavior modification methods were often used. Treatment targeting speech, early language intervention, feeding therapy, and oral motor treatment began to be used about 10 years ago. Inclusion in education and in community life is fairly recent. We have not had even one full generation of individuals with Down syndrome who have had the benefits of a comprehensive approach to speech and language development. We cannot predict how far people can go, with the benefits of early stimulation, treatment to support oral motor skills and speech development, transitional communication systems, improved educational opportunities, improved employment opportunities, and a wide range of social and recreational opportunities in the community.

There are many different approaches to speech and language treatment that can be used, sometimes simultaneously, as part of a comprehensive individually designed program. In early intervention, feeding therapy, stimulation of communicative intent and other language precursors, and oral motor treatment is begun. Sign language, picture communication, or a transitional communication system is introduced at about 8 months to 12 months of age. When the child is using single words (or signs), treatment will assist the child in learning to combine words into multiword utterances. Providing a transitional communication system is very important until the child is neurophysiologically able to speak. Though speech is the most difficult communication system for children with Down syndrome, over 95 percent of children with Down syndrome will use speech as their primary communication system. Total communication (use of sign language plus speech), communication boards, the Picture Exchange Communication System (PECS) (Bondy & Frost, 2001), or computer communication systems may be used as communication systems until the child is ready to transition to speech. We believe a transitional communication system enables the child to continue to progress in language while not yet able to speak, and provides a means of communicating with others to prevent frustration (Kumin et al., 1991). Combinations of systems can be used. For example, a child might learn to sign "juice" but when you and he are at the refrigerator door, you might have three picture magnets on the refrigerator with orange, apple, and grape juice, and the child might use the magnet pictures as a communication board. Parents often fear that using sign- or a picture-based communication system will slow their child's progress toward speech. This has not been found to be true. Actually, the opposite is true. Research has shown that children with Down syndrome will discontinue using the sign when they can say the word so that it is understandable to those around them.

The young child is usually far more advanced in receptive language skills than in expressive language skills, but both areas are usually targeted in therapy. Receptive language therapy may focus on auditory memory and on following directions, which are important skills for the early school years. It will also focus on concept development such as colors, shapes, directions (top and bottom), and prepositions through practice and play experiences. Expressive language therapy may include semantics and expanding the mean length of utterance, and will begin to include grammatical structures (word order) and word endings (such as plural or possessive). Once the young child begins to use single words (in sign or speech), treatment will proceed to stimulate both horizontal and vertical growth in language. Treatment may address single-word vocabulary (semantic skills) in many thematic and whole language activities, such as cooking, crafts, play, and trips. Thus there may be a great deal of horizontal vocabulary growth. Treatment will also target increasing the length of phrases and the combinations of words that the child can use; this is known as increasing the mean length of utterance. There are many meaningful relations that the child learns in two-word phrases (e.g., agent-action, possession, negation), and then further expands into three-word phrases. We have found that a pacing board provides a visual and motoric cueing system that capitalizes on the strengths of children with Down syndrome, and helps children to expand the length of their utterances (Kumin, Councill, & Goodman, 1995). A pacing board is usually a rectangular piece of tag board with separate circles that represent the number of words in the desired utterance (e.g., "throw ball" would have two dots). The pacing system concept can also be implemented by putting a dot under each word in a book.

Pragmatics skills such as asking for help, appropriate use of greetings, requests for information or answering requests as well as role playing different activities of daily living may be addressed. Again, play activities such as dressing and undressing a doll, crafts activities such as making a card, or cooking activities such as making cupcakes may be used. The same activity may target semantic, syntactic, and pragmatics skills (e.g., how many cupcakes should we make, what color frosting should we use, following the directions to make the cupcakes). Many children with Down syndrome learn to read effectively, and this can help in learning language concepts (Buckley, 1993).

During this stage, sounds and specific sound production would be targeted; articulation therapy could begin. But the therapy would also include oral motor exercises and activities on an ongoing basis to strengthen the muscles and improve the coordination of muscles. Intelligibility is the goal of the speech component of therapy.

During the years that the child is in elementary school, there is a great deal of growth in language and in speech. Speech-language therapy may involve collaboration with the teacher and may be based in the classroom. Often, the curriculum becomes the material used for therapy. This makes sense, since school is the child's workplace, and success in school greatly affects self-esteem. Receptive language therapy becomes more detailed and advanced (Miller, 1988), including following directions with multiple parts, similar to the instructions given in school. Receptive language therapy might include comprehension exercises, reading and experiential activities, and specific comprehension of vocabulary, morphology, and syntax. Expressive language therapy focuses on more advanced topics in vocabulary, similarities and differences, morphology, and syntax. Expressive language work might also include work on increasing the length of speech utterances. The pacing board, rehearsal, scaffolds, and scripts have been found helpful in facilitating longer speech utterances.

Curriculum-based language skills are a focus in therapy. During the school years, there is a variety of approaches that can be used in treatment. Therapy may be programmed based on linguistic skills, that is, there may be individual goals for semantics (vocabulary), morphosyntax (language structure), **pragmatics** (social language interaction and conversation), and **phonology** (sounds of the language). This is a bottoms-up approach in which the parts are learned and then combined into the whole. So, a therapy objective may be: "Joan will use the correct ending for plurals 80 percent of the time in sentences," or "Josh will correctly use vocabulary words pertaining to transportation 80 percent of the time in sentences." Therapy may also focus on different channels. The goals for therapy may target auditory skills or speech and oral motor skills, or encoding a language message, or producing a language message. One channel, such as reading, may be used to assist another channel such as expressive language or written language. Therapy may also be approached through the needs of the curriculum. In this approach, vocabulary would be taught based on the vocabulary that the child needs for success in science or social studies. The therapy may be proactive, teaching in advance the language skills that the child will need for the curriculum, or reactive, targeting areas of difficulty as they occur and providing assistance with study skills and strategies to meet classroom expectations or to overcome difficulties when they occur. The SLP can also suggest adaptive and compensatory strategies such as seating in front of the room, or using a peer tutor, visual cue sheets, and the like (Kumin, 2001a).

Whole language is a current approach in which reading, understanding, writing, and expressive language are taught as a whole. This often is based on children's literature and thematic activities accompanying the books (e.g., a book about weather might also involve weather reporting, building a weather station, drawing pictures or taking photographs of different weather conditions, etc.). Whole language does not teach in discrete linguistic units, such as focusing on plurals or verb tenses. Rather, it teaches in larger themes using meaningful multisensory experiences to teach concepts.

Pragmatics becomes very important during this stage; using communication skills in real life in school, at home, and in the community is the goal. Therapy might address social interactive skills with teachers and peers, conversational skills (discourse), how to make requests, how to ask for help to understand material in school, how to clarify what was said when the teacher or other students do not understand what was meant, and so on. As the child matures, the communicative activities of daily living will change. Treatment and/or home practice must keep pace with the child's communication needs at every stage.

Speech skills with emphasis on articulation and intelligibility would be targeted in therapy during this period. An individual analysis of oral motor strengths and challenges is important to determine what specific skills need to be addressed. For example, does the child have low muscle tone or muscle weakness in the oral facial area? Difficulty with motor coordination? Difficulty with motor planning? Are other speech areas such as voice and fluency affecting intelligibility? Each of these areas can be worked on if they are impacting on communication ability for an individual child.

The major difference between inclusion in elementary school and middle school is the need, in middle school, to adjust to different teachers, their expectations, and their teaching styles. The IEP can include assistance with these tasks. Reading skills and writing skills need be sufficient to help the student learn the curriculum material. Various organizational supports can be provided through the IEP. One of the areas in which speech-language pathologists can be helpful is in consulting, or collaborating with the classroom teachers. Together they can determine what kinds of adaptations, scaffolds, and learning assistance will enable the adolescent to learn most effectively.

The middle school and high school student must be able to follow teacher instructions, which may vary from subject to subject. They must be able to adapt to different expectations of teachers in different subject areas. They must be able to understand language of the classroom and curriculum, and be able to shift language tasks. They must be able to decode teacher's cues and other students' cues. They must be able to succeed with class assignments. The students must be able to ask questions and seek clarification and to answer questions and make repairs. In inclusion, higher-level language skills may be needed to meet the educational demands of the curriculum. If this is not possible, alternate goals or alternative skill development must be included in the IEP. The teenage years are a time of social growth. The adolescent must be able to talk about teen topics, to understand idiomatic and abstract language and jokes. One focus in therapy may be to practice conversational skills and to role-play various social situations. Clarity and understandability of speech become more critical.

Speech and language treatment is complex and can include different approaches, a variety of goals, and many different activities. The goal is to find treatment approaches and methods that will enable each child to reach his or her communication potential.

FRAGILE X SYNDROME

Fragile X syndrome is the most common inherited cause of mental retardation. Incidence has been estimated at 1 in 2000 in males and 1 in 4000 in females (Bailey & Nelson, 1995) and at 1 in 4000 over-all (Turner, Webb, Wake, & Robinson, 1996). In addition, about 1 in 250 women and 1 in 800 men are carriers, and could pass the condition on to their children. It is a condition that is greatly underdiagnosed. Symptoms are subtle, and may vary widely from person to person; symptoms may accompany other conditions, making it difficult to identify by symptoms. Though genetic testing is available, it is not done routinely. Estimates are that 80 to 90 percent of people with fragile X syndrome are not correctly identified and diagnosed. It is not unusual for families to have 8 to 10 consultations with different physicians and other specialists before the correct diagnosis is made (Hagerman & Cronister, 1996).

Causes of Fragile X Syndrome

Fragile X syndrome is caused by a defect in the FMR1 gene, which is located on the long arm of the X chromosome. In 1991, scientists identified this gene, which is involved in manufacturing a protein that helps messages travel through the nervous system (Hagerman & Silverman, 1991). The FMR1 protein helps to shape the connections between neurons that underlie learning and memory, so when the protein manufacture is shut down through fragile X syndrome, there is an effect on learning, memory, and communication. People who have a permutation (i.e., the FMR1 gene is damaged but functioning) are known as carriers. Carrier men pass this permutation to all of their daughters. A child of a woman who is a carrier has a 50 percent chance of inheriting the gene. In the general population, the number of COG sequence repeats ranges from 6 to 50. In permutations (in carriers), there are 50 to 200 repeats. In full mutations, there are over 200 COG sequence repeats. A full mutation shuts the FMR1 gene down, and results in fragile X syndrome. Males have XY sex chromosomes, while females have XX sex chromosomes. Males inherit the X chromosome from their mothers and the Y chromosome from their fathers, whereas females inherit an X chromosome from each parent. Since males have only one X chromosome, when they inherit the defective FMR1 gene, they have a full mutation and demonstrate symptoms of fragile X syndrome. Females have two X chromosomes, and that seems to dilute the effects; each body cell needs to use only one of the X chromosomes, so some symptoms appear to be lessened.

Since 1992, there is a genetic test to diagnose fragile X. It is a blood test that can diagnose both permutations and the full mutation present in fragile X. Since it is difficult to diagnose fragile X syndrome from symptoms, physicians recommend that any young child with unexplained developmental delay or mental retardation be tested for fragile X syndrome (Hagerman & Cronister, 1996).

Symptoms of Fragile X Syndrome

Fragile X syndrome is difficult to diagnose by symptoms. The physical and behavioral symptoms that occur in individuals with fragile X syndrome may also be found in individuals in the general population. Physical symptoms of fragile X syndrome may include (see Figure 6-4):

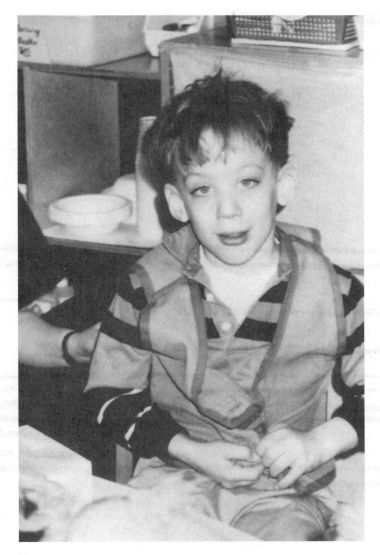

Figure 6-4
Young boy with fragile X syndrome demonstrating typical physical symptoms.

- Long, thin face
- Large ears
- Flat feet
- Hyperextensible joints
- Machrochidism (large testicles in boys)
- Simian crease or Sydney line (single crease on the upper part of the palm)
- Hallucal crease (single crease across the ball of the foot)

Medical and behavioral symptoms may include:

- Otitis media
- Attention deficit and hyperactivity
- Impulsivity
- Sensory integration difficulty
- Autism
- PDD
- Mental retardation
- Learning disabilities
- Seizures
- Anxiety
- Unstable mood
- Emotional problems

There are usually different severity patterns in boys and girls, with the presenting symptoms in boys tending to be more severe. Most boys with fragile X syndrome have mental retardation. Though 30 to 50 percent of girls do have mental retardation, it tends to be milder. The other 50 to 70 percent of girls with fragile X syndrome have normal IQ or learning disabilities. Behavioral problems and emotional problems are common in both groups (Weber, 2000).

Speech and Language Difficulties

There is a wide variety of symptoms and difficulties related to speech and language development, as well as functional communication in daily living (Schopmeyer & Lowe, 1992). Differences between males and females have been noted, with the communication problems being more widespread and more severe in males. Males with fragile X syndrome typically have communication problems (Abbeduto & Hagerman, 1997). The incidence of co-occurrence of fragile X syndrome and autism is higher in males (Bailey, Mesibov, Hatton, Clark, Roberts, & Mayhew, 1998). Males from ages 2 to 7 with fragile X syndrome show significant language delays in semantics and morphosyntax, and difficulties with gestures, reciprocity, and symbolic play skills (Roberts, Mirrett, & Burchinal, 2001). On the Communication and Symbolic Behavior Scale, they show relative strengths in verbal and vocal communication (Roberts, Mirrett, Anderson, Burchinal, & Neebe, 2002). Adolescent and adult males with fragile X syndrome demonstrate speech patterns characterized by fluctuating rate, and frequent perseveration of words, sentences, and topics. Though they may have fairly good intelligibility in single words, they generally have poor intelligibility in conversational speech (Paul, Cohen, Breg, Watson, & Herman, 1984). In language, they generally have delays in vocabulary and morphosyntax (Abbeduto & Hagerman, 1997). Some of the more common speech and language symptoms in males are listed in Table 6-2. In females, the speech and language symptoms tend to be milder. Some of the more common speech and language symptoms in females are presented in Table 6-2.

Treatment for Children with Fragile X Syndrome

Treatment for individuals with fragile X syndrome focuses on targeting each symptom that is manifested in that individual. If mental retardation is evident, special education would help the child learn.

Table 6-2   Speech and Language Characteristics of Children with Fragile X Syndrome

Males	Females
Delayed onset of expressive language	Expressive language difficulties
Syntax difficulty	Auditory memory difficulties
Delays in vocabulary	Difficulty staying on-topic
Receptive/expressive language gap	Use of tangential language
Pediatric verbal apraxia	
Cluttering	
Poor language organization skills	
Reduced speech intelligibility	
Fast, uneven rate of speech	
Echolalia	
Perseveration	
Disturbed speech rhythm	
Hoarse and breathy voice	
Pragmatic difficulties	
Gaze aversion	
Difficulty staying on-topic	
Turn-taking difficulties	

If learning disabilities are evident, treatment would target the learning disability. Medications and specialized treatment methods are used to help control the emotional and behavioral symptoms. Researchers are trying to find new genetic and pharmacological treatments that can address the underlying genetic problem. Currently, there are research treatment initiatives in three areas: gene therapy, gene repair, and psychopharmacology. Gene therapy seeks to insert a functional FMR1 gene into the brain of individuals with fragile X syndrome. Gene repair strategies seek to turn the FMR1 gene back on, so that it can produce the protein for the cell. Psychopharmalogical approaches seek to treat the symptoms and improve daily function for individuals with fragile X syndrome.

Therapeutic approaches target the behavioral, emotional, and communication difficulties experienced by individuals with fragile X syndrome. Many children with fragile X syndrome have sensory integration difficulties, that is, they have difficulty in organizing sensory input from the environment. This may affect the sensory information received through hearing, vision, touch, movement, and balance. It affects how children react to their environment. For example, if a child does not process auditory stimuli accurately, raindrops can sound like bullets, and would be very frightening. The occupational therapist works on sensory integration problems with the child and family.

Behavioral characteristics observed in children with fragile X syndrome may include hand flapping, hand biting, perseveration, poor eye contact, and tantrums (Bailey et al., 1998). Overall behavioral patterns may include short attention span, hyperactivity, difficulty in relating to other people, anxiety, hypervigilance, depression, and autism spectrum disorder. These symptoms make it more difficult to learn in school and to interact socially in the community. Psychologists and special educators will target these symptoms in treatment.

Some children with fragile X syndrome will use sign language or an augmentative communication system to communicate, but most will communicate by using speech. Speech and language development is often severely delayed, especially in males. Perseveration and echolalia may be present. Speech is often difficult to understand because of the presence of rapid rate of speaking, cluttered speech, poor eye contact, and difficulty with staying on-topic. Speech-language pathology treatment will target the specific areas of communication difficulty for the individual. If the child has hypotonia (low muscle tone) in the oral facial muscles, the child would need exercises to help strengthen the muscles to improve speech. If speech is unintelligible, the SLP would need to investigate the reasons for the lack of intelligibility. Is cluttering the problem? Is the child talking too rapidly? The treatment program is always individually designed for the child's strengths and challenges. The treatment program may include:

- Oral motor planning (developmental apraxia of speech) therapy
- Receptive language skills
- Expressive language skills
- Assistive technology for communication
- Conversational skills
- Nonverbal communication skills, including eye contact
- Treatment to decrease rate of speaking
- Treatment for cluttering
- Treatment to reduce perseveration
- Treatment to reduce echolalia

Treatment goals must be individualized, but there are some general strategies that can address the learning and communication challenges of children with fragile X syndrome. Visual cues can be very helpful. For young children, this might include pictures of relevant vocabulary, pictures of requests (help me, juice please), visual schedules to help with transitions, and pictures to help children follow directions. For older children, visual cues for classroom routines and behaviors (quiet, line up), as well as cues to help them learn the curriculum in science and social studies, may be needed. Girls often have difficulty with social situations, and as a result develop anxiety about participating in those situations, avoiding conversations when possible. Lunch and recess are good times to practice social skills. Children with fragile X syndrome seem to learn best in real-life activities and situations. Role playing using props and social scripts can be used if it is not possible to use the real situation.

One of the difficulties in designing treatment programs is that children with fragile X syndrome are often not identified at an early age. It is important to begin treatment early because speech is a motor output system that is based on sensory input and learning from the language environment. Since most infants and toddlers with fragile X syndrome have sensory integration difficulties, they find it difficult to learn from their environment without sensory integration treatment. A comprehensive early intervention language treatment program would involve collaboration between the SLP, occupational therapist (or sensory integration therapy), special educator or developmental specialist, assistive technology specialist, pediatrician, and family. Boys with fragile X syndrome often have complicated communication problems that are affected by physical, oral motor, and speech intelligibility concerns, as well as attentional and behavioral concerns. Girls may have mild speech problems or have good verbal skills, but both girls and boys often have difficulty in pragmatic (social interactive) speech. Speech-language pathology services cannot address all of the complex factors that may be affecting communication in the classroom or the community. A comprehensive language intervention program during the school years would involve collaboration between the SLP, occupational therapist, special educator, regular educator, pediatrician, and family.

With early diagnosis and comprehensive medical and therapeutic treatment, there is hope that the individual with fragile X syndrome can live a full and productive life. Through early intervention and continued communication, psychological, and educational assistance through the school years, children with fragile X syndrome can reach their potential.

Case Study 1: Down Syndrome

Becky is a 9-year-old girl with Down syndrome. Testing soon after birth revealed the etiology to be trisomy 21. Becky was born with cardiac problems (atrial-ventricular septal defect and endocardial cushion defect), which were surgically corrected at 6 months of age. For the first 16 months of life, Becky was breast fed, but experienced some difficulty with sucking early on. Feeding therapy was helpful during this period. Becky did not have difficulty transitioning to a cup or to solid food. It was very difficult to bathe Becky as she did not like to be touched, especially around the mouth, face, and head. So, shampooing her hair became an ordeal for her mother. Early intervention focused on sensory integration and physical therapy, in addition to speech-language pathology services. Becky had chronic fluid in her middle ear, which resulted in a moderate fluctuating conductive hearing loss. Early speech-language pathology services worked on auditory stimulation, turn-taking, oral motor stimulation, and language stimulation through play and musical activities. Becky was taught the signs "more" and "all done" at about 9 months of age, and a total communication program was instituted. Becky began speaking using single words to communicate at age 2. Speech-language pathology treatment focused on the oral motor foundations for articulation and vocabulary development.

At age 3.6, Becky began to combine words into two-word phrases, increasing her communication skills. She was advancing in pragmatics, and was included in a regular preschool program two days weekly and received special education services in a special preschool setting three days weekly. Speech-language pathology treatment targeted names, objects, colors, shapes, numbers, prepositions, and functional vocabulary skills such as social greetings. Becky began kindergarten at age 6, and remained in kindergarten for two years. During this period, she began to read, which helped facilitate vocabulary development. In kindergarten, she had difficulty with transitioning from one activity to another and in following directions. When a functional behavioral assessment was completed, it was determined that communication difficulties were affecting behavior in the classroom. A positive behavior support plan for Becky included use of a picture activity schedule to help with transitioning, and a visual cueing system to help her with following instructions.

In first grade, Becky was on grade level in reading, but had difficulty with mathematics. She learned to add and subtract, but had difficulty following the instructions on worksheets. She also had difficulty paying attention in class and staying focused on the assignments to complete them. A medical and psychological evaluation determined that she had attention deficit disorder, which was treated with medication. The SLP worked with the special education and regular education teacher to adapt worksheets for Becky in class.

Becky is now in third grade. She is included in the regular classroom, and receives special education and speech-language pathology services within the classroom. Becky communicates primarily through using speech, but she is often difficult to understand. Articulation, use of phonological processes, and speech intelligibility are being addressed in treatment. She uses an assistive listening device in class, and has preferential seating. She enjoys social studies and reading, but has difficulty with mathematics and science. In therapy, the SLP helps Becky with the vocabulary that she needs to learn for her subjects. The focus of treatment is on what is needed for the classroom: vocabulary, following instructions, and learning the routines of the class. One of the annual goals addresses speech intelligibility and another addresses grammar, which is difficult for Becky. Testing reveals receptive language scores at age 7.6, and expressive language scores at the age 5 level. Becky speaks in five- to six-word utterances. She is beginning to retell stories that she has read. Socially, she does well with greetings and social language, but has difficulty with requests, idioms, and colloquial expressions.

Case History 2: Fragile X Syndrome

Frank is an 8-year-old boy with fragile X syndrome. At age 3, Frank was not yet speaking. When his parents tried to communicate with him, Frank would look away. He would sometimes use gestures, but it was difficult for his parents to figure out what he was trying to tell them. He often moved his hands in front of his eyes, and seemed to block out the world. He was hyperactive, and had frequent tantrums. He was impulsive and was covered with bumps and bruises from his many daredevil episodes. Frank's parents talked with the pediatrician, who sent them home, telling them that Frank would outgrow this phase. When they did not see positive change after six months, they decided to change pediatricians. The new physician sent them for a developmental evaluation, which included speech-language pathology. The conclusion was that Frank had a developmental delay, and had some symptoms of pervasive developmental disability. Frank began receiving occupational therapy, sensory integration therapy, and speech-language pathology services. Sometimes, the therapies were integrated, and Frank would be working on articulation while he was lying on a big orange ball. He appeared to be more comfortable when he was rolling on the ball or swinging. The movement seemed to help him learn.

By age 5, Frank had made some progress, but was still lagging far behind his peers. He was communicating primarily through pointing. He was using two to three words and some sounds, but was perseverating on those words. He was having great difficulty making sounds and had a limited repertoire of sounds. He had poor lip closure with some drooling. From ages 3 to 5, Frank had six ear infections (serous otitis media) and they seemed to last a long time. Frank's parents were concerned about his development. His mother was worried that he was not getting enough to eat. Frank would only eat macaroni and cheese. If his mom tried to add peas and carrots, he would refuse to eat. Frank was thin, and had a long face and big ears. A more detailed evaluation was suggested by the therapy team. Frank's pediatrician ordered further testing, including DNA analysis. The parents waited anxiously for the results. After two weeks, the genetic testing revealed that Frank had fragile X syndrome.

A referral was made for assistive technology evaluation. Frank began using a Touch Talker communication device. He began with just two pictures, juice and his favorite toy truck. For the first time, people could understand what he was trying to tell them. He did not need to drag his mom to the refrigerator. He could tell her when he was thirsty. Frank began using spoken words along with the device, and appeared more motivated to communicate. The SLP noted that the limited number of sounds that Frank made, his inconsistent sound production, and his effortful attempts at speaking suggested a diagnosis of motor-planning difficulties. She began using specialized methods to teach him to speak that focused on the length and complexity of the words. It is an approach used for children who have been diagnosed with developmental apraxia of speech. This seemed to help Frank. He was more successful in his speech attempts. The combination of using the Touch Talker and speaking enabled him to be understood and communicate his needs. Sensory integration treatment helped Frank, and he began to participate more at school. Frank was enrolled in a special education class within his regular neighborhood school. His favorite activity was center time, because there was a center about transportation. Frank loved airplanes, and he always tried to be the first one at that center. There were books about airplanes, and he would put on the earphones and listen to the story. Sometimes, he would just look at the pictures and turn the pages. He was fascinated by the movements of the propellers. When he played with the toy planes, he would spin the propellers and make whirring sounds. His family often took him to a small local airport, so he could watch the planes. It was difficult to get Frank to leave the airport. He loved those planes!

Presently, at age 8, Frank is using a combination of speech and assistive technology to communicate. It is still difficult to understand his speech, but he is successful at communicating using his augmentative communication device. He is making educational progress. Classroom modifications and adaptations are used to help him learn. Transitions are difficult for him, so he uses picture schedules to help him with transitions in class. When the class has reading time, Frank can participate now. Oral reading is difficult for him, but the teacher has input repeated phrases from books into Frank's augmentative communication device. When the class reads *Chicken Soup with Rice*, Frank pushes the button on his AAC device, and "says" the words right along with the other children. His favorite subject is social studies. He is doing a report now on the Wright brothers, and has been making a paper model of their plane with his dad. Math is difficult for Frank, and the teacher is using visual cues and computer-based learning to help him. Frank's parents still have concerns, but they can see that he is making progress. They hope that he will be able to communicate through his speech. They hope that he will be able to continue learning. They hope he will be able to live and work in his neighborhhod when he grows up. They hope that he has a bright future ahead.

REVIEW QUESTIONS

1. What does a diagnosis of mental retardation mean? What are the severity levels of mental retardation?
2. How can we describe the different levels of support that a person with mental retardation may need?
3. Compare and contrast the speech and language symptoms that often accompany Down syndrome and fragile X syndrome.
4. Compare and contrast treatment for children with Down syndrome and fragile X syndrome in the following areas: phonology, semantics, morphosyntax, pragmatics, speech intelligibility.

REFERENCES

Abbeduto, L., & Hagerman, R. J. (1997). Language and communication in fragile X syndrome. *Mental Retardation and Developmental Disabilities Research Reviews, 3*, 313–322.

Attwood, A. (1988). The understanding and use of interpersonal gestures by autistic and Down's syndrome children. *Journal of Autism and Developmental Disorders, 18*, 241–257.

Bailey, D. B., & Nelson, D. (1995). The nature and consequences of fragile X syndrome. *Mental Retardation and Developmental Disabilities Research Reviews, 1*, 238–244.

Bailey, D., Mesibov, G., Hatton, D., Clark, R., Roberts, J., & Mayhew, L. (1998). Autistic behavior in young boys with fragile X syndrome. *Journal of Autism and Developmental Disorders, 28*, 499–508.

Batshaw, M. L., & Perret, Y. (1992). *Children with disabilities: A medical primer* (3rd ed.). Baltimore: Paul H. Brookes.

Bleile, K. (1982). Consonant ordering in Down's syndrome phonology. *Journal of Communication Disorders, 15*, 275–285.

Bleile, K., & Schwartz, I. (1984). Three perspectives on the speech of children with Down's syndrome. *Journal of Communication Disorders, 17*, 87–94.

Bless, D., Swift, E., & Rosen, M. (1985). Communication profiles of children with Down syndrome. Unpublished manuscript, Waisman Center on Mental Retardation and Human Development, University of Wisconsin.

Bondy, A., & Frost, L. (2001). *A picture's worth: PECS and other visual communication strategies in autism*. Bethesda, MD: Woodbine House.

Bray, M., & Woolnough, L. (1988). The language skills of children with Down's syndrome aged 12 to 16 years. *Child Language Teaching and Therapy, 4*, 311.

Buckley, S. (2000). *Speech and language development for individuals with Down syndrome—An overview*. Portsmouth, UK: Down Syndrome Educational Trust.

Buckley, S. (1993). Language development in children with Down's syndrome: Reasons for optimism. *Down's Syndrome: Research and Practice, 1*, 3–9.

Buckley, S., & Bird, G. (2001). *Speech & language development in individuals with Down syndrome: An overview*. Portsmouth, UK: Down Syndrome Educational Trust.

Buckley, S. (1986) *The development of language and reading skills in children with Down's syndrome*. Portsmouth, UK: Portsmouth Polytechnic Institute.

Cardoso-Martins, C., Mervis, C. B., & Mervis, C. A. (1985). Early vocabulary acquisition by children with Down syndrome. *American Journal of Mental Deficiency, 90*, 177–184.

Chapman, R., Seung, J., Schwartz, S., & Bird, E. R. (1998). Language skills of children and adolescents with Down syndrome II: Production deficits. *Journal of Speech, Language and Hearing Research, 41*, 861–873.

Cohen, W. (Ed.). (1999). Healthcare guidelines for individuals with Down syndrome. Down Syndrome Medical Interest Group. Available at http://www.ds-health.com or http://www.denison.edu. Accessed on 1/24/03.

Crary, M. A. (1993). *Developmental motor speech disorders*. Clifton Park, NY: Delmar Learning.

Devenny, D. A., & Silverman, W. P. (1990). Speech dysfluency and manual specialization in Down's syndrome. *Journal of Mental Deficiency Research, 34*, 253–260.

Dodd, B. (1976). A comparison of the phonological systems of mental age matched, normal, severely subnormal and Down's Syndrome children. *British Journal of Disorders of Communication, 1*, 27–42.

Elliott, D., Weeks, D. J., & Elliott, C. L. (1987). Cerebral specialization in individuals with Down's syndrome. *American Journal on Mental Retardation, 92*, 263–271.

Fowler, A. (1990). Language abilities in children with Down syndrome: Evidence for a specific syntactic delay. In D. Cichetti & M. Beeghley (Eds.), *Children with Down syndrome: A developmental perspective* (pp. 302–328). Cambridge: Cambridge University Press.

Fowler, A. (1995). Linguistic variability in persons with Down syndrome. In L. Nadel & D. Rosenthal (Eds.), *Down syndrome: Living and learning in the community* (pp. 121–131). New York: Wiley-Liss.

Fuchs, D., Fuchs, L., Power, M., & Dailey, A. (1985). Bias in the assessment of handicapped children. *American Educational Research Journal, 22*, 185–187.

Gilham, B. (1979). *The first words programme for mentally handicapped children.* London, UK: George Allen & Unwin.

Hagerman, R. J., & Cronister, A. (1996). *Fragile X syndrome: Diagnosis, treatment and research* (2nd ed.). Baltimore: Johns Hopkins University Press.

Hagerman, R. J., & Silverman, A. C. (1991). *Fragile X syndrome: Diagnosis, treatment and research.* Baltimore: Johns Hopkins University Press.

Heath, M., & Elliott, D. (1999). Cerebral specialization for speech production in persons with Down syndrome. *Brain and Language, 69*, 193–211.

Hopmann, M. R., & Wilen, E. (1993, March). *Visual and auditory processing in children with Down syndrome: Individual differences.* Presented at the Society for Research in Child Development, New Orleans.

Horstmeier, D. (1988). But I don't understand you—The communication interaction of youths and adults with Down syndrome. In S. Pueschel (Ed.), *The young person with Down syndrome.* Baltimore: Paul H. Brookes.

Kent, L., Evans, J., Paul, M., & Sharp, M. (1999). Comorbidity of autism spectrum disorder in children with Down syndrome. *Developmental Medicine and Child Neurology, 41*, 153–158.

Kumin, L. (1994a). Intelligibility of speech in children with Down syndrome in natural settings: Parents' perspective. *Perceptual and Motor Skills, 78*, 307–313.

Kumin, L. (1994b). *Communication skills in children with Down syndrome—A guide for parents.* Bethesda, MD: Woodbine House.

Kumin, L. (1996). Speech and language skills in children with Down syndrome. *Mental Retardation and Developmental Disabilities Research Reviews, 2*, 109–116.

Kumin, L. (1999). Comprehensive speech and language treatment for infants, toddlers, and children with Down syndrome. In T. J. Hassold & D. Patterson (Eds.), *Down syndrome: A promising future, together* (pp. 145–153). New York: Wiley-Liss.

Kumin, L. (2001a). *Classroom language skills for children with Down syndrome: A guide for parents and teachers.* Bethesda, MD: Woodbine House.

Kumin, L. (2001b). Speech intelligibility in individuals with Down syndrome: A framework for targeting specific factors in assessment and treatment. *Down Syndrome Quarterly, 6*, 1–6.

Kumin, L., & Adams, J. (2000). Developmental apraxia of speech and intelligibility in children with Down syndrome. *Down Syndrome Quarterly, 5*, 1–6.

Kumin, L., Councill, C., & Goodman, M. (1994). A longitudinal study of the emergence of phonemes in children with Down syndrome. *Journal of Communication Disorders, 27*, 265–275.

Kumin, L., Councill, C., & Goodman, M. (1995). The pacing board: A technique to assist the transition from single word to multiword utterances. *Infant-Toddler Intervention, 5,* 23–29.

Kumin, L., Councill, C., & Goodman, M. (1996). Comprehensive communication intervention for school-aged children with Down syndrome. *Down Syndrome Quarterly, 1,* 1–8.

Kumin, L., Councill, C., & Goodman, M. (1998). Expressive vocabulary development in children with Down syndrome. *Down Syndrome Quarterly, 3,* 1–7.

Kumin, L., Councill, C., & Goodman, M. (1999). Expressive vocabulary in young children with Down syndrome: From research to treatment. *Infant-Toddler Intervention,* 87–100.

Kumin, L., Goodman, M., & Councill, C. (1991). Comprehensive communication intervention for infants and toddlers with Down syndrome. *Infant-Toddler Intervention, 1,* 275–296.

Leddy, M. (1999). The biological bases of speech in people with Down syndrome. In J. Miller, M. Leddy, & L. A. Leavitt (Eds.), *Improving the communication of people with Down syndrome* (pp. 61–80). Baltimore: Paul H. Brookes.

Leifer, J. S., & Lewis, M. (1984). Acquisition of conversational response skills by young Down syndrome and nonretarded young children. *American Journal of Mental Deficiency, 88,* 610–618.

Loveland, K. A., & Tunali, B. (1991). Social scripts for conversational interactions in autism and Down syndrome. *Journal of Autism and Developmental Disorders, 21,* 177–186.

Luckasson, R., Borthwick-Duffy, S., Buntinx, W., Coulter, D., Craig, E., Reeve, A., Schalock, R., Snell, M., Spitalnik, D., Spreat, S., & Tasse, M. (2002a). *Mental retardation: Definition, classification and systems of supports* (10th edition). Washington, DC: American Association on Mental Retardation.

Mervis, C. (1997, November). *Early lexical and conceptual development in children with Down syndrome.* Presented at the National Down Syndrome Society International Down Syndrome Research Conference on Cognition and Behavior.

Miller, J. (1987). Language and communication characteristics of children with Down's syndrome. In S. Pueschel et al. (Eds.), *New perspectives in Down syndrome.* Baltimore: Paul H. Brookes.

Miller, J. F. (1988). Developmental asynchrony of language development in children with Down syndrome. In L. Nadel (Ed.), *Psychobiology of Down syndrome.* New York: Academic Press.

Miller, J. F. (1992). Lexical development in young children with Down syndrome. In R. Chapman (Ed.), *Processes in language acquisition and disorders.* St. Louis, MO: Mosby Year Book.

Miller, J. F. (1995). Individual differences in vocabulary acquisition in children with Down syndrome. *Progress in Clinical and Biological Research, 393,* 93–103.

Miller, J., & Leddy, M. (1999). Verbal fluency, speech intelligibility, and communicative effectiveness. In J. Miller, M. Leddy, & L. A. Leavitt (Eds.), *Improving the communication of people with Down syndrome* (pp. 81–92). Baltimore: Paul H. Brookes.

Miller, J., Leddy, M., & Leavitt, L. A. (1999). (Eds.). *Improving the communication of people with Down syndrome.* Baltimore: Paul H. Brookes.

Miller, J., Leddy, M., Miolo, G., & Sedey, A. (1995). The development of early language skills in children with Down syndrome. In L. Nadel & D. Rosenthal (Eds.), *Down syndrome: Living and learning in the community* (pp. 115–119). New York: Wiley-Liss.

Mundy, P., Sigman, M., Kasari, C., & Yirmiya, N. (1988). Nonverbal communication skills in Down syndrome children. *Child Development, 59,* 235–249.

NDSS National Down Syndrome Society at www.ndss.org accessed on 1-25-03.

Paul, R., Cohen, D. J., Breg, W. R., Watson, M., & Herman, S. (1984). Fragile X syndrome: Its relation to speech and language disorders. *Journal of Speech and Hearing Disorders, 49,* 326–336.

Pueschel, S. M., Gallagher, P. L., Zastler, A. S., & Pezzulo, J. C. (1987). Cognitive and learning processes in children with Downs syndrome. *Research and Developmental Disabilities, 8,* 21–37.

Roberts, J. E., Mirrett, P., & Burchinal, M. (2001). Receptive and expressive communication development of young males with fragile X syndrome. *American Journal on Mental Retardation, 106,* 216–230.

Roberts, J. E., Mirrett, P., Anderson, K., Burchinal, M., & Neebe, E. (2002). Early communication, symbolic behavior, and social profiles of young males with fragile X syndrome. *American Journal of Speech-Language Pathology, 11,* 295–304.

Roizen, N. J., Wolters, C., Nicol, T., & Blondis, T. (1992). Hearing loss in children with Down syndrome. *Pediatrics, 123,* S 9–12.

Rondal, J. A. (1988). Language development in Down's syndrome: A lifespan perspective. *International Journal of Behavioral Development, 11,* 21–36.

Rosin, P., & Swift, E. (1999). Communication interventions: Improving the speech intelligibility of children with Down syndrome. In J. Miller, M. Leddy, & L. A. Leavitt (Eds.), *Improving the communication of people with Down syndrome* (pp. 133–159). Baltimore: Paul H. Brookes.

Rosin, M., Swift, E., Bless, D., & Vetter, D. K. (1988). Communication profiles of adolescents with Down syndrome. *Journal of Childhood Communication Disorders, 12,* 49–64.

Schalock, R. L., Baker, P. C., & Croser, M. D. (2002). *Embarking on a new century: Mental retardation at the end of the twentieth century.* Washington, DC: AAMR.

Schopmeyer, B., & Lowe, F. (1992). *The fragile X child.* Clifton Park, NY: Delmar Learning.

Shott, S. R. (2000). Down syndrome: Common pediatric ear, nose, and throat problems. *Down Syndrome Quarterly, 5,* 1–6.

Smith, B. L., & Stoel-Gammon, C. (1983). A longitudinal study of the development of stop consonant production in normal and Down's syndrome children. *Journal of Speech and Hearing Disorders, 48,* 114–118.

Sommers, R. K., Patterson, J. P., & Wildgen, P. L. (1988). Phonology of Down syndrome speakers, ages 13–22. *Journal of Childhood Communication Disorders, 12,* 65–91.

Stoel-Gammon, C. (1980). Phonological analysis of four Down's syndrome children. *Applied Psycholinguistics, 1,* 31–48.

Stoel-Gammon, C. (1990). Down syndrome: Effects on language development, *ASHA,* 42–44.

Swift, E., & Rosin, P. (1990). A remediation sequence to improve speech intelligibility for students with Down syndrome. *Language, Speech and Hearing Services in Schools, 21,* 140–146.

Turner, G., Webb, T., Wake, S., & Robinson, H. (1996). Prevalence of fragile X syndrome. *American Journal of Medical Genetics, 64,* 196–197.

Weber, J. D. (Ed.). (2000). *Children with fragile X syndrome: A parent's guide.* Bethesda, MD: Woodbine House.

Weeks, D., Chua, R., & Elliott, D. (Eds.). (2000). *Perceptual-motor behavior in Down syndrome.* Champaign, IL: Human Kinetics.

PART III

Craniofacial Anomalies

Chapter 7

Cleft Lip and Palate

Kathleen Siren, Ph.D., CCC-SLP

CHAPTER OBJECTIVES

Upon completion of this chapter, the student should be able to:

1. Describe the general embryological development of the lip and palate
2. Explain patterns of cleft lip and cleft palate and the classification terms used to describe clefts
3. Discuss both genetic and environmental factors involved in lip and palate clefts
4. List and briefly describe five common syndromes and one sequence that likely involve clefts of the lip and/or palate
5. Describe resonance, articulation, and voice disorders associated with cleft palate or a history of cleft palate
6. Discuss feeding, hearing, and dental difficulties likely for individuals with cleft palate or a history of cleft palate
7. Describe the team approach to management of an individual with a cleft palate, with particular emphasis on the roles of the speech-language pathologist and audiologist
8. Discuss timing of primary and secondary surgeries for cleft lip and cleft palate
9. Provide examples of common surgical techniques for primary cleft palate surgery and for secondary surgical management of velopharyngeal dysfunction
10. Discuss prosthetic management options prior to, or in place of, secondary surgical management for individuals with velopharyngeal dysfunction
11. Discuss possible psychosocial issues affecting individuals born with clefts of the lip and/or palate as well as parents and family members of these individuals

INTRODUCTION

Individuals born with a cleft palate face numerous challenges to normal speech and hearing development. As such, **speech-language pathologists** (SLPs) and audiologists are important members of cleft palate teams. These teams of professionals provide ongoing interdisciplinary assessment and intervention for individuals with a cleft palate or a history of cleft palate. Additionally, speech-language pathologists and audiologists who are not members of a cleft palate team will undoubtedly see clients with a history of cleft palate. These professionals must be able to provide information to the client and family and to make appropriate referrals. This chapter provides an overview of cleft lip and palate, including how and why clefts occur, the effects on speech and hearing, and the team approach to assessment and intervention.

EMBRYOLOGY AND PHYSIOLOGICAL ANOMALIES

Cleft lip and **cleft palate** occur when there is a disruption in development of the oral cavity during gestation of the embryo. To understand how and why clefts occur, it is necessary to have a basic understanding of embryological development of the lip and palate. The following sections will discuss general embryology of the lip and palate; development of the lip and primary palate specifically; development of the secondary palate; and the embryological basis of clefts of the lip and palate.[*]

Embryology of the Lip and Palate

The formation of the facial structures depends upon neural crest cells that develop in the embryo and migrate at different rates during embryological development. Specifically, the first neural crest cells to reach the facial area migrate over the top of the cranial end of the embryo. These cells form the frontonasal process, or frontonasal prominence. This frontonasal process eventually forms the outer nose as well as the middle two-thirds of the upper lip and anterior portion of the palate (primary palate). Other neural crest cells reach the facial area by migrating via a longer route around the primitive facial area. These cells eventually form a series of paired arches. These pairs include one pair, the mandibular arches, each consisting of a lower mandibular process and an upper maxillary process. The paired maxillary processes eventually form the sides of the upper lip. On either side of the embryonic tongue, two palatine processes, or palatal shelves, project medially from the maxillary processes. These palatal shelves eventually form the posterior portion of the palate (secondary palate). These facial processes and palatal shelves merge, or fuse, from the sixth through the 12th weeks of embryological development.

Formation of the Primary Palate (Including the Lip)

During the sixth week of gestation, the frontonasal process and the paired maxillary processes begin to fuse. The formation of the primary palate begins at the incisive foramen with fusion proceeding anteriorly on both sides to form the premaxilla, consisting of the anterior portion of the hard palate and maxilla, and the alveolar ridge. Fusion then proceeds to form the base of the nose. Finally, the frontonasal process and the maxillary processes fuse to form the philtral lines on both sides of the upper lip. This completes the formation of the upper lip.

---

[*]Though students are familiar with the terms *hard palate* and *soft palate*, the distinctions used here will be *primary palate* and *secondary palate*. These terms do not refer to the same structures. The terms *primary palate* and *secondary palate* are based upon embryological development. The embryonic structure called the primary palate consists of the middle portion of the lip and a wedge-shaped portion in the anterior of the palate extending posteriorly to the incisive foramen (a small hole in the bone underlying the alveolar ridge area). The secondary palate is the portion of the palate posterior to the incisive foramen.

Formation of the Secondary Palate

Initially, the palatal shelves hang down vertically on either side of the embryonic tongue. During the seventh or the eighth week of gestation, the palatal shelves rise to a horizontal position. This occurs at nearly the same time that the embryonic tongue begins to drop down. During the eighth to the ninth week, the palatal shelves begin to fuse. This fusion takes place in an anterior to posterior direction. That is, initially the palatal shelves fuse with the primary palate, and then continue to join and fuse with each other from the incisive foramen posteriorly with formation of the uvula occurring last. Additionally, the nasal septum and vomer bone move down and fuse on the superior surface of the palatal shelves. The secondary palate is completely formed somewhere between the 10th and the 12th weeks of gestation.

The Embryology of Clefts

During embryological development, disruptions may occur that impair the fusion of the processes and associated structures. If neural cell migration or palatal shelf movement is disrupted or delayed, clefts can occur where processes and structures do not fuse. Thus, clefts generally follow fusion lines from the incisive foramen out to the periphery (Figure 7-1). Clefts of the lip or primary palate occur when the frontonasal process fails to meet or fuse entirely with the maxillary processes on either or both sides. Clefts of the secondary palate occur when the palatal shelves fail to elevate, join medially, or completely fuse.

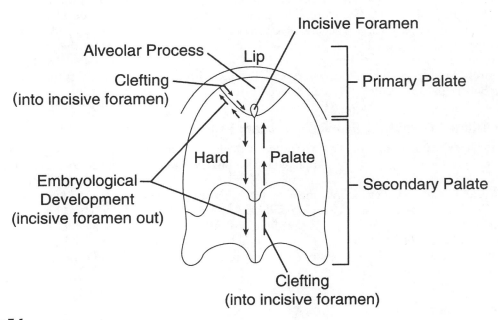

Figure 7-1
Embryological development proceeds from the incisive foramen outward to the periphery. Clefts begin at the periphery and extend inward toward the incisive foramen.

CLASSIFICATION OF CLEFTS

Though clefts generally follow a predictable pattern, describing clefts in different individuals is not an easy task. Clefts can vary along several dimensions. This section discusses general issues related to the classification of clefts.

Clinicians and researchers have proposed numerous classification systems over the years to describe clefts. Most systems were elaborations of the basic dichotomy of cleft lip (with or without cleft palate) versus cleft palate only (Peterson-Falzone, Hardin-Jones, & Karnell, 2001). The most universally accepted system is one proposed by Kernahan and Stark (1958), which classifies clefts based upon embryological development (Kummer, 2001). In Kernahan and Stark's system, clefts of the primary palate are those anterior to the incisive foramen, including clefts of the lip. Clefts of the secondary palate are those posterior to the incisive foramen. Generally, clefts are also classified as either unilateral, on one side, or bilateral, on both sides. Though widely used, the distinction between unilateral and bilateral clefts may not be helpful in describing severity, particularly in cases where unilateral clefts are very wide (Peterson-Falzone et al., 2001). Clefts are also often described as "complete" or "incomplete." A complete cleft is an opening from the periphery completely through to the incisive foramen (Kummer, 2001). An incomplete cleft may be only a slight cleft on the periphery, or it may be a cleft through to the incisive foramen with a minimal band or bridge of tissue at some point along the cleft. Thus, these terms may also not always be useful in describing severity.

In an attempt to describe severity of a cleft, clinicians and researchers have developed several classification systems that are elaborations of these basic dichotomous descriptions. However, unless all future readers of a description are familiar with the classification system used, the descriptors may be meaningless. Additionally, clefts may vary in several dimensions: anterior to posterior, width, and depth (Peterson-Falzone et al., 2001). Therefore, it is best to describe a cleft in as much detail as possible.

The following sections will use general classification terms based on Kernahan and Stark's (1958) system. However, clefts of the lip will be discussed separately from other clefts of the primary palate. The rationale for this is that individuals with clefts of the lip that do not involve the alveolus (or dental arch) rarely have speech problems, whereas individuals with clefts of the alveolus (primary palate) and/or secondary palate often have speech difficulties.

Cleft Lip Without Cleft of the Remaining Primary Palate

Clefts of the lip may range from only a small notch in the lip to a cleft that extends through the philtral lines of the lip to the nostril. A more complete cleft will likely cause flattening or collapse of the nostril on the side of the cleft. Clefts of the lip may be unilateral or bilateral. A unilateral cleft of the lip (with or without additional clefting into the alveolus) more frequently occurs on the left side (Jensen, Kreigorg, Dahl, & Fogh-Anderson, 1988; McWilliams, Morris, & Shelton, 1990). In a bilateral cleft of the lip, the philtral tissue that hangs free is called the prolabium. Occasionally a small bridge of soft tissue extends across an otherwise open cleft. This is called a **Simonart's band.** Clefts of the lip only present cosmetic concerns, but do not generally present serious speech concerns. However, a cleft lip is often accompanied by a cleft through the alveolus.

Cleft of the Primary Palate

Clefts that extend into the alveolus may also range from a small notch to a cleft extending completely through the dental arch. A cleft that extends through the alveolus to the incisive foramen is often called a "complete cleft" or even a "complete cleft lip." Such clefts may also be unilateral or bilateral. When there is a bilateral complete cleft of the lip and alveolus, both the prolabium and premaxilla (the triangular-shaped bone that normally contains the central and lateral maxillary incisors) are unattached and may project anteriorly or appear to be attached to the end of the nose. Figures 7-2 and 7-3 depict infants with unilateral complete clefts of the lip and primary palate. Figure 7-4 shows an infant with a bilateral incomplete cleft of the lip and primary palate. Figure 7-5 illustrates an infant with a bilateral complete cleft of the lip and primary palate.

Due to the course of embryological development, clefts of the alveolus are almost always accompanied by clefts of the lip. However, cleft palate teams have reported cases of alveolar clefting in the absence of lip clefting (Ranta & Rintala, 1989). Moreover, the majority of individuals with clefts of the primary palate also have clefts of the secondary palate.

Cleft of the Secondary Palate

As with clefts of the primary palate, clefts of the secondary palate may also range from minimal to extensive. A defect in the secondary palate may involve only a small notch in the uvula (**bifid uvula**). A bifid uvula is not of concern unless it occurs in conjunction with a submucous cleft palate (discussed below). On the other hand, a complete cleft of the secondary palate extends anteriorly all the way to the incisive foramen. Clefts of the secondary palate may also be unilateral or bilateral. In a unilateral

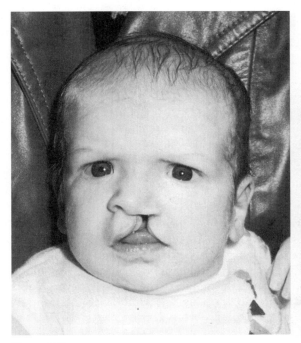

Figure 7-2
Infant with a unilateral complete cleft of the lip and primary palate.

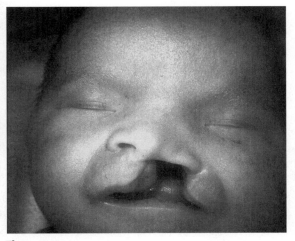

Figure 7-3
Infant with a unilateral complete cleft of the lip and primary palate. Note the wider cleft when compared to the infant in Figure 7-2.

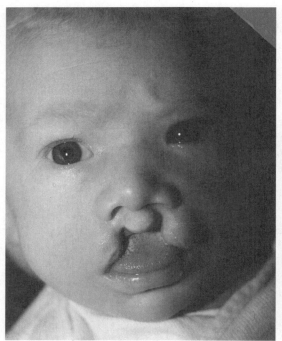

Figure 7-4
Infant with a unilateral complete cleft of the lip and primary palate. Note the wider cleft when compared to the infant in Figure 7-2.

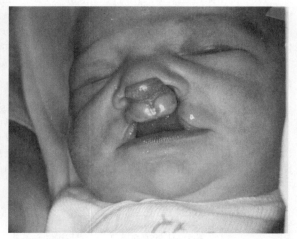

Figure 7-5
Infant with a bilateral complete cleft of the lip. Note the slight forward projections of the prolabium and premaxilla.

cleft, the vomer bone, or bottom part of the nasal septum, generally fuses to the intact palatal shelf. In a bilateral cleft, the vomer bone fails to fuse to either palatal shelf. Figure 7-6 illustrates a child with a bilateral complete cleft of the secondary palate. Figure 7–7 depicts a child with a bilateral complete cleft of the secondary palate in combination with a bilateral complete cleft of the lip and primary palate.

Submucous Cleft of the Secondary Palate

A **submucous cleft palate** is a defect in the underlying structures of the secondary palate without a complete opening between the oral and nasal cavities. Thus, though the surface of the palate in the oral cavity appears to be intact, underlying muscle and bony structures have not entirely fused. Three classic stigmata of a submucous cleft may be identified through oral examination: a bifid uvula, a midline division of the musculature of the soft palate (which may cause the middle of the velum to have a bluish tint), and a notch in the posterior border of the hard palate. Speech-language pathologists (SLPs) must be aware of submucous clefts, as they can cause the same speech problems as overt clefts.

Describing and classifying clefts is not easy. Likewise, determining the cause of clefting is not straightforward. Clefts may have many different causes, or etiologies, and even with similar causes, resulting clefts may be very different across individuals. The following section discusses what is currently known about the etiology of clefts.

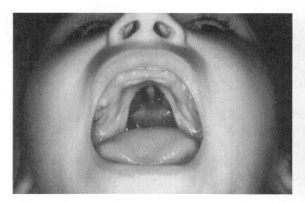

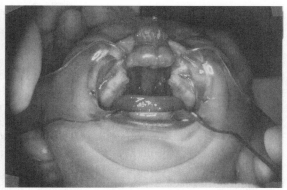

Figure 7-6
Child with a complete bilateral cleft of the secondary palate.

Figure 7-7
Child with a complete bilateral cleft of the secondary palate in combination with a bilateral complete cleft of the lip and primary palate.

ETIOLOGY

As with many physiological traits, no single cause can explain clefting in all or even most individuals. Congenital malformations including clefts may be due to genetic, chromosomal, environmental, multifactorial, or unknown causes. However, both genetics and environmental factors may predispose an individual to clefts of the lip or palate. This section covers three areas: genetic and chromosomal bases of cleft lip and palate; environmental factors involved in clefting; and multifactorial inheritance, the most widely accepted theory regarding the etiology of clefts.

Genetic and Chromosomal Bases of Clefts

In some individuals, disorders that include clefting may be caused by a single, abnormal gene. In many cases, these single-gene disorders appear to be autosomal dominant. Autosomal is a term referring to any chromosome that is not a sex chromosome. Thus, such disorders do not vary by gender. In an **autosomal dominant** disorder, individuals will likely present with the disorder if they receive the abnormal gene from either parent. Additionally, such individuals have a 50 percent chance of passing the abnormal gene on to each of their offspring. Several single-gene, autosomal dominant disorders that include clefts will be discussed in a later section.

In other individuals, clefts may be part of a chromosomal disorder. In a chromosomal disorder, an individual may be missing part of a chromosome or may have an extra chromosome. In some chromosomal disorders, life expectancy may be short or the individual may not be able to produce offspring. In both single-gene and chromosomal disorders, a cleft of the lip and/or palate is often one potential trait in a series of traits that generally characterize a disorder or syndrome.

Environmental Factors Involved in Clefting

An environmental **teratogen** is a chemical or physical substance that may disrupt normal embryological development and, therefore, cause a congenital malformation. Studying the effects of suspected environmental teratogens is difficult because experimenters cannot purposefully expose humans to potentially hazardous substances. However, researchers are able to study individuals who have a history of contact with specific substances. Such studies have highlighted several teratogens that appear to be associated with cleft lip and/or palate. Maternal use of alcohol (Clarren & Smith, 1978; Hanson & Smith, 1975; Jones, Smith, Ulleland, & Streissguth, 1973) and maternal use of cigarettes (or exposure to cigarette smoke) (Ericson, Kallen, & Westerholm, 1979; Khoury, Gomez-Farias, & Mulinare, 1989; Koury, Weinstein, Panny, Holtzman, Lindsay, Farrel, & Eisenberg, 1977; Shaw, Wasserman, Lammer, O'Malley, Murrray, Basart, & Tolarova, 1996; Werler, Lammer, Rosenberg, & Mitchell, 1990) both appear to be linked to an increased risk for clefts in offspring. Additionally, intake of anticonvulsant drugs used to treat epilepsy (Hanson, Myrianthopoulos, Harvey, & Smith, 1976; Meadow, 1968; Owens, Jones, & Harris, 1985) and use of retinoid (Vitamin A) drugs (Fernhoff & Lammer, 1984; Lammer et al., 1985) also appear to increase the risk of clefts. Exposure to organic solvents (Holmberg, Hernberg, Kruppa, Rantala, & Riala, 1982) or pesticides (Gordon & Shy, 1981) also appears to be linked to an increased risk of clefts.

Researchers have also investigated maternal diet and vitamin intake as potentially related to clefts in offspring. Particularly, folic acid deficiency during pregnancy appears to be linked to a decrease in embryonic cell propagation, with resulting congenital malformations such as clefts. Some studies demonstrate a decreased risk of recurrence in subsequent offspring of women who take a folic acid supplement (Tolarova, 1982; Tolarova & Harris, 1995).

Regardless of specific teratogen, the developing embryo is most susceptible to clefts of the lip and/or palate between the fourth and 12th weeks of gestation, the period of time from early neural crest cell migration through the formation of the upper lip and the palate. There do appear to be slight differences between males and females in the timing of embryological fusion. The palatal shelves rise and fuse approximately one week earlier in males (Burdi & Silvey, 1969). The increased time frame for fusion in females may allow for a longer period of time for potential teratogenic agents to affect palatal development. In fact, clefts of the secondary palate occur twice as frequently in females, even though clefts of the lip with or without clefts of the palate occur more frequently in males (Calzolari et al., 1988; Jensen et al., 1988; Shaw, Croen, & Curry, 1991).

Current Theories Regarding the Etiology of Clefts

Currently, the most popular theory to explain clefts is the multifactorial model of inheritance (Fraser, 1970, 1978). This theory holds that clefts are the result of an interaction of several factors, both genetic and environmental. In other words, certain gene combinations may provide a genetic predisposition for a cleft, though a cleft will result only if certain environmental factors are also present. In this model, if enough predisposing genetic and environmental factors are present, the embryo is pushed over a theoretical threshold and a cleft results.

The multifactorial model is used to explain clefts that do not occur as part of a syndrome. Clefts that are present as part of a syndrome generally occur based upon a known pattern of inheritance. The following section discusses some syndromes that have clefts of the lip and/or palate as typical characteristics.

SYNDROMES ASSOCIATED WITH CLEFT LIP AND PALATE

A **syndrome** is a cluster of anomalies that occur together and have a single known, or suspected, cause (Spranger et al., 1982). It is estimated that there are nearly 350 syndromes that involve orofacial clefting. A **sequence**, on the other hand, is a series of secondary anomalies resulting from one initial anomaly. Finally, an **association** is a cluster of anomalies present in two or more individuals, without a known pathogenesis and not identified as either a syndrome or a sequence (Spranger et al., 1982). With repeated identification and a discovered or suspected etiology, associations may later be identified as syndromes or sequences. This section discusses five syndromes and one sequence that involve clefts of the lip and/or palate.[*]

Van der Woude Syndrome

Van der Woude syndrome is an autosomal dominant disorder with the affected gene mapped to chromosome 1. This syndrome is one of the most common syndromes involving clefts of the lip and/or palate. Individuals with this syndrome are likely to have pits in the lower lip either externally or internally, cleft lip, and/or cleft palate (including submucous cleft palate) (Figure 7-8). Individuals may also have neonatal teeth or missing teeth. Speech problems related to the cleft palate are likely. However, the individual's development is likely to be otherwise normal.

Opitz Syndrome

Opitz syndrome may be caused by an autosomal dominant disorder with the affected gene mapped to chromosome 22 (Robin, Opitz, & Muenke, 1996). The syndrome may also be an **X-linked recessive disorder.** X-linked recessive disorders generally affect only males. A carrier female will transmit the disorder to 50 percent of her sons, and 50 percent of her daughters will be carriers. An affected male will pass the gene to 100 percent of his daughters. Opitz syndrome is a common cause of cleft lip with

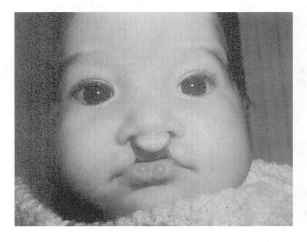

Figure 7-8
An infant with Van der Woude syndrome. Note the bilateral complete cleft of the lip and palate and the lower lip pits.

---

[*]For a more complete listing of craniofacial syndromes involving clefting as of 1991, the student should consult Cohen and Bankier (1991). However, since that time, researchers and clinicians have identified additional syndromes and have reclassified some syndromes and sequences. For a detailed description of syndromes related to communication disorders, the student should consult Shprintzen (1997).

or without cleft palate (Kummer, 2001). Individuals with this syndrome are likely to have **hypertelorism** (widely spaced eyes) and **hypospadias** (malpositioning in the opening of the urethra of the penis in males). Individuals may also have an imperforate anus, undescended testes, and hernias in the area of the groin. In addition to cleft lip with or without cleft palate, these individuals may also have a laryngeal cleft. Those with Opitz syndrome are at risk for learning disabilities, and possibly mental retardation. Voice and feeding problems may result from the laryngeal cleft, and speech problems are likely if cleft palate is present. Figure 7-9 depicts a boy with Opitz syndrome characterized by a bilateral cleft of the lip and palate (repaired) and hypertelorism.

Pierre Robin Sequence

The initiating event for Pierre Robin sequence is interference with mandible (jaw) development during the ninth week of gestation. However, this interference may result from many different causes. Once mandibular growth is restrained, the tongue is likely to remain high in the oral cavity, thus interfering with closure of the secondary palate. Therefore, clefts of the secondary palate are common in individuals with Pierre Robin sequence. These are often described as wide, *U*-shaped clefts, though they may also be *V*-shaped or submucous clefts (LeBlanc & Golding-Kushner, 1992; Shprintzen, 1988). When infants with Pierre Robin sequence are born, their tongues are often in a posterior position, thus blocking the pharynx and airway. Infants generally require individualized treatment to address breathing and feeding difficulties.

Pierre Robin sequence may occur in isolation or may be part of a syndrome. The sequence occurs as part of a syndrome over 50 percent of the time (Tomaski, Zalzal, & Saal, 1995) and has been identified in over 30 syndromes or associations (Gorlin, Cohen, & Levin, 1990). The literature on Pierre Robin sequence is somewhat confusing for three reasons: clinicians and researchers disagree about what features are necessarily associated with the sequence; professionals have changed the name from "syndrome" to "complex" to "sequence"; and clinicians have inconsistently and inaccurately diagnosed

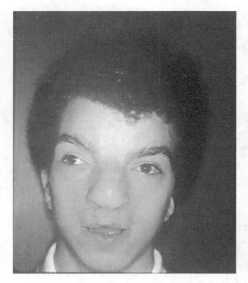

Figure 7-9
A boy with Opitz syndrome (X-linked type). This boy had a bilateral cleft of the lip and palate (repaired at the time of the picture) and hypertelorism.

the sequence due to its co-occurrence with many syndromes (Peterson-Falzone et al., 2001). (For a review of Pierre Robin sequence, including associated syndromes, see St-Hilaire & Buchbinder, 2000.)

Individuals with isolated Pierre Robin sequence will likely have speech problems related to the cleft palate. However, attention to early breathing and feeding issues may delay surgical repair of the palate. This may in turn delay normal phonological development and result in persistent misarticulations (Trost, 1981; Trost-Cardamone & Bernthal, 1993).

Stickler Syndrome

Stickler syndrome is an autosomal dominant disorder with **variable expression.** That is, individuals with this syndrome vary in terms of which structures and functions are affected, and to what extent they are affected. The syndrome may be caused by disruptions in at least four different genes. Individuals with this syndrome are likely to have cleft palate, possibly as part of Pierre Robin sequence; early and progressive osteoarthritis; sensorineural hearing loss; and progressive myopia with risk of retinal detachments (Snead & Yates, 1999). Many individuals also have characteristic craniofacial features including a flat midface (resulting from underdevelopment of the maxillary and mandibular regions), prominent eyes, epicanthal folds (folds of tissue in the inner corners of the eyes), and a long philtrum. Individuals with Stickler syndrome do not appear to be at a greater risk for developmental disabilities. However, speech and language problems are likely due to cleft palate and/or hearing loss.

Velocardiofacial Syndrome

Velocardiofacial syndrome is an autosomal dominant disorder with most cases involving a deletion of part of chromosome 22. The features associated with this syndrome are highly variable. Though more than 160 different anomalies and characteristics have been reported, only the most common are discussed here.

Individuals with velocardiofacial syndrome are likely to have **velopharyngeal insufficiency** either with or without cleft palate. When present, clefts of the secondary palate may occur as part of Pierre Robin sequence. Individuals with velocardiofacial syndrome are also likely to have congenital heart defects. Additionally, certain facial features are often associated with the syndrome. These include, but are not limited to, the following: long face, narrow and downward-slanted eye slits, long maxillary region, wide nasal root, thin upper lip, and small mandible.

Individuals with velocardiofacial syndrome are also likely to have numerous medical problems and developmental disabilities, including language and learning disabilities, mental retardation, and oral-motor dysfunction. Researchers and clinicians have also reported psychiatric problems, in particular schizophrenia (Chow, Bassett, & Weksberg, 1994; Heineman-de Boer, Van Haelst, Cordia-de Haan, & Beemer, 1999; Eliez, Blasey, Schmitt, White, Hu, & Reiss, 2001; Karayiorgou et al., 1995; Pulver et al., 1994).

Most children with velocardiofacial syndrome will exhibit difficulty sucking, and later difficulty chewing and swallowing, due to poor oral motor skills including poor palatal function. Speech disorders are common due to the same factors.

Fetal Alcohol Syndrome

Fetal alcohol syndrome is caused by exposure to alcohol during gestation (Jones & Smith, 1973). This syndrome is one of the common causes of cleft palate associated with Pierre Robin sequence (Kummer,

2001). Individuals with fetal alcohol syndrome may also have cleft lip with or without cleft palate. Most notably, children are small at birth, have microcephaly (small head circumference), short eye slits, a short nose, a flat philtrum, and a thin upper lip, and may have congenital heart defects (Kummer, 2001). Fetal alcohol syndrome may also cause mental retardation (Jones, 1986) as well as significant behavior problems in older children (Streissguth, Aase, Clarren, Randels, LaDue, & Smith, 1991). Speech and language problems may result from developmental disabilities as well as from cleft palate.

CHARACTERISTICS OF CLEFT LIP AND PALATE

In many syndromes other medical conditions require more immediate attention than clefts of the lip or palate. However, whether clefts occur as part of a syndrome or as an isolated occurrence, there are resulting implications for speech, language, hearing, feeding, and often dental development. This section addresses common characteristics associated with clefts.

Individuals with clefts of the lip and/or palate are a heterogeneous group. Not all individuals will have the same characteristics, and individuals with the same characteristics will not have the same degree of difficulty. Even individuals with similar clefts may have very different resulting problems. This section covers the characteristics related to clefts that may adversely impact communication development.

Speech

Since a cleft lip is usually repaired early in infancy, no speech effects generally result. On rare occasion, a repaired lip (particularly if the cleft was bilateral) may be too short for the appropriate production of bilabial sounds (/b, p, m/). However, affected individuals usually can substitute labiodental productions with little perceptual effect on speech production. Rather, most speech problems associated with clefts are related to clefts of the palate.

Individuals with cleft palate are at obvious risk for speech disorders. Most speech disorders resulting from palatal clefts are related to **velopharyngeal dysfunction,** or the inability to utilize the velum and pharynx to close off the oral cavity from the nasal cavity during speech. As with lip clefts, palatal clefts are usually repaired in infancy. However, individuals who have undergone palatal surgery to close a cleft are sometimes left with a velum that is too short to reach the back pharyngeal wall or with velar musculature too weak to achieve velopharyngeal closure. Additionally, a **fistula** (a hole between the oral and nasal cavities) may result if an individual fails to heal properly following surgery, or if future growth of the individual weakens prior suture lines. Any open connection between the oral and nasal cavities will result in difficulties with speech. Speech production problems, particularly those associated with velopharyngeal dysfunction, can be classified into three general categories: resonance, articulation, and voice.

Resonance

Resonance is a difficult term to understand. Though the strict definition of resonance refers to an acoustical phenomenon, it is also often used to refer to a perceived quality of the voice that results from vibration of sound in the pharyngeal, oral, and sometimes nasal cavities during speech. Thus, resonance is a term only applied to speech sounds that are voiced. For most voiced speech sounds in English, vibration of the vocal folds is directed through the pharynx and into the oral cavity. This is accomplished by contact of the velum with the back pharyngeal wall to effectively close off the nasal cavity. By contrast, there are only three speech sounds in English that require nasal resonance: (/m, n, ŋ/). To produce these sounds, an individual relaxes the velum and back pharyngeal wall and allows vocal fold vibration to be directed into the nasal cavity as well. Therefore, if an individual cannot effectively close off the nasal cavity during speech, the resonance of the majority of voiced speech sounds will be affected.

The most common resonance disorder associated with cleft palate is **hypernasality.** In hypernasal speech, vocal fold vibration is directed into the nasal cavity during the production of normally orally resonated sounds. Hypernasality is most obvious perceptually during the production of vowels. This occurs because vowels are voiced, relatively long in duration, and produced with a relatively open vocal tract. Degree of perceived hypernasality will depend to some extent upon size of the opening into the nasal cavity.

Strangely enough, another resonance disorder that can be associated with cleft palate is **hyponasality.** In hyponasal speech, normal nasal resonance is not heard due to a partially occluded or blocked nasal passage. When an individual has a cold, speech is hyponasal due to inflamed tissue and mucus in the nasal passageways. In an individual with a history of a palatal cleft, hyponasality generally results from an obstruction in the nasal cavity or pharynx, such as a deviated septum or hypertrophic adenoids. A type of hyponasality called **cul-de-sac resonance** is also sometimes heard in individuals with a history of cleft palate. Cul-de-sac resonance occurs when acoustic energy is trapped in a pouch with an entrance but no outlet (Kummer, 2001). In individuals with a history of cleft palate, cul-de-sac resonance may occur due to a number of factors, such as a more anterior blockage of the nasal cavity with a deviated septum. The muffled characteristic of cul-de-sac resonance can be simulated if you produce nasal sounds ("me, me, me, me . . .") while pinching your nose. Some individuals with a history of cleft will present with mixed hypernasality and hyponasality. Such an individual may have velopharyngeal dysfunction and some form of nasal resistance.

Hypernasality is clearly a direct result of coupling of the oral and nasal cavities or velopharyngeal dysfunction during speech. However, an individual with either problem may still produce speech that is hyponasal due to structural issues such as those discussed above. Thus, though hyponasality and hypernasality are on opposite ends of the resonance continuum, they are not mutually exclusive. SLPs must remember that the presence of hyponasality in any form in an individual's speech does not rule out velopharyngeal dysfunction.

Though resonance disorders affect perceptual qualities of an individual's speech, such changes in the quality of speech are not likely to have a significant effect on intelligibility. That is, though speech may sound "too nasal" or "not nasal enough" to the listener, the speaker is still generally understood. However, when the oral and nasal cavities are coupled, articulation disorders are also likely, and these may have a significant effect on intelligibility.

Articulation

Articulation disorders are common in individuals with palatal clefts or a history of palatal clefts. As with hypernasality, some articulation disorders are a direct result of poor velopharyngeal structure and function, or an existing palatal cleft or fistula. These articulation disorders include nasal emission and weak-pressure consonants. Other articulation disorders result from an attempt by the individual to overcome the faulty velopharyngeal mechanism. These various articulatory substitutions are called **compensatory articulation.** Still other articulation problems may result from dental anomalies, such as lateralized /s/ production.

Many consonants in English require the buildup of intraoral air pressure for accurate production. These high-pressure consonants include stops, fricatives, and affricatives. In order to build up the required intraoral air pressure, the velopharyngeal mechanism must function appropriately to close off the nasal cavity. Two possible effects on articulation occur when air escapes into the nasal cavity during production of these high-pressure consonants: (1) there is associated nasal emission of air, or (2) the consonants may be produced with weak pressure.

Nasal Emission. **Nasal emission** is the inappropriate escape of air into the nasal cavity during attempted production of high-pressure consonants. Nasal emission may be inaudible or audible. Inaudible nasal emission occurs with no audible evidence of the air leakage. This type of nasal emission is often called "visible nasal emission" because it can be detected when a cold mirror held under the nose fogs up during production of high-pressure consonants. Audible nasal emission can be detected as a soft sound that is heard as air passes through the nose. Sometimes nasal emission meets some resistance either by a narrow velopharyngeal opening or an obstruction in the nose (Kummer, Curtis, Wiggs, Lee, & Strife, 1992; Warren, Wood, & Bradley, 1969). This more turbulent flow of air is sometimes referred to as nasal turbulence or a nasal rustle (McWilliams, 1982; Mason & Grandstaff, 1971). When air is expelled forcibly through the nose during production of these high-pressure sounds, a noisy, sneezelike sound results. This is called a nasal, or nasopharyngeal, snort (Morley, 1970).

Weak-Pressure Consonant. Weak-pressure consonants are another articulation disturbance that may result when individuals with a faulty velopharyngeal mechanism attempt to produce high-pressure consonants. The reduction in available intraoral air pressure for production of these sounds results in consonants that are weak in pressure and intensity and may appear to be completely omitted (McWilliams et al., 1990). Though some investigators and clinicians view weak-pressure consonants as a passive production that is a direct result of velopharyngeal dysfunction (Harding & Grunwell, 1998), others view weak articulation as an active attempt to camouflage the perceptual consequences of velopharyngeal dysfunction (Peterson-Falzone et al., 2001).

The weak production or omission of stops, fricatives, and affricates in an individual's speech is likely to have a significant impact on intelligibility. However, intelligibility is likely to be more severely affected when an individual changes place of production to produce atypical sounds. Such compensatory articulations are discussed next.

Compensatory Articulation. Some articulatory substitutions are clearly compensatory. **Compensatory articulation** productions are many and varied, though they all have one commonality. They are atypical speech sounds produced by the speaker in an attempt to overcome structural or functional inadequacies. When an individual is unable to achieve intraoral air pressure by closing off the nasal cavity from the oral cavity at the velopharyngeal level, that individual may attempt closure at another point along the vocal tract. Generally, place of articulation for high-pressure consonants is changed from an oral location to a pharyngeal or laryngeal location. The individual is then able to take advantage of air pressure in the pharynx before it is lost at the level of the velopharyngeal valve.

Compensatory productions may include glottal stops or pharyngeal stops, fricatives, and affricates as substitutes for the normally produced sounds. **Glottal stops** are produced by a forceful release of air trapped beneath the vocal folds. In individuals with clefts or velopharyngeal dysfunction, glottal stops are often substituted for all stops, though they may also be substituted for fricatives and affricates.

Pharyngeal productions involve the back of the tongue articulating with the pharyngeal wall. **Pharyngeal stops** are typically substituted for velar stops (/k, g/). **Pharyngeal fricatives** are more commonly voiceless and are typically substituted for sibilant sounds (/s/, /z/, /ʃ/ "sh", /ʒ/ "zh", /tʃ/ "ch", /dʒ/ "j"). **Pharyngeal affricates** may also be substituted for sibilant sounds but are more likely substituted only for the affricates (/tʃ/ "ch", /dʒ/ "j") (Kummer, 2001).

Articulation Problems Related to Dental Anomalies.   Some articulation problems result from the dental anomalies typical of individuals with clefts. Crowding of maxillary teeth and/or a narrow palatal arch may result in dentalized or lateralized distortion of sibilants, particularly /s/, or substitution of a mid-dorsum palatal stop for lingua-alveolar and sometimes velar sounds. A **middorsum palatal stop** is produced with the back (dorsum) of the tongue up against the middle of the hard palate.

Articulation disorders are likely in individuals with palatal clefts or a history of palatal clefts. It is important that these individuals be seen regularly by a speech-language pathologist as part of a cleft palate team. Based upon a review of the literature, Peterson-Falzone et al. (2001) report that many individuals with a history of cleft palate will have articulation problems that continue into adolescence. However, they also point out that individuals seen on a regular basis by a cleft palate team are less likely to develop articulation disorders.

Though articulation disorders are many and varied in the cleft population, the relationship between articulation disorders and velopharyngeal dysfunction is relatively clear. However, the relationship between voice disorders and velopharyngeal dysfunction is less clear. The next section addresses voice disorders in individuals with a history of cleft palate.

Voice

Voice disorders are more common in individuals with a history of cleft palate or velopharyngeal dysfunction than they are in the general population. The higher prevalence of voice disorders in the cleft population may be due to several reasons. Some individuals present with a soft, breathy voice. This may simply be due to loss of pressure through the velopharyngeal port (Bernthal & Beukelman, 1977). Or, a soft, breathy voice may be a compensatory strategy to reduce the listener's ability to perceive hypernasality and nasal emission (Bzoch, 1979). Other individuals present with a hoarse or harsh voice. This is probably related to increased strain put on the vocal mechanism. That is, individuals with a small velopharyngeal opening may attempt to achieve closure by increasing muscular and respiratory effort. If these individuals persist with hyperfunctional use of the voice, they may develop vocal nodules. Such hyperfunctional use of the voice sometimes occurs as a result of aggressive speech therapy for individuals with velopharyngeal dysfunction. For this reason, individuals with a faulty velopharyngeal mechanism must be referred for, and receive, the appropriate treatment. Speech therapy should not be undertaken to address velopharyngeal inadequacy when other treatment options are available to address the structural or functional problem.

Language

Though studies throughout the years have resulted in mixed conclusions, children with isolated cleft lip and palate do not appear to be at a higher risk for language delays or disorders. However, when the cleft is associated with a syndrome, developmental and language problems are common and are likely associated with mental retardation or neurological involvement (Kummer, 2001). Still, many factors interact to affect language acquisition and development. Physiological factors such as hearing loss associated with otitis media may impact language acquisition. Additionally, more subtle psychosocial factors, such as multiple hospitalizations, lack of adequate stimulation, and even social isolation, may also influence language development. Further, articulation limitations (in addition to chronic otitis media) may impact phonological development (Harding & Grunwell, 1996; O'Gara & Logemann, 1988). Therefore, the SLP should carefully monitor language development from infancy through the early school years.

Hearing

Individuals with palatal clefts, or a history of clefts, are at high risk for otitis media and conductive hearing loss. This occurs because of the physiological relationship between the velopharyngeal system and the eustachian tube. To explain this, a brief review of anatomy and physiology is necessary. The eustachian tube functions to aerate the middle ear cavity, equalize pressure between the middle ear cavity and external atmospheric pressure, and drain middle ear fluid into the nasopharynx (Peterson-Falzone et al., 2001). The eustachian tube opens to perform these functions. The muscle responsible for opening the eustachian tube is the tensor veli palatini. In its course, the tensor veli palatini attaches to the lateral wall of the eustachian tube, and upon contraction, opens the eustachian tube. In individuals born without compromise to the velopharyngeal system, the tensor veli palatini muscle courses downward to the palate and fans out along the length of the palate. However, in individuals with a palatal cleft, the tensor veli palatini muscle does not have a stable base (the palate), and therefore cannot contract effectively to open the eustachian tube. When the eustachian tube cannot function properly, the middle ear is not ventilated. This may lead to bacterial infection and inflammation of the middle ear, a condition referred to as **otitis media.** The buildup of fluids associated with otitis media results in a temporary conductive hearing loss. In chronic otitis media, permanent damage to the middle ear can result in a permanent conductive hearing loss. In individuals with clefts, the conductive hearing loss is generally bilateral and mild to moderate in degree.

Individuals with clefts are at risk for otitis media from birth, and the risk continues for some individuals through later childhood or early adolescence. Therefore, it is imperative that individuals with clefts, or a history of clefts, are followed by an otolaryngologist and audiologist. Patients should be monitored as early as possible and continuously. When deemed necessary, treatment may involve early myringotomies (surgical punctures of the eardrum to drain fluid). Some patients may also require placement of ventilation tubes inserted into the eardrum as an alternate route for aeration of the middle ear. As a preventative measure, breast milk has been shown to decrease the occurrence of middle ear disease in infants with clefts (Paradise, Elster, & Tan, 1994). Feeding, however, is often a difficult issue in and of itself for children with clefts and their families. The next section will briefly cover feeding difficulties for infants with clefts.

Feeding

Infants with lip and/or palatal clefts are likely to have difficulty with the feeding process. For most infants this occurs because they cannot completely close off the oral cavity to create the necessary negative intraoral pressure required for sucking. Specific problems will vary depending upon type and severity of cleft. Since no single feeding method will work with all infants, modifications must be made on a case-by-case basis. This section presents only general information regarding feeding issues for infants with clefts of the lip only, clefts of the secondary palate only, and clefts of the primary and secondary palate combined.

Infants with cleft lip may only have difficulty achieving adequate closure around the nipple of the bottle or breast. Infants with bilateral lip clefts may have more difficulty than infants with a unilateral lip cleft. However, for most infants with cleft lip, normal feeding is still likely. If the infant is breast fed, the breast will likely conform to fill the lip cleft. The mother may also assist the lip closure with her hand (Kummer, 2001). If the infant is bottle fed, use of a soft, wide-based nipple will likely promote success.

Infants with clefting of the secondary palate only will have difficulty achieving intraoral air pressure for sucking due to air leaking through the open cleft into the nasal cavity. Level of difficulty will depend upon extent of the cleft. However, infants with a cleft of the posterior secondary palate only, particularly if the cleft is narrow, may still be able to achieve adequate pressure for sucking. If the cleft does not extend too far forward, infants will be able to compress the nipple against the hard palate. In breast-fed infants, feeding success is more likely due to the infant's ability to position and compress the breast nipple. In bottle-fed infants, nipple modifications and/or feeder systems that assist milk delivery may be necessary. If the cleft is more extensive, more difficulty is likely for both breast-fed and bottle-fed babies.

Infants with clefting of the primary and secondary palate are likely to have significant difficulty with feeding, particularly if there is also clefting of the lip. These infants are unable to generate negative intraoral air pressure, compress the nipple, or achieve an adequate lip seal. For these infants, a supplemental nursing system and/or a modified feeding device will probably be necessary. In severe cases, orogastric or nasogastric tube feeding may be required. In rare cases, a gastrostomy tube may be needed on a temporary basis.

Since there is no single feeding method that will work for all individuals, infants must be evaluated immediately at birth and followed closely by a pediatrician, nurse, SLP, and/or other professionals as needed. Infants with cleft palate are at high risk for poor weight gain (Carlisle, 1998; Jones, 1988). Additionally, feeding problems must be addressed early since they are likely to have a negative impact on nutrition, sensory and motor stimulation, parent-infant bonding, and oral motor development (Kummer, 2001).

Dental Anomalies

Individuals with cleft lip and palate, or a history of cleft lip and palate, are at-risk for abnormalities of the teeth and jaws. Problems such as missing, crowded, or rotated teeth are particularly likely when clefts pass through the alveolus. In addition, underdevelopment of the midface region may also cause jaw and teeth occlusion problems. A description of these potential problems and possible treatments is too extensive to provide here.[*] However, coordination of management may involve the orthodontist, a pediatric or family dentist, the oral surgeon, and a prosthodontist if necessary. Furthermore, since

---

[*]For more in-depth information on dental anomalies and dental management of individuals with clefts, the student should consult the appropriate chapters in Kummer (2001) or Peterson-Falzone et al. (2001) or the numerous journal articles written on this subject.

dental abnormalities may affect production of speech sounds, a speech-language pathologist should be consulted, and may provide treatment once the structural problems have been addressed.

TEAM ASSESSMENT AND INTERVENTION

The many and varied needs of individuals with clefts of the lip and palate require a team approach to assessment and intervention. This section provides general guidelines for an interdisciplinary approach to evaluation and treatment of individuals with clefts. The role of the SLP will be emphasized.

Rationale for a Team Approach

In 1987, the Surgeon General of the United States recognized that patients with special health care needs required comprehensive, coordinated care by a team of professionals (Surgeon General's Report, 1987). Following this report, the American Cleft Palate-Craniofacial Association (ACPA) received funding from the Maternal and Child Health Bureau to address this need. In response, various professionals participated in a consensus conference in 1991 and published a document outlining evaluation and treatment parameters for individuals with clefts or craniofacial anomalies (American Cleft Palate-Craniofacial Association, 1993). As outlined in this document, a cleft palate team must consist of a surgeon, an orthodontist, an SLP, and at least one other specialist. A craniofacial team must consist of a craniofacial surgeon, an orthodontist, an SLP, and a mental health professional. Additionally, a team must have a coordinator who schedules visits, documents team recommendations, facilitates communication with the patient and family, and ensures implementation of recommendations. In practice, many other professionals may serve on a team in a permanent or consultative role. Table 7-1 lists professionals likely to be included on a cleft palate or craniofacial team. The patient and his or her family are also key members on any team of care. The wishes of the patient and family must be a part of any treatment decisions (Sharp, 1995).

A cleft or craniofacial team is generally required for patient management from birth until an individual is physically grown, typically around age 18 to 20 (Kummer, 2001). Individuals will generally be seen by a team one to two times per year when undergoing treatment. If a team is not located near a patient's community, professional(s) near that individual's home may see the patient for routine care. In this case, local professionals must communicate and consult with the team.

The team approach to assessment and intervention provides many advantages to the patient and family (American Cleft Palate-Craniofacial Association, 1993; Strauss, 1999). The team performs a comprehensive, coordinated evaluation of the whole child in order to make better decisions with respect to the child and the family. Team assessment is generally accomplished with fewer visits and decreased cost as compared to individual evaluations. The single team coordinator who facilitates follow-up and monitors care serves the patient and family better than different individuals scheduling numerous visits. Teams are also generally comprised of experts in various fields who can provide care based upon current, up-to-date information in their field. Finally, teams are generally located in facilities with state-of-the-art equipment and access to educational and psychosocial resources for the patient and the family.

The team approach is also advantageous to the professionals involved. It saves evaluation time, increases interpersonal communication, increases transdisciplinary knowledge, aids collaborative research, and saves time record-keeping (Brogan, 1988; Kummer, 2001). As a required team member, the

Table 7-1 Professionals on a Cleft Palate or Craniofacial Team

Professional	Role on a cleft palate or craniofacial team
Team coordinator (nurse or other professional)	• Schedules patients and plans team meetings • Compiles team recommendations and writes report • Ensures follow-up of recommendations • Represents the team to parents, other professionals, and the community
Plastic surgeon	• Surgically repairs clefts of the lip and palate • Addresses velopharyngeal dysfunction (if surgery indicated) • May perform bone grafts, cranial surgery, or jaw surgery
Oral surgeon	• Performs bone grafts in alveolar cleft area • Performs jaw surgeries
Orthodontist	• Aligns misplaced teeth • Treats dental and jaw malocclusions
Speech-language pathologist (SLP)	• Educates parents regarding speech expectations • Provides information on speech and language stimulation • Evaluates feeding and swallowing • Evaluates speech, language, and resonance • Recommends treatment for disorders identified • Provides therapy as indicated and as appropriate
Psychologist	• Evaluates, and addresses as necessary, the psychosocial needs of the patient and family • Assists in determining readiness for surgical procedures
Social worker	• Helps families deal with issues and stressors related to child's cleft or craniofacial anomaly • May assist with insurance and possible funding sources • May act as team coordinator
Nurse	• Assesses overall physical development • May assist family with feeding in consultation with SLP • Counsels family and answers questions regarding surgical procedures
Pediatrician	• Assesses patient's health, growth, and development • Determines if presurgical medical care is needed
Audiologist	• Tests hearing and middle ear function • Works with otolaryngologist to monitor auditory functioning
Otolaryngologist	• Monitors hearing and middle ear function • Treats middle ear disease if present • Assesses structural aspects of oral and nasal cavities and upper airway • Treats pharyngeal and laryngeal anomalies and upper airway disorders as needed • May perform surgery for velopharyngeal dysfunction

continued

Table 7-1 *(continued)*

Professional	Role on a cleft palate or craniofacial team
Pediatric dentist (pedodontist)	• Provides general care of teeth • Ensures development of good oral hygiene habits • May manage misaligned alveolar segments prior to cleft lip surgery • Manages palatal expansion if necessary to treat malocclusion
Prosthodontist	• Restores or replaces teeth • Develops prosthetic devices for teeth and oral structures • Develops devices to assist with velopharyngeal closure • Develops feeding devices if needed
Geneticist	• Assesses patient's genetic background • Counsels patient and family on recurrence risk for future offspring
Neurosurgeon	• Evaluates and assists surgeon in treating patients with craniofacial syndromes involving cranial and brain anomalies
Ophthalmologist	• Evaluates and treats patients with congenital eye anomalies and vision problems

Source: A. W. Kummer (2001). *Cleft palate & craniofacial anomalies: The effects on speech and resonance.* Clifton Park, NY: Delmar Learning.

SLP can both benefit from, and lend much to, a successful, coordinated team effort. The following section highlights the role of the SLP in team assessment and intervention.

The Role of the Speech-Language Pathologist

For an individual with a cleft palate, one of the main goals of any treatment procedure is accurate speech development. Therefore, an SLP is involved in the team assessment and treatment of an individual with a cleft palate from birth, and will often follow an individual through adolescence or adulthood. Surgeons and prosthodontists will ask the team SLP to assess the individual's speech prior to and following surgical and/or prosthetic procedures. Prosthodontists may have the team SLP present to assess speech production during development and testing of prosthetic devices.

Additionally, another SLP in the child's community may see the child for assessment and/or treatment as needed. In this case, the local SLP must consult with the child's cleft palate management team. If no team is currently managing the child, the SLP should refer the child and family to a cleft palate team.[*] This section will outline the procedures involved in the assessment and treatment of speech-language problems associated with cleft palate.

Assessment

The basic protocol for speech-language assessment of an individual with a cleft or history of cleft is not significantly different from a speech-language evaluation of a child without a cleft. However, the

---

[*]The Cleft Palate Foundation (associated with the American Cleft Palate-Craniofacial Association) is a group dedicated to assisting families and professionals who need information regarding assessment or treatment of individuals with clefts or other craniofacial anomalies. It can provide a list of qualified cleft and craniofacial teams in various areas throughout the country. Its 24-hour toll-free number is (800) 24-CLEFT (800-242-5338). Its web site is http://www.cleft.com.

challenge is in sorting out the contribution of various etiological factors (structural, functional, behavioral). Etiological differentiation is important because speech therapy should never be initiated until the appropriate professionals have addressed all structural and/or functional concerns. The speech-language assessment should include a clinical history, an orofacial examination, an assessment of resonance, an assessment of articulation, an assessment of voice, and a language screening. A language screening will not be discussed here, as students should be familiar with assessment of language skills in children. This section addresses each of the other areas of assessment with attention given only to those aspects specific to individuals with clefts or suspected velopharyngeal dysfunction.

Clinical History. Since an individual with a history of cleft palate is likely to have had extensive prior medical intervention, it is necessary to obtain all possible information in order to assess the individual's current functioning. A thorough clinical history should include information about the following (Peterson-Falzone et al., 2001):

- Surgical history and surgeries planned for the future
- Medical history, including health problems, frequency of middle ear infections, and feeding history
- History of speech-language therapy, including duration, frequency, and type
- Parental perspective, including experiences, expectations, and knowledge

Orofacial Examination. An orofacial examination (oral-peripheral examination) should always be performed on an individual with a cleft palate or history of cleft palate. Students should be familiar with such an examination. Therefore, the following list will be limited to features that may be associated with cleft palate or other craniofacial anomalies (Kummer, 2001; Peterson-Falzone et al., 2001):

- Face: Observe overall structure, symmetry, and muscle tone; observe spacing, size, and structure of eyes; observe shape of nose and note if open-mouth breathing
- Lips: Note lip structure and symmetry; test lip approximation; note presence of internal or external lip pits (Van der Woude's syndrome)
- Teeth: Note bite (occlusion) problems and extra or misplaced teeth; note presence of dental appliances
- Tongue: Judge tongue size relative to oral cavity; note any tongue growths or deviations
- Hard palate: Note contour and width; examine carefully for fistulae; palpate for notch in border (may suggest submucous cleft)
- Tonsils: Note size if present
- Soft palate: Note symmetry, examine for bifid uvula or bluish tone midline (may suggest submucous cleft); examine for fistulae, observe velar movement during sustained phonation ("ah")
- Pharyngeal walls: Note any movement during sustained phonation

Assessment of Resonance. Assessment of resonance involves three steps. First, the SLP must determine if resonance is normal or not. Second, if resonance is judged to be abnormal, the SLP should note the type of abnormal resonance. Third, once type of abnormal resonance is determined, the SLP should estimate degree of severity.

Determining normal versus abnormal resonance is not always an easy task. Nasality in speech occurs along a continuum and is affected by factors such as dialect. Additionally, resonance disorders in an individual may be subtle, may be difficult to distinguish from abnormal voice characteristics, and may be complicated by the presence of unusual articulation errors. Appropriate stimulus materials will help the clinician determine both presence and type of abnormal resonance. The following list provides examples of stimulus items and procedures most helpful in identifying different resonance disorders:

- Hypernasality: The individual should produce words or sentences with vowels and low-pressure consonants (e.g., "Why are you where we were?"). The SLP should listen for increased nasality, particularly during vowel production.
- Hyponasality: The individual should produce words or sentences with nasal consonants and vowels (e.g. "My mama knew many men."). The SLP should listen for decreased nasality, particularly during nasal consonants and adjacent vowels.

During assessment, an SLP may note both hypernasality and hyponasality in the same individual. This likely indicates velopharyngeal dysfunction with other structural complications. As mentioned previously, the SLP should not interpret the presence of hyponasality as a sign that the individual is able to achieve appropriate velopharyngeal closure. Additionally, if hyponasal speech has a "muffled" quality, cul-de-sac resonance should be noted.

Assessment of resonance should also include a conversational speech sample. Some individuals with small velopharyngeal gaps are able to achieve fairly normal resonance during short productions. However, during conversational speech, resonance disorders may become more obvious.

Once the SLP identifies the presence of hypernasality or hyponasality, degree of severity should be estimated. Some clinicians use a numbered rating scale while others use terms such as "mild," "moderate," "severe." If hyponasality is evident, presence or absence of mixed nasality or cul-de-sac resonance may also be noted.

Assessment of Articulation.   An articulation assessment should include word or sentence productions as well as a sample of conversational speech. Since individuals with cleft palate may have developmental or phonological errors, an articulation assessment should include all speech sounds. However, in order to identify atypical articulation disorders prevalent in this population (nasal emission, weak-pressure consonants, and compensatory articulation substitutions), the SLP may need to focus on production of high-pressure consonants. High-pressure consonants include stops (/p, b, t, d, k, g/), fricatives (/f, v, θ, ð, s, z, ʃ, ʒ, h/), and affricates (/ʧ, ʤ/). Two formal articulation tests are available that specifically focus on these consonants. These are the Iowa Pressure Articulation Test, a part of the Templin-Darley Tests of Articulation (Templin & Darley, 1960), and the Bzoch Error Pattern Diagnostic Articulation Tests (Bzoch, 1979). However, these tests are limited to single-word productions. Clinicians should also have the individual produce sentences when possible. It is best if stimulus sentences focus on one articulatory placement at a time. Additionally, it may be easier to sort out articulation disorders utilizing voiceless sounds. For example, the sentence "Try to tell Teddy" assesses the voiceless lingua-alveolar stop.

To test for inaudible nasal emission, the SLP should hold a cold mirror under the client's nose during production of high-pressure consonants. Since no air should be directed out the nose, if the mirror fogs the SLP can tentatively diagnose inaudible nasal emission.

Assessment of Voice.   Procedures for a voice screening or voice evaluation will not be discussed here. However, some individuals may use a soft voice to mask resonance and articulation disorders. Additionally, some individuals may develop hyperfunctional use of the voice as a response to an inadequate velopharyngeal mechanism. Thus, differential diagnosis of voice disorders is important for this population.

Intervention

An SLP on a cleft palate team will have an immediate role in early intervention for a child born with a cleft lip and/or palate. This will initially involve parent education. This education should include (Peterson-Falzone et al., 2001):

- Information about the impact of a cleft on the speech structure, and therefore communication development of the child
- Information and guidance in speech and language stimulation techniques
- Information about possible compensatory articulation productions and guidance to avoid reinforcement of these sounds
- Information about expected speech performance after surgical procedures
- Referral for early speech-language intervention if needed

Once information is provided to the parents, the SLP on a cleft palate team continues in an active role in the ongoing surgical, dental, and prosthetic management of the individual. In addition to this involvement in ongoing team treatment of an individual, an SLP may see an individual with a history of cleft for individual speech therapy. However, it is more likely that an SLP in the child's community will provide this therapy. The local SLP must consult with, and report to, the cleft palate team managing the individual in order for treatment to be most effective.

A caveat is in order, particularly for beginning SLPs who may one day find themselves face to face with a client with hypernasality and nasal emission. If an individual produces speech with any of the resonance or articulation characteristics associated with velopharyngeal dysfunction, the SLP should assume that the individual has an underlying structural or functional inadequacy. In this case, the individual should be referred to a cleft-palate team or an otolaryngologist with experience evaluating velopharyngeal function. Speech therapy should never be initiated with an individual who does not have an intact velopharyngeal system. Such therapy will be frustrating at best, futile more likely, and may cause a secondary voice disorder. Individuals with velopharyngeal dysfunction are best treated with surgical or prosthetic management.

There are times when speech therapy for resonance disorders may be provided. However, such therapy is usually only provided on a trial basis by an SLP with experience with the cleft population. This is also true for articulation disorders such as nasal emission and weak-pressure consonants that are secondary to velopharyngeal dysfunction. Therefore, therapy for these speech disorders will not be discussed here. However, an SLP may be called upon to provide therapy to an individual who produces compensatory articulations.

Compensatory articulation productions generally develop because the individual cannot achieve adequate intraoral air pressure to produce the sounds normally. Therefore, the speaker moves place of production posterior to the velopharyngeal area. Though such productions are atypical and may sound odd to a listener, they may result in better use of airflow and therefore improve intelligibility (Kummer, 2001). Therefore, therapy to eliminate compensatory articulation in individuals with an inadequate velopharyngeal mechanism is not advised, particularly if surgery to correct the velopharyngeal dysfunction is planned.

However, there are three instances when therapy for compensatory articulations is warranted. First, in the rare case where velopharyngeal function is unclear, and compensatory articulations are the only speech characteristic, therapy is mandatory. If correction of the compensatory articulation results in normal speech, no additional treatment is necessary. On the other hand, if correction of the compensatory articulation results in articulation that is appropriate in place, but produced with nasal emission, further surgical or prosthetic management of the individual may be needed. Second, if velopharyngeal function is judged to be normal, and compensatory articulations continue, therapy is also necessary. Such productions may now be a learned part of speech production, even in the absence of velopharyngeal dysfunction. Third, even if surgery to correct velopharyngeal dysfunction is planned, if the SLP finds the individual is highly stimulable to correct place of production and the resulting correct productions do not have nasal emission, therapy should be initiated prior to surgery. In this case, following successful speech therapy, surgery may be reconsidered or at least revised. Researchers have found that an increase in oral articulation is often accompanied by an increase in velopharyngeal movement (Henningsson & Isberg, 1986; Ysunza, Pamplona, & Toledo, 1992). The following are suggestions to modify place of production for specific compensatory articulations (Kummer, 2001):

Glottal stops as substitutes for oral stops:

- Have child whisper syllable to prevent glottal closure
- Have child produce stops slowly followed by /h/ before the vowel (i.e., t-ha for ta)

Pharyngeal stops as substitutes for oral stops:

- Have child yawn to get base of tongue down and velum up; then have child use anterior articulation during the yawn (for bilabial and lingua-alveolar stops)
- Have child begin with /ŋ/ ("ng") and push tongue back to produce velar stops

Pharyngeal fricatives as a substitute for sibilant sounds:

- Have child produce fricative sounds first with the nostrils occluded and then with the nostrils open to get a feel for oral versus pharyngeal airflow
- For /s/ production, have child close the teeth and produce a hard /t/; gradually increase duration of sound (/tsssssss/); then eliminate initial /t/
- For /ʃ/ ("sh") production, have child close the teeth, round the lips, and produce a big sigh; work on increasing air pressure
- For /tʃ/ ("ch") production, have child close the teeth and produce a hard /t/ or a loud sneeze

Middorsum palatal stops:

- Have child bite on a tongue blade between the canine and molar teeth and depress the midtongue; then have child produce lingua-alveolar sounds in front of the blade and produce velar sounds behind the blade

Though an SLP may provide therapy on an individual basis, most SLPs who work with individuals with a history of cleft palate do so as members of a cleft palate team. As a required member of a cleft palate or craniofacial team, the SLP has an important and ongoing role in the assessment and intervention for individuals with clefts.

SURGICAL AND PROSTHETIC MANAGEMENT

In addition to the SLP, the surgeon is another required member of cleft palate and craniofacial teams. Plastic or oral surgeons often work in conjunction with SLPs, orthodontists, and other team members to decide appropriate care of the individual with a cleft. This section discusses general surgical procedures related to clefts of the lip and palate.

There are many different theories regarding timing of surgery and many different surgical procedures. Therefore, this section presents broad guidelines and general standards used in the United States for lip and palate repair. The terms *primary surgery* and *secondary surgery* will be used. These do not correspond to primary palate and secondary palate, but refer to initial surgery (primary surgery) and follow-up surgery (secondary surgery), whether related to clefts of the lip, primary palate, or secondary palate. This section will discuss primary and secondary surgery for cleft lip, primary surgery for cleft palate, secondary surgery for velopharyngeal dysfunction, nonsurgical prosthetic management for velopharyngeal dysfunction, and orthognathic surgery.

Primary and Secondary Surgery for Clefts of the Lip

The initial, or primary, surgery to repair cleft lip (**cheiloplasty**) is usually performed when the infant is between 1 and 3 months of age. However, surgeons often follow the "rule of tens," which states that an infant should weigh at least 10 pounds, be at least 10 weeks of age, and have a hemoglobin of 10 gm before surgery is performed (Wilhelmsen & Musgrave, 1966). Prior to the formal lip surgery, particularly for wide clefts, some surgeons attempt to bring the lip into better alignment. This presurgical management may involve taping the lip, utilizing an extraoral or intraoral dental appliance, or pulling the segments of the lip together in a modified surgical procedure.

Two major surgical techniques are widely used to repair a unilateral cleft lip. These are the Millard rotation-advancement technique (Bardach, 1994; Millard, 1958, 1976) and the Randall-Tennison triangular-flap procedure (Bardach & Salyer, 1987; Randall, 1959, 1990; Tennison, 1952). Modifications of both techniques are also used to surgically repair bilateral cleft lip (Millard, 1977; Noordhoff, 1994).

Most children with a cleft lip also undergo additional, or secondary, surgery around age 6 or more. This surgery is largely cosmetic in that it is undertaken to improve lip symmetry, improve nose appearance and symmetry, and reduce scar tissue. Secondary surgery is generally delayed until early school age so that it does not interfere with midfacial growth.

Primary Surgery for Clefts of the Palate

The initial, or primary, surgery to repair cleft palate is usually performed when the infant is between 6 months and 1 year of age, though surgery may be performed earlier or later. Over the past several decades, cleft palate team members have debated timing of primary palatal surgery. Early surgery appears to favor better speech results, but may be more likely to restrict growth of the maxilla and midfacial region. As more longitudinal data are collected, more precise guidelines may be developed.

Veloplasty, or delayed hard palate closure, attempts to address concerns about midfacial growth while still providing a workable speech mechanism (Schweckendiek & Kruse, 1990). This procedure closes the velum at a young age, usually around 6 months, but delays closing the hard palate until around age 4 or 5 following some midfacial growth. An intraoral appliance is generally used to cover the hard palate opening. It is unclear whether or not this procedure enhances midfacial growth, and whether or not it poses a threat to communication development (Peterson-Falzone et al., 2001). Veloplasty continues to be evaluated, though it has not gained wide acceptance. Most surgeons still attempt to completely close the palatal cleft, a procedure called **palatoplasty.**

The oldest and still most widely used technique for palatoplasty is the Von Langenbeck repair (Trier & Dreyer, 1984). Another widely used technique is the Wardill-Kilner V-Y pushback closure. These repairs attempt to close the palate, but do not address reconstructing the levator sling.[*] More recently developed techniques attempt to reconstruct the levator sling. Two such techniques are the two-flap palatoplasty, or levator retropositioning, and the Furlow Z-plasty (Furlow, 1986). To close unilateral or bilateral clefts of the primary palate, or complete clefts of the secondary palate, surgeons may combine procedures, utilizing one technique for hard palate closure and another technique for soft palate closure (Peterson-Falzone et al., 2001).

Approximately 20 percent of individuals who undergo primary palatoplasty will still have velopharyngeal dysfunction or velopharyngeal inadequacy following surgery. The resulting velopharyngeal dysfunction may be caused by anatomical factors such as a velum that is too short due to scarring or may be caused by neuromuscular factors such as poor muscle insertion. Regardless of cause, these individuals must undergo some form of secondary management, often in the form of surgery.

Secondary Surgery for Velopharyngeal Dysfunction

In order to diagnose velopharyngeal dysfunction, the child must be able to produce connected speech. For most children, this occurs around age 3. Therefore, secondary surgery does not usually take place until the child is around ages 3.5 to 4.

One surgical approach to address velopharyngeal dysfunction is velar augmentation or repositioning of the velar muscles. This approach utilizes many of the same surgical techniques used for primary palatoplasty. The advantage of such an approach is that the result is a velopharyngeal mechanism with the approximate structure and function present had there not been a cleft (Peterson-Falzone et al., 2001). More commonly, a secondary surgical procedure is utilized that changes the physiology of the velopharyngeal mechanism. This procedure might be a pharyngeal flap, pharyngeal wall augmentation, or sphincter pharyngoplasty.

Pharyngeal Flap

During a **pharyngeal flap** procedure, a flap of tissue is dissected from the pharyngeal wall, brought forward, and sutured into the velum. This provides a bridge of tissue in the middle of the velopharyngeal port. Pharyngeal flaps can be either inferiorly or superiorly based. Openings are left on both sides of the flap so that normal nasal breathing, as well as production of nasal speech sounds, can occur. During speech, the lateral pharyngeal walls must move medially toward the flap, effectively closing off the velopharyngeal port for non-nasal sounds. Thus, patients are candidates for this procedure only if they have good lateral pharyngeal wall movement (Argamaso et al., 1980).

---

[*]In individuals with normal palatal development, the levator veli palatini muscle fuses in the middle of the velum on both sides to form the levator sling, which contracts to assist velopharyngeal closure. In individuals with cleft palate, the levator veli palatini instead inserts into the back of the hard palate.

Pharyngeal Wall Augmentation

Pharyngeal wall augmentation is another procedure surgeons utilize to address velopharyngeal dysfunction following primary palatal surgery. During this procedure, the surgeon injects a substance or material into the posterior pharyngeal wall in an attempt to bring the wall forward. This "bulge" then fills part of the velopharyngeal gap. With adequate velar movement and enough lateral pharyngeal wall movement, the individual can achieve velopharyngeal closure. Though many substances have been used in the past, surgeons commonly use silicone or Silastic implants (Blocksma, 1963, 1964) and, more recently, injectable collagen (Remacle, Bertrand, Eloy, & Marbaix, 1990).

Sphincter Pharyngoplasty

A third surgical procedure to achieve velopharyngeal closure is **sphincter pharyngoplasty** (Jackson, 1985; Orticochea, 1968, 1997). In this procedure, bilateral flaps from the posterior faucial pillars are dissected, rotated, and sutured to an inferiorly based pharyngeal flap. Once healing occurs, a small round opening remains in the center of the pharynx. This small sphincter closes during speech with contraction of the levator palatini and palatopharyngeus muscles. This procedure may be most useful with individuals with poor lateral pharyngeal wall movement.

Prosthetic Management for Cleft Palate and Velopharyngeal Dysfunction

In some individuals with cleft palate or velopharyngeal dysfunction, surgical management is not an option. In this case, prosthetic management is a good alternative. This section discusses prosthetic management for cleft palate and velopharyngeal dysfunction.

When an individual with cleft palate or velopharyngeal dysfunction cannot undergo surgery, or must wait to undergo surgery, the **prosthodontist** may develop prosthetic devices to aid an individual in achieving velopharyngeal closure for speech. There are three basic types of speech appliances: a palatal obturator, a speech bulb obturator, and a palatal lift. The prosthodontist may develop combinations of these devices as necessary for patients.

Palatal Obturator

A **palatal obturator** is a device used to cover a palatal cleft or, more likely, a palatal fistula. A fistula is a hole between the oral and nasal cavities that may result from a surgical suture that did not heal properly, or a suture that opened when growth took place. A palatal obturator looks and fits much like a dental retainer, though it has additional acrylic on top to cover the palatal opening.

Speech Bulb Obturator

A **speech bulb obturator** is used to address velopharyngeal dysfunction when the velum is too short to reach the back pharyngeal wall. A speech bulb is a removable device that fits on the teeth. However, the important part of a speech bulb is the posterior extension, on the end of which is an acrylic mass or bulb. The bulb functions to partially occlude the velopharyngeal space. Individuals then utilize lateral pharyngeal wall movement to completely close the space during non-nasal speech production.

Palatal Lift Device

A **palatal lift** device may be used to address velopharyngeal dysfunction. It also attaches to the teeth and extends in a posterior fashion. However, a palatal lift device involves a rigid posterior extension that serves to lift the velum up and back against the posterior pharyngeal wall. With a palatal lift, the velum is constantly held in a position to achieve velopharyngeal closure. Therefore, a palatal lift is generally only used with individuals who have neurological impairment of velar movement.

In determining treatment options for patients, the prosthodontist works closely with the surgeon. Choice of appropriate initial and follow-up surgical procedures, as well as possible prosthetic device development, is dependent upon a careful and complete evaluation of the patient. This involves accurate assessment of velopharyngeal function by physiological evaluation and measurement. Additionally, the SLP will be consulted to assess speech prior to, and following, any treatment procedure. Often the SLP, plastic surgeon, and/or prosthodontist will also work with an oral surgeon for surgeries that involve bony structures. Examples of such orthognathic surgery are described in the next section.

Orthognatic Surgery

Since clefts may affect underlying bony tissues as well as soft tissues, **orthognatic surgery,** or surgery that involves the bones of the upper and lower jaw, is often necessary. Two common types of orthognathic surgery for individuals with palatal clefts are alveolar bone grafting and maxillary advancement.

Alveolar Bone Grafting
Alveolar bone grafting may be necessary due to absence of bone, particularly in alveolar clefts. This surgery attempts to restore the continuity of the alveolus so that the child is less likely to develop crossbite or have missing teeth. Additionally, gaps in the alveolus may result in an oronasal fistula. Timing of surgery to address alveolar gaps is also a source of controversy. Alveolar bone grafting may be done early, often at the same time as primary palatal surgery, and prior to the eruption of the teeth. This is called primary bone grafting. In some individuals, this surgery is postponed until permanent teeth begin to erupt. This is called secondary bone grafting.

Maxillary Advancement
Maxillary advancement surgery may be necessary due to underdevelopment of the midface region. Various midface advancement surgeries attempt to establish an appropriate upper and lower jaw relationship and improve facial appearance. Maxillary advancement surgery is usually postponed until early adolescence when mandibular growth has occurred.

Though surgical management is but one part of the treatment for individuals with clefts, it is an important one. Appropriate surgery combined with other necessary treatment will have a positive impact on a child's self-image and on how that child functions in the family, and eventually in school and society. The following section discusses psychosocial issues related to individuals with clefts and their families.

PSYCHOSOCIAL ISSUES

One of the main concerns of parents-to-be is "Will my child be okay?" The birth of a baby who is "different" is therefore a shock to new parents. Because of the nature of cleft lip and cleft palate, early medical intervention is necessary, which further complicates life with a newborn. As the child grows, the child and the family must deal with both personal issues and societal pressures related to having a craniofacial anomaly. The child must deal with such issues through the school years and beyond. This section will examine psychosocial issues related to clefts of the lip and palate and will address the following topics: initial concerns of the parents, the effect of continued medical management, self-image and socialization, and school adjustment and performance. Discussion of these issues will be limited to children with isolated clefts of the lip and/or palate. Children who have other craniofacial anomalies or associated syndromes will likely have additional and more complex psychosocial issues.

Current technology allows some parents to know more about their child before birth. Prenatal imaging techniques such as ultrasound may detect clefts of the lip and some multiple anomaly disorders. Prenatal chromosomal or genetic analysis such as amniocentesis can identify many syndromes. It is likely that studies will begin to look at the psychosocial impact of such knowledge on parents and families (Peterson-Falzone et al., 2001). Currently, however, most literature still focuses on parents' reaction to the birth of a child with a cleft.

Initial Concerns of the Parents

Several reports have documented the various reactions of parents to learning that their infant has a cleft. These reactions may include shock, grief, anger, guilt, depression, and/or fear (Barden, Ford, Jensen, Rogers-Salyer, & Salyer, 1989; Carreto, 1981; Pope, 1999). For some parents, a period of mourning follows as they adjust to the unexpected situation (van Staden & Gerhardt, 1995). Because a cleft lip is visible, parental reactions may be severe (Natsume, Suzuki, & Kawai, 1987). However, some research suggests that reactions may also be severe when a "nonvisible" palatal cleft is present (Endriga & Speltz, 1997). Adverse effects on the marriage and other family and social relationships might seem likely, though research findings are inconclusive.

Almost immediately, parents of a child with a cleft must begin to deal with management issues. Feeding the infant, usually a pleasant interaction, may be difficult and stressful. The need for explanation and support to relatives and other family members may also take a toll on parents. Additionally, parents must begin to face the extensive medical interventions necessary for their child during the first year of life and beyond.

The Effect of Continued Medical Management

Infants with clefts of the lip and/or palate face one, and often two, surgeries within the first year of life. The first surgery and subsequent hospitalization is a period of high stress for the parents. Though hospital stays are generally more family-friendly today, with less isolation of the child from family, the potential negative effects on parent-infant bonding and family life should still be considered (Peterson-Falzone et al., 2001). The child will most likely require additional surgeries and treatments throughout childhood and adolescence. This is particularly true of a child with a cleft palate. Continued contact with health professionals, and continued emotional and financial demands on the family, may result in the perception of cleft palate as a "chronic medical condition" (Kummer, 2001). Thus, the stress on the family does not end with the first surgery, and may have a cumulative adverse effect (Tobiasen, 1990, 1993).

Self-Image and Socialization

Stressors to the child and family continue through the toddler and preschool years. However, during this period of time, the child's self-image is largely developing based upon the parents' behaviors and attitudes (Eliason, 1991). Once a child enters school, self-image and socialization issues take on a more significant role and become more complex (Peterson-Falzone et al., 2001).

Secondary lip surgery to improve appearance does not generally occur until at least age 6. Likewise, secondary surgery for remaining palatal clefts and/or velopharyngeal incompetence also does not occur until the child is older. Therefore, as children with a history of clefts enter school, they may still look and/or sound different than their peers. Though findings are somewhat inconsistent, children who have had clefts of the lip and/or palate tend to have a more negative self-concept and lowered self-esteem compared to peers with no history of physical anomalies (Broder & Strauss, 1989; Kapp-Simon, 1986). These children are also more likely to be teased by their peers (Jones, 1984; Noar, 1991; Turner, Thomas, Dowell, Rumsey, & Sandy, 1997). Children with a history of clefts do not typically have as many friends as other age-matched children and, as they get older, tend to be more concerned about interpersonal relationships (Kummer, 2001). All of these findings vary by disorder, gender, and age, and are largely influenced by the support the child receives, particularly from family. Self-esteem and socialization issues also have an influence on the child's academic success.

School Adjustment and Performance

Academic achievement is a major focus for children and their families from the time the child enters school throughout the school years. The effects of clefts on academic achievement are difficult to sort out, and are influenced by self-esteem and socialization issues, as well as by societal and cultural views of clefts.

Children with clefts, as a group, achieve below expectations academically when achievement is compared to intellectual skill level (Broder, Richman, & Matheson, 1998; Richman & Eliason, 1982). However, this may be due to several interacting factors. Children with craniofacial anomalies have a higher incidence of learning disabilities compared to the general population (Broder et al., 1998; Endriga & Kapp-Simon, 1999). Additionally, academic achievement may be influenced by the expectations of others (Broder & Strauss, 1989; Tobiasen, 1987). Teachers may underestimate the intellectual skills and abilities of individuals with craniofacial anomalies. Further, both parents and teachers may expect less academically of these individuals. This may result in lower academic aspirations for the child and less favorable evaluations by the teachers (Richman & Eliason, 1982).

Individuals with cleft palate are also more likely to have serious reading disabilities (Richman & Millard, 1997). However, children with a history of cleft may lack self-confidence reading aloud in class, which may adversely affect teacher evaluations and thus stigmatize students as reading disabled (Kummer, 2001). Overall, peers and teachers perceive children with clefts as more inhibited in the classroom (Richman & Eliason, 1982).

There are several variables that interact to affect achievement in school. These include intelligence, language abilities, speech and hearing abilities, the presence or absence of learning disabilities, self-concept, social adjustment to school, and the expectations of peers, parents, and teachers (Peterson-Falzone et al., 2001). It is therefore imperative that cleft palate teams have a psychologist or similar professional address these issues with children and their families. Providing assistance to the child and family will maximize the possibility of the child functioning optimally in the family, school, and community.

Case Study 1: Samuel

Samuel was born with a bilateral complete cleft of the secondary palate. At 9 months of age, he underwent surgery to repair the cleft. When Samuel was 2 years old, his family moved to a rural area. He did not begin to speak until he was 2.5 years old. When Samuel began to produce words, he left out many of the sounds. Samuel's parents realized that he was not producing as many sounds or words as he should, but they attributed it to lasting trauma from his early surgery. His parents assumed Samuel would eventually learn all his sounds. At age 4, Samuel entered a preschool. Samuel's teacher could not understand him and suggested that Samuel's parents take him to see an SLP. A local SLP assessed Samuel and diagnosed a severe articulation disorder. She noted that Samuel omitted all stop, fricative, and affricate consonants. However, she noted accurate production of vowels as well as liquid, glide, and nasal consonants. She immediately began therapy to address Samuel's numerous sound omissions.

Therapy focused on placement of the articulators to produce sounds. Though Samuel was able to imitate articulator placement for sound production, he appeared to struggle when attempting to produce the sounds. Because the preschool teacher and Samuel's preschool classmates could not understand him, and because Samuel seemed frustrated by this, his parents withdrew him from preschool. Samuel continued to receive speech therapy three times a week for six months. At the end of six months, Samuel was still omitting stops, fricatives, and affricates in his speech. Furthermore, his voice was now taking on a harsh, rough quality. The SLP suggested that Samuel's parents have him evaluated by an otolaryngologist to determine whether or not he had vocal nodules.

The otolaryngologist did observe small bilateral vocal nodules on Samuel's vocal folds, but suggested the parents have Samuel evaluated by a cleft palate team. The parents insisted that Samuel's cleft palate had already been repaired. However, they took Samuel to the nearest city's cleft palate team. Following a complete evaluation by the team, it was determined that Samuel had velopharyngeal insufficiency due to a short velum. Though Samuel's speech was judged to be mildly hypernasal, the main characteristic of his speech was inability to produce high-pressure consonants due to leakage of air into the nasal cavity. It was assumed that Samuel had developed a secondary voice disorder due to hyperfunctional use of the laryngeal muscles in attempting to produce high-pressure sounds in therapy. It was recommended that Samuel undergo secondary surgery to create a pharyngeal flap. However, the cleft palate team recommended that the family postpone secondary surgery until additional midfacial growth had occurred. In the meantime, Samuel was fitted for a speech bulb obturator.

On Samuel's 5th birthday, he was seen by the cleft palate team prosthodontist to be fitted for the speech bulb obturator. During fitting, the prosthodontist modified size and placement of the acrylic bulb as the cleft palate team SLP listened to Samuel's speech to judge nasality. When nasality was judged to be normal, the speech bulb obturator was completed. Samuel quickly adjusted to the new appliance. His speech was no longer mildly hypernasal and he gradually began to "acquire" stops, fricatives and affricates. When Samuel was 9 years old, he underwent surgery to create a permanent pharyngeal flap. At that point his speech was normal.

Case Study 2: Gretchen

Gretchen was a 4-year-old girl whose parents brought her to an SLP for an articulation evaluation. Gretchen's parents reported that she often produced strange gargling and spitting sounds when she spoke. The SLP discovered that Gretchen had been born with a cleft palate, but this had been repaired when Gretchen was 9 months old. During the speech evaluation the SLP noted that Gretchen produced pharyngeal stops as substitutes for bilabial and lingua-alveolar stops, and glottal stops as substitutes for lingua-velar stops. Likewise, Gretchen produced pharyngeal fricatives as substitutes for labiodental, interdental, and lingua-alveolar fricatives, and glottal fricatives as substitutes for lingua-palatal fricatives. Additionally, Gretchen substituted glottal affricates for the lingua-palatal affricates. The SLP noted normal resonance. However, due to Gretchen's history and presenting articulation characteristics, the SLP referred her to an otolaryngologist for an evaluation. Following an examination, the otolaryngologist reported that Gretchen's velopharyngeal mechanism appeared to be functioning normally. Therefore, the SLP recommended articulation therapy.

In therapy, the SLP worked on placement of stop consonants. The SLP had a difficult time getting Gretchen to change place of articulation. When Gretchen did use a more front place of articulation, it appeared difficult for her to make an audible stop consonant sound. Due to Gretchen's history of cleft palate, as well as her difficulty with therapy, after six months the SLP referred Gretchen to a cleft palate team. Gretchen underwent several tests and examinations. Her evaluation included a videotaped X-ray image of movement of the velopharyngeal mechanism during speech (a procedure called **video-flouroscopy**) and measurement of oral and nasal airflow during speech to get an idea of size of velopharyngeal port opening (a procedure called pressure-flow technique). The cleft palate team concluded that Gretchen had minor velopharyngeal dysfunction due to a slightly short velum. Velopharyngeal dysfunction was only evident during attempts to accurately produce high-pressure consonants. When Gretchen attempted accurate production of these sounds, the velopharyngeal mechanism required the tightest closure, and a small amount of air leakage into the nasal cavity was evident. The cleft palate team advised Gretchen and her parents of their finding and recommended pharyngeal wall augmentation. After more testing to determine exact injection site, this procedure was performed. Following pharyngeal wall augmentation, Gretchen still produced pharyngeal and glottal stops, fricatives, and affricates. She was referred back to her SLP. This time, with a fully functional velopharyngeal mechanism, Gretchen was successful in therapy. She was dismissed from therapy after three months.

REVIEW QUESTIONS

1. How do the structures referred to in this chapter as *primary palate* and *secondary palate* compare to the structures commonly referred to as "hard palate" and "soft palate"? Why are the terms *primary palate* and *secondary palate* preferable when discussing clefts?

2. Why do you think the multifactorial model of inheritence is the most popular theory to explain clefts?

3. Suppose you are involved in a debate about best age for primary surgery to correct a palatal cleft. What age do you choose and why? Suppose you must argue for surgery during the first three months of life. What will be your main points? Next, suppose you must argue for postponing surgery until early adolescence. What will be your main points now?

4. Secondary surgery for individuals with a history of cleft lip is performed for a different reason than secondary surgery for individuals with a history of cleft palate. Compare and contrast the two types of secondary surgery.

5. Describe different options for secondary management of velopharyngeal dysfunction. For whom, and at what age, are the various surgical options best? For whom, and at what age, are the various prosthetic options best? For whom, and at what age, is speech therapy best?

6. Discuss how it is possible for an individual with velopharyngeal dysfunction to be both hypernasal and hyponasal.

7. Explain why individuals with a history of cleft palate often produce a lateralized /s/.

8. Nasal emission and weak pressure consonants are often described as "passive" articulation errors whereas compensatory articulation is often described as an "active" articulation strategy. Why are these terms used? Is a "passive" error or an "active" strategy preferable? (Consider such factors as intelligibility, habit formation, need for speech therapy, etc.)

9. Is it possible to assess resonance and articulation in a child who is producing only one-word utterances? If so, what will be your strategy? Provide examples of stimulus items.

10. Suppose you are a speech-language pathologist and an individual with a history of a cleft palate is referred to you. The individual presents with hypernasality, audible nasal emission of high-pressure consonants, and a hoarse voice. What might be the cause of the voice disorder? How will you differentially diagnose the resonance disorder from the voice disorder?

REFERENCES

American Cleft Palate-Craniofacial Association. (1993). Parameters for evaluation and treatment of patients with cleft lip/palate or other craniofacial anomalies. *Cleft Palate Craniofacial Journal, 30*(Suppl.), 1–16.

Argamaso, R. V., Shprintzen, R. J., Strauch, B., Lewin, M., Daniller, A., Ship, A., & Croft, C. (1980). The role of lateral pharyngeal wall movement in pharyngeal flap surgery. *Plastic and Reconstructive Surgery, 66*, 214–219.

Bardach, J. (1994). Unilateral cleft lip. In M. M. Cohen (Ed.), *Mastery of plastic and reconstructive surgery* (Vol. 1, pp. 548–565). Boston: Little, Brown.

Bardach, J., & Salyer, K. (1987). *Surgical techniques in cleft lip and palate.* Chicago: Year Book.

Barden, C., Ford, M., Jensen, A. G., Rogers-Salyer, M., & Salyer, K. E. (1989). Effects of craniofacial deformity in infancy on the quality of mother-infant interactions. *Child Development, 60*, 819–824.

Bernthal, J. E., & Beukelman, D. R. (1977). The effect of changes in velopharyngeal orifice area on vowel intensity. *Cleft Palate Journal, 14*(1), 63–77.

Blocksma, R. (1963). Correction of velopharyngeal insufficiency by silastic pharyngeal implant. *Plastic and Reconstructive Surgery, 31*, 268–274.

Blocksma, R. (1964). Silicone implants for velopharyngeal incompetence: A progress report. *Cleft Palate Journal, 1*, 72–81.

Broder, H. L., Richman, L. C., & Matheson, P. B. (1998). Learning disability, school achievement, and grade retention among children with cleft: A two-center study. *Cleft Palate-Craniofacial Journal, 35*, 127–131.

Broder, H. L., & Strauss, R. P. (1989). Self-concept of early primary school age children with visible or invisible defects. *Cleft Palate Journal, 26*, 114–117.

Brogan, W. F. (1988). Team approach to the treatment of cleft lip and palate. *Annals of the Academy of Medicine, Singapore, 17*(3), 335–338.

Burdi, A. R., & Silvey, R. G. (1969). Sexual differences in closure of the human palatal shelves. *Cleft Palate Journal, 6*, 1–7.

Bzoch, K. R. (1979). Measurement and assessment of categorical aspects of cleft palate speech. In K. R. Bzoch (Ed.), *Communicative disorders related to cleft lip and palate*. Boston: Little, Brown.

Calzolari, E., Milan, M., Cavazzuti, G. B., Cocchi, G., Gandini, E., Magnani, C., Moretti, M., Garani, G. P., Salvioli, G. B., & Volpato, S. (1988). Epidemiological and genetic study of 200 cases of oral cleft in the Emilia Romagna region of Northern Italy. *Teratology, 38*, 559–564.

Carlisle, D. (1998). Feeding babies with cleft lip and palate. *Nursing Times, 94*(4), 59–60.

Carreto, V. (1981). Maternal responses to an infant with cleft lip and palate: A review of the literature. *Maternal-Child Nursing Journal, 10*, 197–206.

Chow, E. W. C., Bassett, A. S., & Weksberg, R. (1994). Velo-cardio-facial syndrome and psychotic disorders: Implications for psychiatric genetics. *American Journal of Medical Genetics, 54*, 107–112.

Clarren, S. K., & Smith, D. W. (1978). The fetal alcohol syndrome. *New England Journal of Medicine, 298*, 1063–1067.

Cohen, M. M., Jr., & Bankier, A. (1991). Syndrome delineation involving orofacial clefting. *Cleft Palate-Craniofacial Journal, 28*, 119–120.

Eliason, M. J. (1991). Cleft lip and palate: Developmental effects. *Journal of Pediatric Nursing, 5*, 107–113.

Eliez, S., Blasey, C. M., Schmitt, E. J., White, C. D., Hu, D., & Reiss, A. L. (2001). Velocardiofacial syndrome: Are structural changes in the temporal and mesial temporal regions related to schizophrenia? *American Journal of Psychiatry, 158*(3), 447–453.

Endriga, M. C., & Kapp-Simon, K. A. (1999). Psychological issues in craniofacial care: State of the art. *Cleft Palate-Craniofacial Journal, 36*, 3–11.

Endriga, M. C., & Speltz, M. L. (1997). Face-to-face interaction between infants with orofacial clefts and their mothers. *Journal of Pediatric Psychology, 22*, 439–453.

Ericson, A., Kallen, B., & Westerholm, P. (1979). Cigarette smoking as an etiologic factor in cleft lip and palate. *American Journal of Obstetrics and Gynecology, 135*, 348–351.

Fernhoff, P. M., & Lammer, E. J. (1984). Craniofacial features of isotretonoin embryopathy. *Pediatrics, 105*, 595–597.

Fraser, F. C. (1970). The genetics of cleft lip and palate. *American Journal of Human Genetics, 22*, 336–352.

Fraser, F. C. (1978). The multifactorial threshold concept—uses and misuses. *Teratology, 14*, 267–280.

Furlow, L., Jr. (1986). Cleft palate repair by double opposing Z-plasty. *Plastic and Reconstructive Surgery, 78*(6), 724–738.

Gordon, J. E., & Shy, C. M. (1981). Agricultural chemical use and congenital cleft lip and/or palate. *Archives of Environmental Health, 36*, 213–221.

Gorlin, R. J., Cohen, M. J., & Levin, L. S. (1990). *Syndromes of the head and neck* (3rd ed.). New York: Oxford University Press.

Hanson, J. W., Myrianthopoulos, N. C., Harvey, M. A. S., & Smith, D. W. (1976). Risks to the offspring of women treated with hydantoin anticonvulsants with emphasis on the fetal hydantoin syndrome. *Journal of Pediatrics, 89*, 662–668.

Hanson, J. W., & Smith, D. W. (1975). Fetal alcohol syndrome: Experience with 41 cases. *Journal of Pediatrics, 87,* 285–290.

Harding, A., & Grunwell, P. (1996). Characteristics of cleft palate speech. *European Journal of Disorders of Communication, 31,* 331–357.

Harding, A., & Grunwell, P. (1998). Active versus passive cleft-type speech characteristics. *International Journal of Language and Communication Disorders, 33*(3), 329–352.

Heineman-de Boer, J. A., Van Haelst, M. J., Cordia-de Haan, M., & Beemer, F. A. (1999). Behavior problems and personality aspects of 40 children with velo-cardio-facial syndrome. *Genetic Counseling, 10*(1), 89–93.

Henningsson, G. E., & Isberg, A. M. (1986). Velopharyngeal movement patterns in patients alternating between oral and glottal articulation: A clinical and cine radiological study. *Cleft Palate Journal, 23,* 1–9.

Holmberg, P. C., Hernberg, S., Kruppa, K., Rantala, K., & Riala, R. (1982). Oral clefts and organic solvent exposure during pregnancy. *International Archives of Occupational and Environmental Health, 50,* 371–376.

Jackson, I. T. (1985). Sphincter pharyngoplasty. *Clinics in Plastic Surgery, 12*(4), 711–717.

Jensen, B. L., Kreigorg, S., Dahl, E., & Fogh-Anderson, P. (1988). Cleft lip and palate in Denmark, 1976–1981: Epidemiology, variability, and early somatic development. *Cleft Palate Journal, 25*(3), 258–269.

Jones, J. E. (1984). Self-concept and parental evaluation of peer relationships in cleft lip and palate children. *Pediatric Dentistry, 6,* 132–138.

Jones, K. L. (1986). Fetal alcohol syndrome. *Pediatric Development, 8*(4), 122–126.

Jones, K. L., & Smith, D. W. (1973). Recognition of the fetal alcohol syndrome in early infancy. *Lancet, 2*(7836), 999–1001.

Jones, K. L., Smith, D. W., Ulleland, C. N., & Streissguth, A. P. (1973). Pattern of malformation in offspring of chronic alcoholic mothers. *Lancet, 1,* 1267–1271.

Jones, W. B. (1988). Weight gain and feeding in the neonate with cleft: A three-center study. *Cleft Palate Journal, 25*(4), 379–384.

Kapp-Simon, K. A. (1986). Self-concept of primary-school-age children with cleft lip, cleft palate, or both. *Cleft Palate Journal, 23,* 24–27.

Karayiorgou, M., Morris, M. A., Morrow, B., Shprintzen, R. J., Goldberg, R. B., Borrow, J., Gos, A., Nestadt, G., Wolyniec, P. S., Lasseter, V. K., Eisen, H., Childs, B., Kazazian, H. H., Kucherlapati, R., Antonarakis, S. E., Pulver, A. E., & Housman, D. E. (1995). Schizophrenia susceptibility associated with interstitial deletions of chromosome 22q11. *Proceedings of the National Academy of Sciences of the United States of America, 92,* 7612–7615.

Kernahan, D. A., & Stark, R. B. (1958). A new classification system for cleft lip and cleft palate. *Plastic and Reconstructive Surgery, 22,* 435.

Khoury, M. J., Weinstein, A., Panny, S., Holtzman, N. A., Lindsay, P. K., Farrel, K., & Eisenberg, M. (1977). Maternal cigarette smoking and oral clefts: A population-based study. *American Journal of Public Health, 77,* 623–625.

Khoury, M. J., Gomez-Farias, J., & Mulinare, J. (1989). Does maternal cigarette smoking during pregnancy cause cleft lip and palate in offspring? *American Journal of Diseases in Children, 143,* 333–337.

Kummer, A. W. (2001). *Cleft palate & craniofacial anomalies: The effects on speech and resonance.* Clifton Park, NY: Delmar Learning.

Kummer, A. W., Curtis, C., Wiggs, M., Lee, L., & Strife, J. L. (1992). Comparison of velopharyngeal gap size in patients with hypernasality, hypernasality and nasal emission, or nasal turbulence (rustle) as the primary speech characteristic. *Cleft Palate-Craniofacial Journal, 29*(2), 152–156.

Lammer, E. J., Chen, D. T., Hoar, R. M., Agnish, N. D., Benke, P. J., Braun, J. T., Curry, C. J., Fernhoff, P. M., Grix, A. W., Lott, I. T., Richard J. M., & Sun, S. C. (1985). Retinoic acid embryopathy. *New England Journal of Medicine, 313,* 837–841.

LeBlanc, S. M., & Golding-Kushner, K. J. (1992). Effect of glossopexy on speech sound production in Robin sequence. *Cleft Palate-Craniofacial Journal, 29,* 239–245.

Mason, R. M., & Grandstaff, H. L. (1971). Evaluating the velopharyngeal mechanism in hypernasal speakers. *Language, Speech, and Hearing Services in the Schools, 2*(4), 53–61.

McWilliams, B. J. (1982). Cleft palate. In G. Shames & E. Wiig (Eds.), *Human communication disorders.* Columbus, OH: C. E. Merrill.

McWilliams, B. J., Morris, H. L., & Shelton, R. L. (1990). *Cleft palate speech* (2nd ed.). Philadelphia: B. C. Decker.

Meadow, S. F. (1968). Anticonvulsant drugs and congenital abnormalities. *Lancet, 2,* 1269.

Millard, D. R. (1958). A radical rotation in single harelip. *American Journal of Surgery, 95,* 318–322.

Millard, D. R. (1976). *Cleft craft: The evolution of its surgeries.* Vol. I: *The unilateral deformity.* Boston: Little, Brown.

Millard, D. R. (1977). *Cleft craft: The evolution of its surgeries.* Vol. II: *The bilateral deformity.* Boston: Little, Brown.

Morley, M. E. (1970). *Cleft palate and speech* (7th ed.). Baltimore: Williams & Wilkins.

Natsume, N., Suzuki, T., & Kawai, T. (1987). Maternal reactions to the birth of a child with cleft lip and/or palate. *Plastic and Reconstructive Surgery, 79,* 1003–1004.

Noar, J. H. (1991). Questionnaire survey of attitudes and concerns of patients with cleft lip and palate and their parents. *Cleft Palate-Craniofacial Journal, 28,* 279–284.

Noordhoff, M. S. (1994). Bilateral cleft lip. In M. Cohen (Ed.), *Mastery of plastic and reconstructive surgery.* Vol. 1. Boston: Little, Brown.

O'Gara, M. M., & Logemann, J. A. (1988). Phonetic analyses of the speech development of babies with cleft palate. *Cleft Palate Journal, 25*(2), 122–134.

Orticochea, M. (1968). Construction of a dynamic muscle sphincter in cleft palates. *Plastic and Reconstructive Surgery, 41,* 323–327.

Orticochea, M. (1997). Physiopathology of the dynamic muscular sphincter of the pharynx. *Plastic and Reconstructive, Surgery, 100*(7), 1918–1923.

Owens, J. R., Jones, J. W., & Harris, F. (1985). Epidemiology of facial clefting. *Archives of Disease in Childhood, 60,* 521–524.

Paradise, J. L., Elster, B. A., & Tan, L. (1994). Evidence in infants with cleft palate that breast milk protects against otitis media. *Pediatrics, 94,* 853–860.

Peterson-Falzone, S. J., Hardin-Jones, M. A., & Karnell, M. P. (2001). *Cleft palate speech* (3rd ed.). St. Louis: Mosby.

Pope, A. W. (1999). Points of risk and opportunity for parents of children with craniofacial conditions. *Cleft Palate-Craniofacial Journal, 36,* 36–39.

Pulver, A. E., Nestadt, G., Goldberg, R., Shprintzen, R. J., Lamacz, J., Wolyniec, P. S., Morrow, B., Karayiorgou, M., Antonarakis, S. E., Housman, D., & Kucherlapati, R. (1994). Psychotic illness in patients diagnosed with velo-cardio-facial syndrome and their relatives. *Journal of Nervous and Mental Disease, 182,* 476–478.

Randall, P. (1959). A triangular flap operation for the primary repair of unilateral clefts of the lip. *Plastic and Reconstructive Surgery, 23,* 331–347.

Randall, P. (1990). Long-term results with the triangular flap technique for unilateral cleft lip repair. In J. Bardach & H. L. Morris (Eds.), *Multidisciplinary management of cleft lip and palate* (pp. 173–183). Philadelphia: W. B. Saunders.

Ranta, R., & Rintala, A. (1989). Unusual alveolar clefts: Report of cases. *Journal of Dentistry for Children, 56,* 363–365.

Remacle, M., Bertrand, B., Eloy, P., & Marbaix, E. (1990). The use of injectable collagen to correct velopharyngeal insufficiency. *Laryngoscope, 100,* 269–274.

Richman, L. C., & Eliason, M. J. (1982). Psychological characteristics of children with cleft lip and palate: Intellectual, achievement, behavioral, and personality variables. *Cleft Palate Journal, 19,* 249–257.

Richman, L. C., & Millard, T. L. (1997). Cleft lip and palate: Longitudinal behavior and relationships of cleft conditions to behavior and achievement. *Journal of Pediatric Psychology, 22,* 487–494.

Robin, N. H., Opitz, J. M., & Muenke, M. (1996). Opitz G/BBB syndrome: Clinical comparisons of families linked to Xp22 and 22q, and a review of the literature. *American Journal of Medical Genetics, 62*(3), 305–317.

St-Hilaire, H., & Buchbinder, D. (2000). Maxillofacial pathology and management of Pierre Robin sequence. *Otolaryngology Clinics of North America, 33*(6), 1241–1256.

Schweckendiek, W., & Kruse, E. (1990). Two-stage palatoplasty: Schweckendiek technique. In J. Bardach & H. L. Morris (Eds.), *Multidisciplinary management of cleft lip and palate* (pp. 315–320). Philadelphia: W. B. Saunders.

Sharp, H. M. (1995). Ethical decision-making in interdisciplinary team care. *Cleft Palate Craniofacial Journal, 32*(6), 495–499.

Shaw, G., Wasserman, C., Lammer, E., O'Malley, C., Murray, J., Basart, A., & Tolarova, M. (1996). Orofacial clefts, parental cigarette smoking, and transforming growth factor-alpha gene variants. *American Journal of Human Genetics, 58,* 551–561.

Shaw, G. M., Croen, L. A., & Curry, C. J. (1991). Isolated oral cleft malformations: Associations with maternal and infant characteristics in a California population. *Teratology, 43,* 225–228.

Shprintzen, R. J. (1988). Pierre Robin, micrognathia, and airway obstruction: The dependency of treatment on accurate diagnosis. *International Anesthesiology Clinics, 26,* 84–91.

Shprintzen, R. J. (1997). *Genetics, syndromes, and communication disorders*. Clifton Park, NY: Delmar Learning.

Snead, M. P., & Yates, J. R. (1999). Clinical and molecular genetics of Stickler syndrome. *Journal of Medical Genetics, 36*(5), 353–359.

Spranger, J., Benerischke, K., Hall, J. G., Lenz, W., Lowry, R. B., Opitz, J. M., Pinsky, L., Schwarzacher, H. G., & Smith, D. W. (1982). Errors of morphogenesis: Concepts and terms. Recommendations of an international working group. *Journal of Pediatrics, 100*(1), 160–165.

Strauss, R. P. (1999). The organization and delivery of craniofacial health services: The state of the art. *Cleft Palate-Craniofacial Journal, 36*(3), 189–195.

Streissguth, A. P., Aase, J. M., Clarren, S. K., Randels, S. P., LaDue, R. A., & Smith, D. F. (1991). Fetal alcohol syndrome in adolescents and adults [see Comments]. *Journal of the American Medical Association, 265*(15), 1961–1967.

Surgeon General's Report. (1987, June). *Children with special needs*. Washington, DC: Office of Maternal and Child Health, U.S. Department of Health and Human Services, Public Health Service.

Templin, M. C., & Darley, F. L. (1960). *The Templin-Darley tests of articulation* (2nd ed.). Iowa City: Bureau of Educational Research and Service, University of Iowa.

Tennison, C. W. (1952). Repair of unilateral cleft lip by the stencil method. *Plastic and Reconstructive Surgery, 9*, 115–120.

Tobiasen, J. M. (1987). Social judgments of facial deformity. *Cleft Palate Journal, 24*, 323–327.

Tobiasen, J. M. (1990). Psychosocial adjustment to cleft lip and palate. In J. Bardach & H. L. Morris (Eds.), *Multidisciplinary management of cleft lip and palate* (pp. 820–825). Philadelphia: W. B. Saunders.

Tobiasen, J. M. (1993). Clefting and psychosocial judgment: Influence of facial aesthetics. *Advances in Management of Cleft Lip and Palate: Clinics in Plastic Surgery, 20*, 623–631.

Tolarova, M. (1982). Periconceptional supplementation with vitamins and folic acid to prevent recurrence of cleft lip. *Lancet, 2*, 217.

Tolarova, M., & Harris, J. (1995). Reduced recurrence of orofacial clefts after periconceptional supplementation with high-dose folic acid and multivitamins. *Teratology, 51*, 71–78.

Tomaski, S. M., Zalzal G. H., & Saal, H. M. (1995). Airway obstruction in Pierre Robin sequence *Laryngoscope, 105*, 111–115.

Trier, W., & Dreyer, T. (1984). Primary von Langenbeck palatoplasty with levator reconstruction: Rationales and technique. *Cleft Palate Journal, 21*(4), 254–262.

Trost, J. E. (1981). Articulatory additions to the classical description of the speech of persons with cleft palate. *Cleft Palate Journal, 18*, 193–203.

Trost-Cardamone, J. E., & Bernthal, J. E. (1993). Articulation assessment and procedures and treatment decisions. In K. T. Moller & C. D. Starr (Eds.), *Cleft palate: Interdisciplinary issues and treatment* (pp. 307–366). Austin: Pro-Ed.

Turner, S. R., Thomas, P. W. N., Dowell, T., Rumsey, N., & Sandy, J. R. (1997). Psychological outcomes amongst cleft patients and their families. *British Journal of Plastic Surgery, 50*, 1–9.

van Staden, F., & Gerhardt, C. (1995). Mothers of children with facial cleft deformities: Reactions and effects. *South American Journal of Psychology, 25*(1), 39–46.

Warren, D. W., Wood, M. T., & Bradley, D. P. (1969). Respiratory volumes in normal and cleft palate speech. *Cleft Palate Journal, 6,* 449–460.

Werler, M. M., Lammer, E. J., Rosenberg, L., & Mitchell, A. A. (1990). Maternal cigarette smoking during pregnancy in relation to oral clefts. *American Journal of Epidemiology, 132,* 926–932.

Wilhelmsen, H. R., & Musgrave, R. H. (1966). Complications of cleft lip surgery. *Cleft Palate Journal, 3,* 223–231.

Ysunza, A., Pamplona, C., & Toledo, E. (1992). Change in velopharyngeal valving after speech therapy in cleft palate patients. A videonasopharyngoscopic and multi-view videofluoroscopic study. *International Journal of Pediatric Otorhinolaryngology, 24*(1), 45–54.

PART IV

Disorders Secondary
to Environmental Factors

Chapter 8

Substance Abuse

Tracie Bullock Dickson Ph.D., CCC-SLP

CHAPTER OBJECTIVES

Upon completing this chapter, the reader should be able to:

1. Describe substance abuse as a consistent abusive pattern of drug use that can significantly impact daily living
2. Describe substance dependence as the continued use of drugs even when significant problems are overtly evident to the user
3. Understand the impact of substance abuse on the fetus in the areas of fetal growth and development
4. Understand the possible effects of substance abuse on neurobehavioral, neuromotor, physical, cognitive, and language development
5. Understand the pivotal role that a caregiving environment plays in the development of young children

INTRODUCTION

Drug abuse in pregnant women is a widespread and serious problem in the United States (Chasnoff, 1988). History reveals that there have always been women who have used illegal drugs such as cocaine, heroin, and methamphetamines, and legal drugs such as tobacco, alcohol, and prescription drugs during pregnancy. Society and economics generally dictate what will be the social drug of choice for substance abusers, and statistics reveal that cocaine and alcohol are the most pervasively used drugs in the United States. The popularity and addictive properties of cocaine and the ease of consuming alcohol continue to generate considerable concerns at the local and national levels. Abuse of drugs or addiction during pregnancy is a serious health and social problem with unique challenges for researchers, developmental specialists, health care professionals, social services, and the mother. With the large numbers of women abusing substances during pregnancy, researchers, policy makers, and service providers persistently work to determine how to address the problem of infants and toddlers exposed to drugs, including alcohol.

Current research lacks a consistent pattern of outcomes for young children with cocaine exposure (Nulman et al., 2001; Betancourt, Fischer, Giannetta, Malmud, Brodsky, & Hurt, 1999). More consistent and definitive patterns of developmental disability in alcohol-exposed infants have been documented (Streissguth, 1997). However, cocaine use during pregnancy places these children at-risk for negative outcomes (Sparks, 1993). This chapter assumes that children with prenatal substance exposure are at-risk for developmental delays. Categorization of these children within a deficit paradigm unfairly and wrongly assumes that all children with substance exposure will suffer negative outcomes (Chavkin, 2001). The problem of substance abuse in adults and its effects on children is complex, with many confounding variables (Chasnoff, 1988) that make it difficult to make definitive claims regarding substance exposure in young children.

Results of previous studies indicate that some drugs, such as cocaine, used during pregnancy do not consistently negatively impact the fetus (Betancourt et al., 1999), though popular belief leads one to believe that cocaine is a dangerous **teratogen** leading to devastating developmental disabilities (Leckman, Mayes, & Hodgins, 2001). As stated earlier, that belief is largely unsubstantiated (Leckman, Mayes, & Hodgins, 2001; Gittler & McPherson, 1990). A teratogenic agent is one that causes developmental disabilities or malformations. Early research on the effects of cocaine, especially crack cocaine, on young children grew out of the belief that these babies would require special education resources and other health care and social services (Leckman, Mayes, & Hodgins, 2001, Besharov, 1990). This fact turned out to be a tenuous claim. In fact, when these children are provided with stable and nurturing environments, along with early intervention services, their development more closely emulates that of their non-drug exposed peers (Black, Schuler, & Nair, 1993). However, other confounding variables, such as maternal tobacco and alcohol use, as well as environmental factors have a more significant impact on development. Women who abuse drugs during pregnancy or abuse cocaine are typically users of other substances such as alcohol. Therefore, these children are at-risk for a myriad of problems that can result in developmental delays.

Alcohol, a dangerous and powerful teratogen, is known to cause developmental delays, birth defects, mental retardation, and congenital malformations. Alcohol is considered to be the most dangerous substance to abuse during pregnancy, as it can have devastating long-term and irreversible consequences. Today, alcohol is known to be the leading cause of mental retardation in the United States (Abel & Sokol, 1987). Children exposed to alcohol can be diagnosed with **fetal alcohol syndrome (FAS)** or **fetal alcohol effect (FAE).** FAS is a profound birth defect with specific patterns of disability manifested in physical growth and development, physical anomalies, behavior, and central nervous system damage (Streissguth, 1997). FAE is a diagnosis given when some, but not all, of the deficits associated with FAS are present.

Given the current public health concerns, researchers and service providers want to understand the effects of maternal substance abuse on the fetus and the possible outcomes of children including cognition, language, motor skills, and neurological and physical growth and development. This chapter provides a framework for understanding the specific problems related to cocaine and alcohol abuse during pregnancy and subsequent outcomes, concomitant environmental and family issues, and assessment and intervention procedures for speech-language pathologists.

DEFINITION OF SUBSTANCE ABUSE

The term **substance abuse** is used to describe a consistent abusive pattern of drug use that can lead to significant problems in one's personal and social life. It can further compromise the abuser's health, economic status, and occupational status. According to Doweiko (1999), substance abuse is the continued use of a mood-altering chemical that causes harm to the user and/or others. Furthermore, it can lead to social, financial, employment, or health problems. Substance abuse progresses to substance dependency with continued use (Doweiko, 1999).

Substance dependence is the continued use of drugs, including alcohol, even when significant problems related to the abuse are evident. Individuals continue to use the substance despite significant substance-related cognitive, behavioral, and physiological problems (Doweiko, 1999). Drug dependency is characterized by a greater tolerance and/or increased need for larger amounts of the abused substance to attain the desired effect, withdrawal symptoms that may occur when use is decreased, and an inability to stop using the drug without professional intervention. Like substance abuse, a person with drug dependency may spend an extraordinary amount of time involved in drug-seeking activity, which consequently leads to withdrawal from social, occupational, and family obligations. Generally, people with substance dependency will continue to engage in drug-taking behaviors even when they are aware of the physical, social, and psychological problems created by their drug use.

TRENDS IN DRUG ABUSE

According to the National Institute on Drug Abuse (1999), cocaine continues to be the primary drug of choice in the United States along with alcohol. Use of other illicit drugs such as heroin, ecstasy, and methamphetamine is on the rise. Abuse of and/or dependency on prescription drugs has also increased. Numerous studies have been performed in an attempt to determine the incidence of prenatal drug and alcohol exposure in children; however, due to the instability of the testing population, procedures, and materials, specific figures have yet to be determined.

The number of infants exposed to drugs ranged from 13 to 181 per 1000 births in 1990 (Ondersma, Malcoe, & Simpson, 2001). During 1992–1993, the National Institute on Drug Abuse (NIDA) conducted the National Pregnancy and Health Survey, a nationwide hospital survey to determine the extent of substance abuse among pregnant women in the United States. This survey still provides the most recent national hospital-based data available. The survey examined the reported use of alcohol, tobacco, and illegal drugs such as cocaine and marijuana, as well as differences among ethnic groups. While approximately 4 million women were determined to have given birth that year, the survey found that 221,000 of them used illegal drugs during their pregnancies, with marijuana and cocaine being the most commonly used drugs. Approximately 119,000 women reported the use of marijuana and 45,000 reported the use of cocaine. The survey further estimated that 222,000 babies were born to these women. Overall, illegal substance abuse was estimated to be higher among all African American women, both pregnant and nonpregnant. However, the number of white women using drugs during pregnancy was estimated to be higher at 113,000, followed by African American women at 75,000 and Hispanic women at 28,000. When surveying use of legal drugs, estimates of alcohol use were also reportedly higher among white women, followed by African American women and, lastly, Hispanic women. Whites also had the highest rates for tobacco use, followed by African Americans, then Hispanic women. Though statistics vary across populations, drug abuse knows no ethnic or economic boundaries.

In 1998 the Substance Abuse and Mental Health Services Administration (SAMHSA) reported results of the 1997 National Household Survey on Drug Abuse and estimated that 1.5 million Americans used illicit drugs during the month prior to the administration of the survey (SAMHSA, 1998). Approximately 3.3 percent of pregnant women ages 15 to 44 were determined to have used illicit drugs one month prior to being surveyed. SAMHSA estimated that over a million Americans were users of cocaine. Further, 265,000 in that group were determined to use crack cocaine. They also found that the use of cocaine was highest for the 18 to 20 age group.

Despite the results of previous surveys, these figures are likely to be underestimated because drug users are sometimes unwilling to divulge their drug-using histories or may not provide a complete and accurate history. Also, only a limited number of infants are tested for prenatal drug exposure. Often, many infants are not tested because maternal drug abuse is not suspected, and the baby may appear to be fine. In addition, maternal drug use is only detectable for a few days preceding use. If the mother used illicit drugs at other times throughout the pregnancy, this would not be evident on the test results. Therefore, the incidence of prenatal drug exposure in infants is assumed to be underestimated.

State and federal policy makers have become increasingly concerned with the overall cost of substance abuse treatment and prevention programs. Prevention of cocaine or crack use during pregnancy could save $352 million per year, according to a study conducted by Lester, LaGasse, and Seifer (1998). They estimated that because some children may experience developmental delays and learning difficulties, additional special education costs of $352 million per year will be required nationwide. The researchers reported that this figure is probably an underestimation because it is based only on new cases each year, and does not account for a cumulative effect.

As stated earlier, drug abuse and dependency can occur in women and men. Women who abuse drugs during pregnancy are at-risk for a complicated pregnancy, labor, and delivery, and furthermore place their unborn child at significant risk for compromised fetal development and developmental delays later in life. Researchers really do not have a clear picture of the amount of a drug that may cause developmental problems in young children, so it is generally accepted that drugs should not be taken during pregnancy except under the direction of a physician. The term **prenatal drug exposure** refers to mothers who use legal or illegal substances during pregnancy without the consent of a physician. It is difficult to identify clearly postnatal outcomes in children with cocaine exposure because of the confounding variables that complicate such research. Confounding variables include polydrug use, the amount of drugs taken, the trimester, and inconsistent maternal histories (Bergin, Cameron, Fleitz, & Patel, 2001).

THE BIOLOGICAL ACTION OF COCAINE

Prior to discussing the effects of cocaine exposure, it is first necessary to understand what cocaine is, how it affects the user, and how it is passed from the mother to the fetus during pregnancy. It is also important to note that an unborn life is called a fetus from the end of the eighth week of pregnancy to the moment of birth, and is distinguished from the embryo.

Cocaine has pronounced effects on both the peripheral and central nervous systems. Cocaine is a substance that increases neurological activity in the brain and the spinal cord when it enters the bloodstream because it alters chemical activity in the brain. The brain contains substances or chemical messengers called neurotransmitters that help transmit nerve impulses across nerve synapses. Cocaine affects the activity of three neurotransmitters that researchers have associated with addiction: dopamine, epinephrine, and norepinephrine. Dopamine is a neurotransmitter that is similar to adrenaline. It is involved in brain activities that control movement, emotional response, and the ability to experience pleasure and pain. Epinephrine is associated with vasoconstriction and raising blood pressure. Norepinephrine is also associated with emotional regulation, and an increased amount of norepinephrine is associated with mania. Cocaine may also affect another neurotransmitter called serotonin. Serotonin plays a role in emotional processing and sleep regulation, and it is also a vasoconstrictor. Vasoconstriction is a condition in which the blood vessels constrict or become narrow, thereby reducing the flow of blood and oxygen to the heart and brain.

Cocaine produces its effects by altering the flow of neurotransmitters, affecting appropriate levels needed in the central nervous system. Normally, when a neuron is stimulated it releases neurotransmitters into the synaptic cleft. The synaptic cleft is the space between two neurons. When the neurotransmitter is released into the synaptic cleft, it causes a specific excitatory biological effect. After the chemical is released into the synaptic cleft and the appropriate neural signal is transmitted, it must then be deactivated. Deactivation occurs through a process called reuptake that stops the action of the chemical. Reuptake is the process by which a neuron returns certain amounts of a neurotransmitter back to the neuron that released it. This action decreases the amount of neurotransmitters in the synaptic cleft, which decreases the excitatory action. Cocaine increases the levels of these neurotransmitters in the central nervous system by preventing reuptake, thereby leaving more of the chemical or higher levels in the synapse, which produces an increased degree of stimulation and/or excitability in the nervous system. In other words, cocaine impairs the central nervous system's ability to deactivate stimulatory processes, resulting in the accumulation of the neurotransmitters at the synapses.

With the use of cocaine, a remarkable activation of the peripheral nervous system excitatory and inhibitory effects occurs, as well as stimulation in the central nervous system. This activation causes the most noticeable acute effects of the drug, that is, tachycardia, hypertension, and vasoconstriction. In effect, cocaine can cause tachycardia and hypertension, both of which can be life threatening. **Tachycardia** is a rapid heartbeat, and **hypertension** is increased blood pressure. In addition, cocaine can also cause **vasoconstriction** to occur. The result is a reduction in the flow of blood and oxygen, which then requires the heart to work harder to pump blood throughout the body. One of the most dangerous side effects of cocaine use is that it can rapidly lead to heart failure, stroke, and, in rare cases, sudden death.

When dopamine accumulates in synaptic clefts, it activates dopaminergic systems. This activation is crucial to the sense of euphoria that follows the ingestion of cocaine, and also accounts for the strong addictive qualities of the drug. Many cocaine users attempt to obtain the initial intense euphoric high of the drug. All of these conditions may affect pregnancy, labor and delivery, fetal growth, and fetal neurological maturation. The cocaine has the same effect on the central and peripheral nervous systems of the fetus, causing placental vasoconstriction, decreased blow flow to the fetus, and increased uterine contractions.

Adults who use cocaine also experience various physical side effects such as constricted blood vessels, increased heart rate, elevated temperature and blood pressure, and euphoria. The euphoria leads to overstimulation, with increased energy output and compromised mental clarity. Physical effects depend on the route of administration and the rate of absorption by the body. Some users of cocaine report feelings of restlessness and irritability, impaired vision, visual hallucinations, anxiety, aggression, paranoia, food cravings, poor attention/concentration, and tremors. Individuals with long-term dependency may experience excessive weight loss, skin problems, and coughs. Individuals who are long-term users of crack cocaine have poor appetites and are often very undernourished, gaunt in appearance, and unkempt. With increased use and tolerance, many users fail to achieve the same level of pleasure felt with the first use of the drug. Fatigue and depression are often experienced after the feeling of euphoria comes to an end. Cocaine has powerful neurological and psychological reinforcing properties that cause users to continue to use the drug even when they are aware of the unpleasant side effects.

When a pregnant woman uses cocaine, the drug rapidly crosses the placenta and is slowly processed by the fetus and may, in fact, accumulate in the fetus. Therefore, the fetus is exposed to significant levels of cocaine for long periods of time (Keller & Snyder-Keller, 2000). The placenta is the lining of the uterine wall that envelops the fetus and passes life-sustaining nutrients from the mother to the fetus. After transfer from the mother to the fetus, cocaine achieves peak levels in fetal circulation within 3 minutes and remains in the system of the fetus for quite some time (Gingras, Weese-Mayer, Hume, & O'Donnell, 1992). Hence, cocaine transfers rapidly into the fetus and may increase the potential for adverse fetal effects with subsequent developmental delay in young children. Once in the fetal system, cocaine blocks reuptake of the neurotransmitters, resulting in excitatory physiologic effects similar to those seen in the mothers (Chan et al., 1992).

THE EFFECTS OF COCAINE ON THE FETUS AND INFANT, AND LONG-TERM OUTCOMES

As stated previously, prenatal drug exposure may have a significant, though not clearly defined, negative effect on the fetus, infant, and developing child. At present, conflicting information is available regarding the long-term effects of substance exposure, but researchers continue to study the development of exposed children through school age. It is clear, however, that these children must certainly be considered at-risk for developmental and learning problems. Service providers and other professionals must understand that maternal substance abuse during pregnancy does not automatically lead to infants with developmental delays.

Intrauterine Effects of Cocaine

Since cocaine crosses the placenta in pregnant mothers (Behnke & Davis-Eyler, 1993), negative fetal effects might be expected. Vasoconstriction resulting in decreased oxygen to the uterus and placenta may lead to restricted nutrients to the fetus (Hurt, Malmud, Betancourt, Brodsky, & Giannetta, 2001). This vascular compromise stemming from cocaine exposure during early gestation could cause birth defects as well as complications of labor and delivery. Cocaine use during pregnancy may also lead to serious destructive lesions in the fetal brain, specifically cerebral infarction and intracranial hemorrhage, which may result in restricted blood flow to the developing brain (Hurt et al., 2001). Research supports the notion that neurological correlates are possible with fetal cocaine exposure (Dixon & Bejar, 1989; Chiriboga, 1998; Chiriboga, Burst, Bateman, & Hauser, 1999). Cocaine abuse in pregnant women is also reported to be associated with abruptio placenta, intrauterine growth retardation, congenital malformations (Behnke & Eyler, 1993), and an abnormal fetal heart rate (Mehta et al., 2001). These effects are summarized in Box 8-1.

Box 8-1   Intrauterine Effects of Cocaine Exposure

Abruptio placenta	Intrauterine growth retardation
Intracranial hemorrhages	Cerebral infarctions
Congenital malformations	Abnormal fetal heart rate

Abruptio placenta occurs when the placenta separates from the uterine wall and is delivered before the infant is born. This condition causes the neonate to be deprived of oxygen, which can lead to serious medical complications for the newborn. **Intrauterine growth retardation** is a condition that occurs when the fetus is deprived of oxygen and other nutrients, resulting in a low fetal weight and decreased size. The incidence of low birth weight has been reported in approximately 20 percent of infants born to cocaine-abusing mothers. Additionally, the mean birth weight of drug-exposed infants is significantly lower than that of nonexposed control infants delivered at term (38 to 40 weeks) (Chasnoff, Griffith, MacGregor, Drikes, & Burns, 1989). **Congenital malformations** are defects seen in the physical development of the fetus (Ornoy, 2002). Some researchers documented congenital anomalies of the urinary system, cardiac malformations, skull defects, and defects in the vascular system (Behnke & Eyler, 1993). However, a consistent pattern of congenital malformations is not yet identified, and no increased incidence or risk of malformations has been substantiated (Behnke, Eyler, Garvan, & Wobie, 2001). The pregnancy may be further compromised by an increased risk of miscarriage (at less than 16 weeks' gestation) and an elevated risk for fetal death.

The Effects of Cocaine on the Infant

Infants with cocaine exposure are at-risk for sustaining neurobehavioral and neuromotor deficits (Coles & Platzman, 1993; Fetters & Tronick, 1996). Neurobehavioral deficits are associated with state regulation and neuromotor deficits refer to motor skill development. Not all infants will experience neurologically based effects of cocaine exposure.

Neurobehavioral Effects in the Infant

Researchers have not identified a specific pattern of neurobehavioral effects in young children with cocaine exposure (Morrow, Bandstra, Anthony, Ofir, Xue, & Reyes, 2001), and some researchers indicate there is no specific link between in utero exposure and neurodevelopment (Frank, Augustyn, Knight, Pell, & Zuckerman, 2001). What is certain is that the caregiving environment influences neurobehavioral development in young children (Black et al., 1993; Rodning, Beckwith, & Howard, 1991). Nevertheless, impaired neurobehavioral functioning *may* be identified in children with cocaine exposure (Hurt, Giannetta, Brodsky, Malmud, & Pelham, 2001; Singer, Arendt, Minnes, Farkas, & Salvator, 2000; Coles & Platzman, 1993). As stated earlier, the biological action of cocaine alters central nervous system function (Espy, Francis, & Riese, 2000), which may lead to later neurodevelopmental problems; some newborns experience withdrawal symptoms that may further impact on neurobehavioral outcomes (Eyler, Behnke, Garvan, Woods, Wobie, & Conlon, 2001).

Specific neurobehavioral effects that may be seen in infants exposed to cocaine are poor state regulation (i.e., overstimulation, tremulousness, jitteriness, irritability) (Singer et al., 2000), decreased attention or level of alertness (Bandstra, Morrow, Anthony, Accornero, & Fried, 2001), poor sleeping habits (Scher, Richardson, & Day, 2000), and increased crying (White-Traut, Studer, Meleedy-Rey, Murrary, Labovsky, & Kahn, 2002).

Infants exposed to cocaine may have increased difficulty regulating their internal state of being and organizing a transition from one state to another. They may remain longer in emotional states such as crying or irritability with difficulty calming themselves or allowing themselves to be consoled by a caregiver. These infants may also have increased difficulty regulating sleep-wake cycles, remaining in sleep states longer and thus increasing their vulnerability to overstimulation when awake. Transitions from one emotional state to another may be abrupt, causing heightened emotional states that are difficult to calm. Because of their inability to calm themselves effectively or be consoled by a caregiver these infants may experience jitteriness and irritability and require intervention measures to calm hypersensitive emotional states.

In addition to poor internal state control, infants exposed to drugs may be hypersensitive to sensory stimulation. Negative reactions such as increased and prolonged crying may be seen with tactile/kinesthetic stimulation, auditory stimulation, and visual stimulation. The infant may experience difficulty integrating these incoming sensory stimuli, causing overstimulation and making daily care routines difficult. Hypersensitivity to sensory stimulation may require intervention by appropriate health care professionals such as occupational therapists.

Level of alertness or attention and orientation are behavioral states often measured in infants (Bayley, 1993). Young infants generally shift from states of sleep to increased levels of attention during alert states. It is during this alert state that young children are stimulated to learn and attend to incoming auditory and visual stimuli. Infants are left in their cribs for varying amounts of time to attend to visual stimuli such as mobiles or auditory stimuli such as quiet music. Drug-exposed infants may experience decreased levels of alertness, affecting their ability to learn, and less quiet sleep, increasing levels of irritability. They may be unable to attend to visual and/or auditory stimuli without becoming overstimulated. This overstimulation, again, leads to increased irritability and periods of crying.

Lester and Tronick (1994) outlined four areas most affected by prenatal drug exposure seen in infants: attention, arousal, affect, and action. Deficits in attention refer to reduced visual and auditory ability to process information from the environment; deficits in arousal are associated with poor sleep patterns, crying, and stimulation from external stimuli; affect is associated with development of social and emotional behaviors; and action relates to motor function. Lester and Tronick (1994) concluded that drug-exposed infants may experience difficulties in one or all of these developmental domains. Auditory processing and arousal and attention deficits are also identified in infants with cocaine exposure (Mayes, Bornstein, Chawarska, & Granger, 1995). These deficits may serve as an early identifying marker for risk of language delay and auditory processing difficulties.

Neuromotor/Physical Effects of Cocaine on the Infant

Infants with cocaine exposure may experience motor deficits (Arendt, Angelopoulso, Salvator, & Singer, 1999), but the effects of cocaine on motor development are small (Fetters & Tronick, 1996). Again, the trimester timing of exposure and other social factors are crucial in linking motor and physical deficits with cocaine exposure (Swanson, Strissguth, Sampson, & Olson, 1999). Infants with cocaine exposure may experience a poor suck reflex, resulting in feeding problems and general delays in motor development. There is a possible increased incidence of upper body **hypotonia** in younger infants that is thought to normalize after a few months (Belcher et al., 1999). Nevertheless, this seemingly temporary deficit may lead to delayed ability to control head movements and coordinate trunk control at critical points in time. Both of these motor skills are necessary for babies to sit up, crawl, and walk.

Prematurity and **low birth weight** (LBW) are commonly seen in babies with substance exposure and are strong risk factors for compromised development. A baby with a low birth weight is born weighing less than 5.5 pounds. LBW is not a diagnosis, but a label that categorizes children at risk for similar disabilities. LBW can result from intrauterine growth retardation and/or prematurity. Babies born with a low birth weight are at high risk generally because of their premature birth. Premature birth can result in serious illness at birth, feeding problems, developmental delays such as cerebral palsy, mental retardation, vision impairment, hearing impairment, learning disabilities, and behavioral problems. The lower the birth weight and the more prematurely a baby is delivered the greater the risk that the baby will experience adverse developmental outcomes. The effects of cocaine in the infant are summarized in Box 8-2.

Long-Term Effects of Prenatal Cocaine Exposure

Again, it is important to note that prenatal drug exposure does not automatically predispose a child to experience long-term effects. Maternal influence plays a larger role in outcomes over time (Accornero, Morrow, Bandstra, Johnson, & Anthony, 2002). Researchers are clear that many drug-exposed children look much like their nonexposed peers, and very little information substantiates any claim that long-term effects will be certain (Frank et al., 2001). The important point is that there is no typical developmental profile of a child exposed to drugs in utero, but prenatal cocaine exposure does put a child at-risk for long-term developmental delays and disabilities (Chapman, 2000a, 2000b). Though the research is unclear, researchers have identified possible long-term characteristics in children with prenatal substance exposure (Singer, Hawkins, Huang, Davillier, & Baley, 2001). It is important to reiterate that many mothers use multiple drugs that may also affect development. Tobacco (Brook, Brook, & Whiteman, 2000), alcohol, and marijuana (Fried, Watkinson, & Gray, 1999) are the most common, and are associated with long-term developmental problems. Children with prenatal cocaine exposure are at-risk for experiencing long-term cognitive (Chapman, 2000a) and speech and language (Bland-Stewart, Seymour, Beeghly, & Frank, 1998) delays. Long-term consequences are primarily dependent upon the history of prematurity, birth weight, head circumference, exposure to other substances, and environmental factors (see Box 8-3).

Cognitive Deficits with Prenatal Cocaine Exposure

Researchers have found that prenatal cocaine exposure puts children at-risk for experiencing long-term cognitive deficits (van Baar & de Graaff, 1994; Morrison, Cerles, Montaini-Klovdahl, & Skowron, 2000) when assessed using measures to evaluate IQ. However, researchers also found that both biological and environmental factors are linked to intellectual development in these children (Chasnoff, Anson, Hatcher, Stenson, Iaukea, & Randolph, 1998; Chiriboga, 1998), and some children may not experience cognitive deficits at all (Hurt, Malmud, Betancourt, Braitman, Brodsky, & Giannetta, 1997). However, those children who experience deficits in cognition may display difficulties in the areas of problem solving, concentration, memory, and attention. Specific deficits are difficult to identify because of varying profiles related to prenatal cocaine exposure.

Box 8-2 Effects of Cocaine Exposure in Infants

Poor state regulation	Sleeping difficulties
Feeding problems	Altered crying patterns
Prematurity	Small head circumference
Low birth weight	Poor motor performance
Poor caregiving environment	HIV/AIDS, hepatitis, venereal diseases
Poor attachment or bonding	

Box 8-3   Long-Term Effects of Cocaine Exposure

Speech and language delay	Neurobehavioral problems
Learning problems	Behavior problems
Motor problems	Impact of the environment

Toddlers with prenatal cocaine exposure may experience impaired representational play and disorganized play skills. Play provides insight into cognitive/mental development in young children (Betancourt et al., 1999). Mental organization or representational skills during play is important for later more complex cognitive functioning. Children with prenatal cocaine exposure may demonstrate simple play schemes with less pretend play, less purposeful play, and less exploration. Decreased attention may cause children to interact briefly with toys, demonstrated by picking them up and quickly throwing them down and moving on to another toy. There may be no integration or use of several toys to engage in complex play schemes (Howard, Beckwith, Rodning, & Kropenske, 1989). As substance-exposed children get older their play behaviors improve, though they may continue to use less imaginative play structures in more restricted ways, resulting in less rich play schemes (Rivers & Hedrick, 1992).

In addition to possible impaired play skills, according to some researchers drug-exposed toddlers may also demonstrate poor problem-solving skills and less sustained attention (Bandstra et al., 2001), though these claims are contradicted by other researchers (Betancourt et al., 1999).

Speech and Language Delays in Cocaine-Exposed Children

Cocaine exposure may put young children at-risk for speech and language delays (Singer, Arendt, Minnes, Salvator, Siegel, & Lewis, 2001; Angelilli, Fischer, Delaney-Black, Rubinstein, Ager, & Sokol, 1994; Johnson, Seikel, Madison, Foose, & Rinard, 1997) though no identifiable pattern of language or speech delay is identified in this population. Furthermore, research that examines language development in young children with cocaine exposure is limited. Again, language and speech development also depends on other social factors such as economic status and access to quality education, among other factors. Nevertheless, possible speech and language delays must be considered when discussing this population.

Bland-Stewart et al. (1998) found that young children with cocaine exposure exhibited delays in semantic development, though they did not identify deficits in language structure, cognition, or general language abilities. Other researchers also identified expressive and receptive language deficits (Bender, Word, Diclemente, Crittenden, Persaud, & Ponton, 1995; Johnson, Seikel, & Madison, 1997; Delaney-Black et al., 2000a). Dixon, Thal, Potrykus, Dickson, and Jacoby (1997) examined early language development in young children born to substance-abusing mothers and found significant delays in all aspects of language. In this study, the older children performed more poorly than the younger children, which suggested that language delays might become more distinct as children grow older. Phonological processes and/or delays have also been identified in these children (Bullock, 1994; Johnson et al., 1997; Madison, Johnson, Seikel, Arnold & Schultheis, 1998).

Language development is significantly correlated with a child's environment (Thyssen van Beveren, Little, & Spence, 2000). When children live in a drug-abusing, chaotic environment, their language skills as well as their ability to learn will be impacted. Most researchers point out that other substances such as tobacco (Johnson, 2000) and alcohol (Schonfeld, Mattson, Lang, Delis, & Riley, 2001) significantly impact language development. These factors must be taken into consideration when interpreting results and analyzing language development in young children with cocaine exposure.

As you can see, children born with prenatal cocaine exposure have the potential to present with many developmental disorders and delays. These issues can greatly impede their functional abilities, especially those involving language, cognition, and motor skills. Therefore, intervention by trained professionals is essential to meet the needs of these children in an effort to help them overcome the functional and social barriers.

FETAL ALCOHOL SYNDROME

Children born with prenatal alcohol exposure are at-risk for a myriad of delays in all areas of development, especially physical, cognitive, emotional, behavioral, and social maturity (Batshaw & Conlon, 1997; Kozma & Stock, 1993; Wunsch, Conlon, & Scheidt, 2002). These deficiencies greatly impede their functional abilities, especially those involving receptive and expressive language and communication. This section will discuss fetal alcohol syndrome (FAS), the causes, characteristic traits, and the effects of the substance on the fetus and child. It will also discuss assessment techniques and intervention plans essential to enhance development of the affected children.

Definition and Incidence of Fetal Alcohol Syndrome

Fetal alcohol syndrome is the leading cause of mental retardation in children worldwide (Kozma & Stock, 1993). According to Wunsch et al. (2002), the incidence of fetal alcohol syndrome is 1 to 5/1000 live births. Maternal alcohol consumption during pregnancy has the potential to cause birth anomalies that impede development, many of which can remain for life. Children who display developmental delays, which include physical and cognitive deficiencies, as well as central nervous system dysfunction and significant cognitive impairment as a result of prenatal alcohol exposure, are diagnosed with fetal alcohol syndrome. FAS has long-term consequences that include behavior disorders and language impairments. Central nervous system dysfunction is the most severe impeding factor in children with FAS. Some children exhibit average or low-average intelligence with learning disabilities, while others have varying degrees of mental retardation and learning disabilities (Richard & Hoge, 1999; Sparks, 1993; Wunsch et al., 2002). Those children who display less severe impairments and do not exhibit all of the physical signs of FAS are classified as having fetal alcohol effect (FAE) (see Figures 8-1 and 8-2). Individuals with FAE often present with subtle impairments or deficiencies in memory and fine motor skills and experience difficulty with reading and mathematics (Batshaw & Conlon, 1997). The specific criteria used to diagnosis FAS will be discussed in the following section.

Characteristics of Fetal Alcohol Syndrome

Children exposed to alcohol in utero are often born with low birth weight and delayed or aberrant nervous system development. As a result, physical, social, and cognitive problems are common. Delays in these areas can then impact future educational and learning ability as well as increase the risk of a hearing impairment. The diagnosis of FAS is a clinical judgment, which means that the disorder is not identified through laboratory tests. Fetal alcohol syndrome is diagnosed according to three specific criteria.

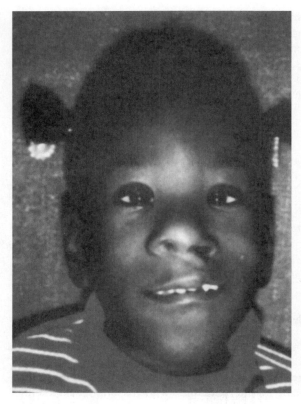

Figure 8-1
A young girl with fetal alcohol syndrome, whose mother drank heavily throughout her entire pregnancy.

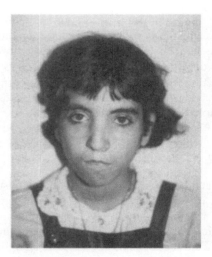

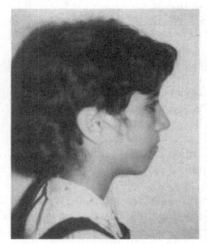

Figure 8-2
A young girl with fetal alcohol effects, whose mother drank heavily only during the last trimester.

Infants with FAS exhibit prenatal and postnatal growth deficiency, central nervous system dysfunction, and craniofacial abnormalities (Batshaw & Conlon, 1997; Kozma & Stock, 1993; Richard & Hoge, 1999; Weinberg, 1997).

Craniofacial Abnormalities in Fetal Alcohol Syndrome

Children with fetal alcohol syndrome exhibit facial anomalies that include **microcephaly** (a small head), narrow eyelids, and widely spaced eyes. In addition, they have a short palpebral fissure, which is the crease in the eye between the upper and lower eyelids, and the philtrum (the groove in the midline of the lips) and maxilla appear flat. A thin upper lip and a short, upturned nose are also prominent characteristics. Underdevelopment of the midface is also common, as well as small teeth with malocclusions, and a high incidence of cleft lip and/or palate. Subsequently, many of these facial characteristics impede speech and language development. Though some of the craniofacial characteristics diminish as the child reaches adolescence, microcephaly usually remains a permanent feature of FAS. Finally, some children with FAS have pinna and middle ear malformations, which increase the chance of recurrent **otitis media,** as well as conductive (due to physical anomalies) and sensorineural (resulting from CNS dysfunction) hearing loss (Batshaw & Conlon, 1997; Church, Eldis, Blakley, & Bawle, 1997; Kozma & Stock, 1993; Richard & Hoge, 1999; Weinberg, 1997; Wunsch et al., 2002).

Prenatal and Postnatal Growth Deficiency in Fetal Alcohol Syndrome

Infants with prenatal alcohol exposure are usually born following a term pregnancy. However, 80 percent of these babies have low birth weight (LBW), and 70 percent suffer from acute eating disorders, which often result in a diagnosis of failure to thrive due to LBW and failure to receive adequate nutrition. These children frequently have microcephaly, with head circumferences below the 5th percentile (Batshaw & Conlon, 1997). In addition, short stature and cervical vertebral defects are also characteristics of FAS. These children usually remain in the lower one-third percentile throughout their childhood in height, weight, and head circumference. In addition, minor joint and limb abnormalities, and vision complications, such as strabismus, nystagmus, and myopia, may also be present in children with FAS (Batshaw & Conlon, 1997; Richard & Hoge, 1999; Sparks, 1993; Wunsch et al., 2002).

Central Nervous System Dysfunction in Fetal Alcohol Syndrome

The effect of alcohol on central nervous system (CNS) development and functioning varies with each child. **Mental retardation** is the most serious and most common disability associated with FAS. However, the effects of alcohol and extent of intellectual impairment vary with each individual. Some children experience mild to severe mental retardation, while others display learning disabilities, but function at the lower end of average intelligence (Becker, Warr-Leeper, & Leeper, 1990; Kozma & Stock, 1993; Richard & Hoge, 1999).

As a result of CNS dysfunction, infants with prenatal alcohol exposure are often agitated and restless, and have abnormal sleep patterns. In addition, infants frequently display hypotonia and thus exhibit a poor sucking response, which impedes ability to receive adequate nutrition. Tremors may also be present in infants with prenatal alcohol exposure.

During childhood and early adolescence, delayed motor development, poor fine motor skills, and behavioral/emotional problems are often present as a result of CNS dysfunction. These can include, but are not limited to, oppositional and defiant behaviors, an inability to govern behavior, a strong will, persistent anxiousness, and seizures. CNS damage in school-age children can also be manifested in executive function deficits, slower reaction time, latent responses, attention deficits, hyperactivity, and poor memory skills. These characteristics, combined with varying degrees of mental retardation, and/or learning disabilities, compromise all areas of academic performance (Richard & Hoge, 1999; Schonfeld et al., 2001; Sparks, 1993; Wunsch et al., 2002).

Speech and Language Difficulties in Fetal Alcohol Syndrome

Speech and language disorders are also associated with FAS in both receptive and expressive domains. For example, children with FAS frequently exhibit resonance disorders, most often in the form of **hypernasality.** Subsequently, their speech may sound as though they are talking through their nose rather than their mouth. The presence of a cleft palate further enhances hypernasality. Articulation delays may also be present due to structural anomalies or delayed development of the speech mechanism. Hypotonia plays a factor in oral-motor development as well, which also compromises articulation (Batshaw & Conlon, 1997; Richard & Hoge, 1999).

Language difficulties are common among children with FAS, and can be manifested in many different forms. These can include delayed language acquisition or impaired language with cognitive impairment due to mental retardation. This means that children may experience delays or difficulties in the acquisition of language skills and concepts, as well as social interaction skills. Receptive language deficits encompass a multitude of developmental delays, some of which include learning, problem-solving, and reading comprehension difficulties. As a result, many children with FAS will experience difficulties grasping concepts in school. Those who are of lower average intelligence often experience learning disabilities, which promote setbacks in the academic setting. In addition, central auditory processing (CAP) disorders are common, which further impede the children's ability to decipher meaning and process incoming stimuli and information. Language disorders, slower reaction times, and subsequent misunderstanding are difficulties associated with FAS as well. In addition, these children often require extra instruction and assistance, particularly during reading and mathematics.

Furthermore, **executive function** difficulties, which include planning, sequencing, problem solving, reasoning, and self-monitoring skills, affect decision making, routine activities, and social interactions, and often contribute to behavioral problems as well. Children with FAS are often unable to determine cause/effect relationships or provide a rational solution to various problems. All of these areas affect academic performance (Richard, & Hoge, 1999; Schonfeld et al., 2001; Sparks, 1993; Wunsch et al., 2002).

Difficulties with syntactic, pragmatic, and semantic structures of language are also frequent. For example, children with fetal alcohol syndrome may experience difficulty with acquisition of the syntactic structure of language. They may fail to discriminate between proper sentence structure and word order, or use of irregular verbs, adverbs, and adjectives. Semantics are also affected, as children with FAS often fail to understand concepts and meanings at typical acquisition ages. This impedes communication ability and can cause greater difficulty in academic as well as social settings.

Impaired pragmatic, or social development and interaction skills are also prevalent among children with FAS. Many children with FAS experience social difficulties, and often fail to understand social cues from others. For example, they may be boisterous and talkative, and fail to give others a chance to speak. In addition, uncomfortable situations often arise when these children fail to read social cues that would otherwise inhibit or promote them to respond appropriately in various social contexts.

Assessment

Early assessment and intervention begins by educating pregnant women about the dangers of substance abuse and providing early treatment and prenatal care if necessary. Health care professionals should be prepared to refer mothers to appropriate professionals to ensure that they provide the best opportunities for their babies to grow and develop. The earlier the mother is able to stop substance dependency, the better, thereby decreasing the developmental risks for her baby. In addition, if the mother has undesirable living arrangements, a social worker could assist her with stabilizing her life, finding a more secure home, and identifying social resources as necessary. Virtually all mothers, including those who use drugs, really want the best for their children. When families are given the opportunities and support to provide the best, they will usually be compliant and follow recommendations. However, when intervention during pregnancy is not possible, intervention for the baby and family should be started as soon as a baby is born. Children and their families may be assessed in the hospital, public health clinics, early intervention programs, or private physician referrals.

There is no specific developmental assessment protocol for young children with prenatal substance exposure. A developmental assessment early in infancy is one of the most important issues, and should be family centered. The assessment must include the developmental needs of both the child and the family. Family needs must be identified because that is the foundation for the infant's development. Early diagnosis of any developmental delays and family risk factors will prepare professionals to provide adequate intervention services as soon as possible. When possible, service providers should use a team assessment model to ensure a collaborative assessment plan.

A case history should be part of any developmental assessment with suspected substance exposure. The history should attempt to establish the family's history of cocaine use and identify any signs of developmental delay. Often, these children will be in the custody of individuals other than the biological parents. As a result, this information may be difficult to obtain, but it can be supplemented by other sources if possible. It is desirable to establish the cocaine history of the biological mother such as determining if there was a drug problem and what the drug use pattern/habit was during pregnancy. As discussed earlier, cocaine abusers typically use other drugs, legal and illegal, and it is important to gather this information as well.

Neonates and infants may experience impaired state regulation and sensory integration (e.g., attention, interaction, self-regulation), feeding problems, jitteriness, impaired motor performance, and poor attachment or bonding. They may also experience impaired sleep-wake cycles, which compounds the above problems. Sparks (1993, 2000) suggested that test measures be used that evaluate triggers for stress and frustration, positive response to calming techniques, energy levels, tolerance for handling, and what supports should be put into place to facilitate adequate functioning. Developmental assessments in the area of behavior, state regulation, and motor skills are important for infants.

Standardized and/or criterion-referenced developmental assessment measures are appropriate to use with infants and children with a history of cocaine exposure. Play-based assessment measures are also appropriate. Some acceptable evaluation tools for infants are the Neonatal Behavior Assessment Scales (Brazelton, 1984) and the Bayley Scales of Infant Development-II (Bayley, 1993). In neonates and infants all developmental areas should be assessed, including motor skills, neurobehavioral skills, cognitive skills, and socio-emotional skills. More than one assessment measure should be used, as all tests may not be as comprehensive as this population requires.

As children grow older it becomes important to assess speech and language skills as well as play skills. Again, standardized assessment measures such as the Preschool Language Scale (Zimmerman, Steiner, & Pond, 1992) or the Clinical Evaluation of Language Fundamentals-Preschool (Wiig, Secord, & Semel, 1992) may be appropriate. Language assessments should address any deficits in the areas of pragmatics, semantics, syntax, morphology, and phonology. Sparks (2000) suggested that caregiver interaction with the child must also be evaluated and this can be done through videotaping the caregiver and child during an interactive activity.

In many instances, children with a history of cocaine exposure may experience multiple developmental delays and should be evaluated by appropriate professionals such as occupational therapists, physical therapists, SLPs, vision specialists, audiologists, nutritionists, psychologists, social workers, and physicians. Early intervention programs such as Early Head Start and Head Start are designed to provide collaborative, coordinated multidisciplinary assessment services as well as an analysis of family needs. Family risk factors that should be assessed by the appropriate professionals include health care, parenting training, job training and assistance locating employment, mental health and substance abuse counseling and/or treatment, transportation, respite care, and public assistance. These family risk factors will undermine any early intervention program for the child and can impede a child's development if not addressed. Most states have regulated early intervention programs that may provide these comprehensive services through a case management system.

Finally, professionals should refrain from using pejorative labels such as *drug-exposed baby* or *crack baby* or diagnosing infants and children as delayed or disabled. Infants should be diagnosed as at-risk to obtain early intervention services.

Intervention

Intervention plans should be family centered to include the child and family. All parents want the best for their children and should be the center of any intervention plan. Intervention goals should be based on professional findings and the therapeutic outcomes that the family desires. When designing intervention plans, goals should be developed in coordination with the families.

Early intervention goals for infants in the first month of life should address attention, arousal, affect, and motor skills. Goals for attention should address visual and auditory ability such as visual and auditory tracking. Goals for arousal should address sleep patterns. Therapeutic goals to address affect should facilitate the development of social and emotional behaviors and attachment and bonding, decreasing increased reaction to stimulation, and decreasing irritability. Goals to address action relate to motor function and could include posture, handling, feeding, and sensory-motor integration. Feeding therapy goals should be designed to decrease oral sensitivity and defensiveness and to facilitate adequate suck/swallow reflexes to ensure adequate nutritional intake. **Physical therapists** and **occupational therapists** assist with handling and positioning and motor skills. Occupational therapists may be involved in feeding therapy.

As infants grow older motor performance should continue to be addressed by a physical therapist. Physical therapists can design activities to address issues with muscle tone in the limbs and trunk, positioning, and handling. Speech-language pathologists can begin to facilitate early communication skills such as gestures, attentional interactions, infant vocalizations, rituals, and game playing in infants by promoting appropriate infant-caregiver dyads.

Intervention beyond infancy may be needed in children with a history of substance exposure. The goal of intervention for toddlers and preschoolers should continue in all developmental domains. These children may require a structured, predictable classroom environment with decreased environmental stimulation. Early intervention programs with toddlers and preschoolers should be collaborative and comprehensive with developmental services for all specialists. Services should address motor, neurological, neurobehavioral, language, cognition, hearing, vision, and any medical needs.

In any early intervention program, parent education and training is the foundation for success. Parents should be encouraged to observe professionals providing therapeutic services and be provided with hands-on training to facilitate carryover. Early intervention programs should address not only the needs of the child but also those of the family, and assist them in getting any needs met. Family members should also be taught to advocate for services for their children. Parents can provide appropriate environments and early developmental activities with the proper training.

Lastly, professionals should avoid stereotyping families who have children with a history of drug exposure. Professionals must be sensitive to the special needs and sometimes overwhelming challenges of these families and be willing to provide therapy with an unbiased frame of mind.

CONCLUSION

Children born with prenatal substance exposure are at-risk for many developmental delays. These children are at-risk because researchers have concluded that not all young children will experience developmental delays as a result of substance exposure. Very often, substance abusers use many different kinds of drugs, making it difficult to establish a specific profile in affected young children. Many of these potential developmental delays are directly linked to the field of speech-language pathology. Professionals in the field must familiarize themselves with the many possible developmental effects, especially those concerning language and cognition, in order to provide maximum intervention services that are tailored to meet the needs of individual children and their families.

Case Study 1: Fetal Alcohol Syndrome

Karen, age 28, the mother of four children under age 6, arrived at the hospital in early labor during her seventh month of pregnancy. At the time of delivery Karen was enrolled in a residential alcohol treatment facility designed to assist pregnant mothers who are dependent on alcohol and in danger of losing custody of their children. Karen was ordered into the alcohol treatment program by the courts when she was two months' pregnant because she frequently left her children alone in their apartment for long periods of time while she went out for various reasons. Up until her enrollment into the treatment program Karen had not received any prenatal care. Furthermore, she admitted to drinking hard alcohol prior to her pregnancy and she reported that her drinking had increased significantly after she discovered she was pregnant. She indicated that she began drinking heavily because she became severely depressed over the thought of having another child and being unemployed and unmarried. Karen said that she only drank beer while she was pregnant and did not associate beer drinking with alcoholism.

Karen gave birth to a little girl, Drew, who was born prematurely at 30 weeks' gestation. At birth, Drew weighed 3 pounds, 2 ounces, and was classified as having a very low birth weight, indicating intrauterine growth retardation. The baby exhibited characteristics of microcephaly and she also had very distinct facial characteristics such as wide-spaced eyes, a flattened philtrum, and a very thin upper lip.

Drew's premature birth was complicated by respiratory problems secondary to underdeveloped lung capacity, which placed her at-risk for inadequate oxygen supply to the brain and other vital organs. To counteract this problem Drew was placed on a respirator to assist with her breathing, and she remained in the neonatal intensive care unit (NICU) until her general health status began to stabilize. At about 3 weeks of age she was removed from the respirator and transferred to the regular nursery. However, a weak suck reflex attributed to generalized hypotonia continued to compromise feeding, leading to slow weight gain, so Drew was subsequently placed on a nasogastric tube to supplement her oral feedings. Drew's stay in the nursery was further complicated by neurobehavioral alterations such as irritability indicated by increased inconsolable crying and abnormal sleep patterns. Furthermore, Drew experienced tremors that were thought to be symptoms of withdrawal.

Drew was treated by an SLP during the eight weeks she was in the NICU and the regular nursery. While Drew was in the NICU, the SLP's primary goal was to transition the baby off of the nasogastric tube and to encourage only oral feedings. Once Drew was transferred to the regular nursery, the SLP engaged the baby in intense feeding therapy to improve oral muscular strength, to facilitate a stronger suck reflex, and to coordinate suck-swallow-breathing patterns. She also implemented sensory stimulation and calming techniques to decrease irritability during feeding. The SLP also worked closely with a respiratory therapist to monitor oxygen levels using a pulse oximeter during feeding. Since Drew exhibited hypotonia, the SLP consulted with a physical therapist and an occupational therapist to facilitate improved positioning and posture during feeding.

Since Drew was obviously at-risk for global developmental delays she would qualify for early intervention services through the state's developmental disabilities office. Upon her discharge from the hospital she was assigned to a caseworker who worked toward setting up home-based speech therapy through the state infant and toddler intervention program. Home therapy began one month postdischarge when Drew was 3 months of age. In addition to being followed once a week by an early interventionist, Drew continued to receive oral motor and feeding therapy by an SLP twice weekly. In addition to the feeding difficulties, the SLP also observed that Drew was not attaining early social communication skills so therapy was initiated to facilitate these behaviors. Also, the SLP recommended a transdisciplinary-based assessment so that Drew could begin receiving home-based therapy for continuing gross and fine motor delays and any emerging cognitive deficits. By the time Drew was 4 months of age a comprehensive therapeutic support program had been initiated that would follow her until she transitions out of early intervention at age 3.

Initially, Drew's mother was overwhelmed with the array of services. An individualized family service plan was developed to coordinate services for Drew and to provide additional supports for the mother, which enabled her to cope with the situation much better. It was anticipated that Drew would receive home-based services until she was 12 months, at which time she would be reassessed for an appropriate center-based early intervention program.

Case Study 2: Prenatal Cocaine Exposure

Isabella is a 2.5-year-old toddler who was abandoned by her biological mother in an urban public hospital shortly after her birth. In the advanced stages of labor of a full-term pregnancy, the mother admitted herself into the hospital under an alias and left the hospital within hours after giving birth. Because this mother was in the hospital for such a short period of time hospital officials had little knowledge regarding the baby's background. The mother delivered the baby shortly after her admission and the hospital was able to get a sample of the mother's blood and urine before she left the hospital. Furthermore, officials did determine that the mother received no prenatal care during pregnancy. It was also noted that the mother's erratic behavior indicated that she was impaired by possible drug use. In addition, she was undernourished, unclean, and displayed no interest in her health status other than to deliver the baby. Lab reports on the mother revealed significant blood levels of cocaine and alcohol. Her long-term substance abuse history remained unknown.

The baby was born full term with a birth weight of 5 pounds, 2 ounces. Her hospital course was unremarkable except that a significant amount of cocaine and alcohol were detected per lab reports. The baby remained in the hospital under observation for three weeks and was subsequently adopted by a loving and stable family with a 5-year-old little girl. Her adoptive family named her Isabella.

Isabella was determined to be at-risk for developmental delays because of her birth history and qualified for early intervention services through the state infant and toddler program. She began receiving home-based early intervention services at 4 months of age and was seen by an early interventionist twice a week. The early interventionist developed an individualized family service plan designed to provide cognitive and language stimulation as well as fine and gross motor activities. The early interventionist followed Isabella in a home-based setting until she was 18 months of age. Isabella was observed to adequately progress cognitively and her motor skills fell within the normal range as well. The early interventionist began to become concerned about possible language delays because Isabella did not seem to achieve language milestones expected of an 18-month-old toddler. A hearing evaluation revealed hearing sensitivity to be within normal limits. The early interventionist recommended that Isabella receive a comprehensive speech and language evaluation to determine eligibility for center-based early intervention services.

Isabella was visited by an SLP to conduct a speech and language evaluation in the home. The Preschool Language Scale-3 (PLS), a standardized test, was administered to assess language skill and to determine eligibility for infant and toddler services. In addition, a language sample was collected while engaging the child with the examiner and then with the caregivers. On the PLS, Isabella's scores fell slightly below the 10th percentile and the language sample revealed commensurate delays. Because Isabella did not exhibit delays in at least two developmental domains she did not qualify for Early Head Start services even though the SLP recommended center-based intervention services that included speech therapy to address language delays. However, Isabella's parents were able to locate a private center that offered language intervention services. Isabella received language services to address language delays and the parents were encouraged to continue to provide a language-rich home by reading to Isabella, talking to her during caregiving routines, naming objects and people, and keeping her busy with peer play groups. Isabella began to make positive progress with her language skills once the SLP's recommendations were implemented.

REVIEW QUESTIONS

1. What is the difference between substance abuse and substance dependency?

2. Discuss why not all children with a history of cocaine exposure will experience developmental delays.

3. Discuss at least two possible language outcomes in children with prenatal cocaine exposure.

4. Identify four neurobehavioral deficits that may be found in infants with prenatal cocaine exposure.

5. Why is the caregiving environment so important for developing young children?

6. What is the difference between fetal alcohol syndrome and fetal alcohol effects?

7. Discuss CNS impairments in young children with fetal alcohol syndrome.

8. What are the facial characteristics in young children with fetal alcohol syndrome?

9. Why is it difficult to specifically link developmental delays to substance exposure?

10. Compare and contrast neurological correlates between children with fetal alcohol exposure and prenatal cocaine exposure.

REFERENCES

Abel, E. L., & Sokol, R. J. (1987). Incidence of fetal alcohol syndrome and economic impact of FAS-related anomalies. *Drug Alcohol Dependency, 19*, 51–70.

Accornero, V. H., Morrow, C. E., Bandstra, E. S., Johnson, A. L., & Anthony, J. C. (2002). Behavioral outcome of preschoolers exposed prenatally to cocaine: Role of maternal behavioral health. *Journal of Pediatric Psychology, 27*(3), 259–269.

Angelilli, M. L., Fischer, H., Delaney-Black, V., Rubinstein, M., Ager, J. W., & Sokol, R. J. (1994). History of in utero cocaine exposure in language-delayed children. *Clinical Pediatrics, 33*(9), 514–516.

Bandstra, E. S., Morrow, C. E., Anthony, J. C., Accornero, V. H., & Fried, P. A. (2001). Longitudinal investigation of task persistence and sustained attention in children with prenatal cocaine exposure. *Neurotoxicology and Teratology, 23*, 545–559.

Batshaw, M. L., & Conlon, C. J. (1997). Substance abuse. In M. L. Batshaw (Ed.), *Children with disabilities* (pp. 143–148). Baltimore: Paul H. Brookes.

Bayley, N. (1993). *Bayley Scales of Infant Development* (2nd ed.). New York: Psychological Corporation.

Becker, M., Warr-Leeper, G. A., & Leeper, H. A. (1990). Fetal alcohol syndrome: A description of oral motor, articulatory, short-term memory, grammatical, and semantic abilities. *Journal of Communication Disorders, 23*, 97–124.

Behnke, M., & Davis-Eyler, F. (1993). The consequences of prenatal substance use for the developing fetus, newborn, and young child. *International Journal of the Addictions, 28*(13), 1341–1391.

Behnke, M., Eyler, F. D., Garvan, C. V., & Wobie, K. (2001). The search for congenital malformations in newborns with fetal alcohol exposure. *Pediatrics, 107*(5), 1341–1391.

Belcher, H. M. E., Shapiro, B. K., Leppert, M., Butz, A. M., Sellers, S., Arch, E., Kolodner, K., Pulsifer, M., Lears, M. K., & Kaufmann, W. E. (1999). Sequential neuromotor examination in children with intrauterine cocaine/polydrug exposure. *Developmental Medicine & Child Neurology, 41*, 240–246.

Bender, S. L, Word, C. O., Diclemente, R. J., Crittenden, M. R., Persaud, N. A., & Ponton, L. E. (1995). The developmental implications of prenatal and/or postnatal crack cocaine exposure in preschool children: A preliminary report. *Developmental and Behavioral Pediatrics, 16*(6), 418–424.

Bergin, C., Cameron, C. E., Fleitz, R. S., & Patel, A. V. (2001). Measuring prenatal drug exposure. *Journal of Pediatric Nursing,16*(4), 245–255.

Beshavarov, D. J. (1990). Crack children in foster care: Re-examining the balance between children's rights and parents' rights. *Children Today*, 21–35.

Betancourt, L., Fischer, R., Giannetta, J., Malmud, E., Brodsky, N. L., & Hurt, H. (1999). Problem-solving ability of inner-city children with and without in utero cocaine exposure. *Developmental and Behavioral Pediatrics, 20*(6), 418–424.

Black, M., Schuler, M., & Nair, P. (1993). Prenatal drug exposure: Neurodevelopmental outcome and parenting environment. *Journal of Pediatric Psychology, 18*(5), 605–620.

Bland-Stewart, L. M., Seymour, H. N., Beeghly, M., & Frank, D. A. (1998). Semantic development of African-American children prenatally exposed to cocaine. *Seminar in Speech and Language, 19*(2), 167–186.

Brazelton, T. B. (1984). *Neonatal Behavioral Assessment Scale* (2nd ed). Philadelphia: Lippincott.

Brook, J. S., Brook, D. W., & Whiteman, M. (2000). The influence of maternal smoking during pregnancy on the toddler's negativity. *Archives of Pediatric and Adolescent Medicine, 154*(4), 381–385.

Bullock, T. J. (1994). Phonological development in children of substance abusing mothers. *Echo, 2,* 21–24.

Chan, K., Dodd, P. A., Day, L., Kullama, L., Ervin, M. G., Padbury, J., & Ross, M. G. (1992). Fetal catecholamine, cardiovascular, and neurobehavioral response to cocaine. *American Journal of Obstetrics and Gynecology, 167*(6), 1616–1623.

Chapman, J. K. (2000a). Developmental outcomes in two groups of infants and toddlers: Prenatally cocaine exposed and noncocaine exposed, Part 1. *Infant-Toddler Intervention, 10*(1), 19–36.

Chapman, J. K. (2000b). Developmental outcomes in two groups of infants and toddlers: Prenatally cocaine exposed and noncocaine exposed, Part 2. *Infant-Toddler Intervention, 10*(2), 81–96.

Chasnoff, I. J. (1988). Drug use in pregnancy: Parameters of risk. *Pediatric Clinics of North America, 35,* 1403–1412.

Chasnoff, I. J., Anson, A., Hatcher, R., Stenson, H., Iaukea, K., & Randolph, L. A. (1998). Prenatal exposure to cocaine and other drugs: Outcome at four to six years. *Annals of the New York Academy of Science, 846,* 314–328.

Chasnoff, I. J., Griffith, D. R., MacGregor, S., Drikes, K., & Burns, K. A. (1989). Temporal patterns of cocaine use in pregnancy. *Journal of the American Medical Association, 261,* 1741–1744.

Chavkin, W. (2001). Cocaine and pregnancy—Time to look at the evidence. *Journal of the American Medical Association, 285*(2), 1626.

Chiriboga, C. A. (1998). Neurological correlates of fetal cocaine exposure. *Annals of the New York Academy of Science, 846,* 109–125.

Chiriboga, C. A., Brust, C. M., Bateman, D., & Hauser, W. A. (1999). Dose-response effect of fetal cocaine exposure on newborn neurologic function. *Pediatrics, 103*(1), 79–81.

Church, M.W., Eldis, F., Blakley, B.W., & Bawle, E.V. (1997). Hearing, language, speech, vestibular, and dentofacial disorders in fetal alcohol syndrome. *Alcoholism: Clinical and Experimental Research, 21*(2), 227–237.

Coles, C.D., & Platzman, K.A. (1993). Behavioral development in children prenatally exposed to drugs and alcohol. *International Journal of the Addictions, 28*(13), 1393–1433.

Delaney-Black, V., Covington, C., Templin, T., Kershaw, T., Nordstrom-Klee, B., Ager, J., et al. (2000a). Expressive language development of children exposed to cocaine prenatally: Literature review and report of a prospective cohort study. *Journal of Communication Disorders, 33,* 463–481.

Delaney-Black, V., Covington, C., Templin, T., Ager, J., Nordstrom-Klee, B., Martier, S., Leddick, L., Czerwinski, R. H., & Sokol, R. J. (2000b). Teacher-assessed behavior of children prenatally exposed to cocaine. *Pediatrics, 106*(4), 782–791.

Dixon, S. D., & Bejar, R. (1989). Echoencephalographic findings in neonates associated with maternal cocaine and methamphetamine use: Incidence and clinical correlates. *Journal of Pediatrics, 115,* 770–778.

Dixon, S., Thal, D., Potrykus, J., Dickson, T. B., & Jacoby, J. (1997). Early language development in children with prenatal exposure to stimulant drugs. *Developmental Neuropsychology, 13*(3), 371–396.

Doweiko, H. (1999). *Concepts of chemical dependency* (4th ed.). Pacific Grove, CA: Brooks/Cole.

Espy, K. A., Francis, D. J., & Riese, M. (2000). Prenatal cocaine exposure and prematurity: Neurodevelopmental growth. *Developmental and Behavioral Pediatrics, 21*(4), 262–270.

Eyler, F. D., Behnke, M., Garvan, C. W., Woods, N. S., Wobie, K., & Conlon, M. (2001). Newborn evaluations of toxicity and withdrawal related to prenatal cocaine exposure. *Neurotoxicology and Teratology, 23,* 399–411.

Fetters, L., & Tronick, E. Z. (1996). Neuromotor development of cocaine-exposed and control infants from birth through 15 months: Poor and poorer performance. *Journal of Pediatrics, 98*(5), 938–943.

Frank, D. A., Augustyn, M., Knight, W. G., Pell, T., & Zuckerman, B. (2001). Growth, development, and behavior in early childhood following prenatal cocaine exposure: A systematic review. *Journal of the American Medical Association, 285*(12), 1626–1628.

Fried, P. A., James, D. S., & Watkinson, B. (2001). Growth and pubertal milestones during adolescence in offspring prenatally exposed to cigarettes and marijuana. *Neurotoxicology and Teratology, 23,* 431–436.

Gingras, J. L., Weese-Mayer, D. E., Hume, R. F., & O'Donnell, K. J. (1992). Cocaine and development: Mechanisms of fetal toxicity and neonatal consequences of prenatal cocaine exposure. *Early Human Development, 31,* 1–24.

Gittler, J., & McPherson, M. (1990). Prenatal substance abuse: An overview of the problem. *Children Today, 19*(4), 3–8.

Howard, J., Beckwith, L., Rodning, C., & Kropenske, V. (1989). The development of young children of substance abusing parents: Insights from seven years of intervention and research. *Zero to Three, 9*(5), 8–12.

Hurt, H., Giannetta, J., Brodsky, N. L., Malmud, E., & Pelham, T. (2001). Are there neurologic correlates of in utero cocaine exposure at age 6 years? *Journal of Pediatrics, 138*(6), 911–913.

Hurt, H., Malmud, E., Betancourt, L., Braitman, L. E., Brodsky, N. L., & Giannetta, J. (1997a). Children with in utero cocaine exposure do not differ from control subjects on intelligence testing. *Archives of Pediatric and Adolescent Medicine, 151*(12), 1237–1241.

Hurt, H., Malmud, E., Betancourt, L., Brodsky, N. L., & Giannetta, J. (1997b). A prospective evaluation of early language development in children with in utero cocaine exposure and in control subjects. *Journal of Pediatrics, 130*(2), 310–322.

Hurt, H., Malmud, E., Betancourt, L. M., Brodsky, N. L., & Giannetta, J. M. (2001). A prospective comparison of developmental outcome of children with in utero cocaine exposure and controls using the Battelle Developmental Inventory. *Developmental and Behavioral Pediatrics, 22*(1), 27–34.

Johnson, J. M., Seikel, A., & Madison, C. L. (1997). Standardized test performance of children with a history of prenatal exposure to multiple drugs/cocaine. *Journal of Communication Disorders, 31,* 231–244.

Johnson, J. M., Seikel, J. A., Madison, C. L., Foose, S. M., & Rinard, K. D. (1997). Standardized test performance of children with a history of prenatal exposure to multiple drugs/cocaine. *Journal of Communication Disorders, 30*(1), 45–72.

Keller, R. W., & Snyder-Keller, A. (2000). Prenatal cocaine exposure. *Annals of the New York Academy of Science, 909,* 217–232.

Kozma, C., & Stock, J. S. (1993). What is mental retardation? In R. Smith (Ed.), *Children with mental retardation* (pp. 32–33). Bethesda, MD: Woodbine House.

Leckman, E. B., Mayes, L. C., & Hodgins, H. S. (2001). Perceptions and attitudes toward prenatal cocaine exposure in young children. *Child Psychiatry and Human Development, 31*(4), 313–328.

Lester, B. M., & Tronick, E. Z. (1994). The effects of prenatal cocaine exposure on child outcome. *Infant Mental Health Journal, 15*(2), 107–119.

Lester, B. M., LaGasse, L. L., & Seifer, R. (1998). Cocaine exposure and children: The meaning of subtle effects. *Science, 282*(5389): 633–634.

Madison, C. L., Johnson, J. M., Seikel, J. A., Arnold, M., & Schultheis, L. (1998). Comparative study of the phonology of preschool children prenatally exposed to cocaine and multiple drugs and non-exposed children. *Journal of Communication Disorders, 31*(3), 231–243.

Mayes, L. C., Bornstein, M. H., Chawarska, K., & Granger, R. H. (1995). Information processing and developmental assessments in 3-month-old infants exposed prenatally to cocaine. *Pediatrics, 95*(4), 539–545.

Mehta, S. K., Super, D. M., Salvator, A., Singer, L., Connuck, D. Fradley, L. G., et al. (2001). Heart rate variability in cocaine-exposed newborn infants. *American Heart Journal, 142*(5), 828–832.

Morrison, D. C., Cerles, L., Montaini-Klovdahl, L., & Skowron, E. (2000). Prenatally drug-exposed toddlers: Cognitive and social development. *American Journal of Orthopsychiatry, 70*(2), 278–283.

Morrow, C. E., Bandstra, E. S., Anthony, J. C., Ofir, A. Y., Xue, L., & Reyes, M. L. (2001). Influence of prenatal cocaine exposure on full-term infant neurobehavioral functioning. *Neurotoxicology and Teratology, 23,* 533–544.

National Institute on Drug Abuse. (1999). NIDA Research Report Series, *Cocaine abuse and addiction,* NIH Pub. No. 99-4342. Washington, DC.

Nulman, I., Rovet, J., Greenbaum, R., Loebstein, M., Wolpin, J., Pace-Asciak, P., & Koren, G. (2001). Neurodevelopment of adopted children exposed in utero to cocaine: The Toronto Adoption Study. *Clinical Investigative Medicine, 24*(3), 129–137.

Ondersma, S. J., Malcoe, L. H., & Simpson, S. M. (2001). Child protective services' response to prenatal drug exposure: Results from a nationwide survey. *Child Abuse & Neglect, 25,* 657–668.

Ornoy, A. (2002). The effects of alcohol and illicit drugs on the human embryo and fetus. *Israel Journal of Psychiatry and Related Sciences, 39*(2), 120–132.

Richard, G. J., & Hoge, D. R. (1999). Fetal alcohol syndrome. In *The source for syndromes.* East Moline, IL: LinguiSystems.

Rivers, M., & Hedrick, D. (1992). Language and behavioral concerns for drug-exposed infants and toddlers. In L. M. Rossetti (Ed.), *Developmental problems of drug-exposed infants* (pp. 63–73). Clifton Park, NY: Delmar Learning.

Rodning, C., Beckwith, L., & Howard, J. (1991). Quality of attachment and home environments in children prenatally exposed to PCP and cocaine. *Development and Psychopathology, 3,* 351–366.

Scher, M. S., Richardson, G. A., & Day, N. L. (2000). Effects of prenatal cocaine/crack and other drug exposure on electroencephalographic sleep studies at birth and one year. *Pediatrics, 105*(1), 39–48.

Schonfeld, A. M., Mattson, S. N., Lang, A. R., Delis, D. C., & Riley, E. P. (2001). Verbal and non-verbal fluency in children with heavy prenatal alcohol exposure. *Journal of Studies on Alcohol, 62,* 239–246.

Singer, L. T., Arendt, R., Minnes, S., Farkas, K., & Salvator, A. (2000). Neurobehavioral outcomes of cocaine-exposed infants. *Neurotoxicology Teratology, 22*(5), 653–666.

Singer, L. T., Arendt, R., Minnes, S., Salvator, A., Siegel, C., & Lewis, B. A. (2001). Developing language skills of cocaine-exposed infants. *Pediatrics, 107*(5), 1057.

Singer, L. T., Hawkins, S., Huang, J., Davillier, M., & Baley, J. (2001). Developmental outcomes and environmental correlates of very low birthweight, cocaine-exposed infants. *Early Human Development, 64*(2), 91–103.

Sparks, S. N. (1993). *Children of prenatal substance abuse.* Clifton Park, NY: Delmar Learning.

Sparks, S. N. (2000). Prenatal substance use and its impact on young children. In T. L. Layton, E. Crais, & L. R. Watson (Eds.), *Handbook of early language impairment in children: Nature* (pp. 287–316). Clifton Park, NY: Delmar Learning.

Streissguth, A. (1997). *Fetal alcohol syndrome: A guide for families and communities.* Baltimore: Paul H. Brookes.

Substance Abuse and Mental Health Services Administration. Preliminary Results from the 1997 National Household Survey on Drug Abuse. SAMHSA, 1998.

Swanson, M. W., Streissguth, A. P., Sampson, P. D., & Olson, H. C. (1999). Prenatal cocaine and neuromotor outcome at four months: Effect of duration of exposure. *Journal of Developmental Behavioral Pediatrics, 20*(5), 325–334.

Thyssen van Beveren, T., Little, B. B., & Spence, M. J. (2000). Effects of prenatal cocaine exposure and postnatal environment on child development. *American Journal of Human Biology, 12*(3), 417–428.

van Baar, A., & de Graaff, B. M. (1994). Cognitive development at preschool-age of infants of drug-dependent mothers. *Developmental Medicine and Child Neurology, 36*(12), 1063–1075.

Weinberg, N. Z. (1997). Cognitive and behavioral deficits associated with parental alcohol use. *Journal of the American Academy of Child and Adolescent Psychiatry, 36*(9), 1177–1187.

White-Traut, R., Studer, T., Meleedy-Rey, P., Murrary, P., Labovsky, S., & Kahn, J. (2002). Pulse rate and behavioral state correlates after auditory, tactile, visual, and vestibular intervention in drug exposed neonates. *Journal of Perinatology, 22,* 291–299.

Wiig, E., Secord, W. A., & Semel, E. (1992). *Clinical Evaluation of Language Fundamentals-Preschool.* San Antonio, TX: Psychological Corporation.

Wunsch, M. J., Conlon, C. J., & Scheidt, P. C. (2002). In M. L. Batshaw (Ed.), *Children with disabilities* (5th ed., pp. 111–113). Baltimore: Paul H. Brookes.

Zimmerman, I. L., Steiner, V. G., & Pond, R. E. (1992). *Preschool Language Scale-3.* San Antonio, TX: Psychological Corporation.

PART V

Communication Disorders Secondary
to Psychiatric Disorders

Chapter 9

Psychiatric Disorders in the Speech-Language Impaired Youngster

Marie Kerins, Ed.D., CCC-SLP

Upon completing this chapter, the reader should be able to:

1. Paraphrase the federal definition of emotional disturbance and provide at least one reason why some professionals do not like it
2. Name the four major psychiatric areas involved in speech and language disorders
3. List several speech and language characteristics observed in each of the four categories
4. Provide several descriptors associated with internalizing and externalizing behaviors
5. List five other professionals likely to be on the multidisciplinary team and give their functions
6. State one of the most widely used classification systems for psychiatric disorders
7. Describe what a functional behavior assessment is
3 Describe three commonly used intervention strategies for individuals with pragmatic language deficits

INTRODUCTION

The **speech-language pathologist** (SLP) must understand the connection between speech and language development/disorders and psychiatric disorders. Language is intricately and intimately tied to socio-emotional development, frequently making a differential diagnosis between a psychiatric disorder and a speech-language disorder difficult to discern. Over the past 30 years, researchers have demonstrated that a relationship between the two areas exists (Baker & Cantwell, 1987; Baltaxe & Simmons, 1988; Camarata, Hughes & Ruhl, 1988; Prizant, Audet, Burke, Hummel, Maher, & Theodore, 1990). Today most professionals recognize that a relationship exists, but struggle to reach a consensus on the degree of influence one has over the other. The argument over degree may remain, but language and socio-emotional development are woven so closely that knowledge of these interactions is vital for understanding, assessment, and treatment of the individual with characteristics of psychiatric disorders and speech and language disorders.

This chapter begins by reviewing definitions used in identifying children with emotional and behavioral problems. Then four of the most commonly found psychiatric disorders in children and adolescents that occur with speech and language disorders are described in greater detail. The disorders will be described according to general characteristics, speech-language characteristics, and other relevant details often associated with the psychiatric disorder. The latter part of the chapter provides an overview of assessment procedures, followed by interventions used by SLPs.

SCHOOL-AGE POPULATION

School-age children are identified and provided services under the federal law that ensures an appropriate education to all children based upon individual ability and need. This is commonly known as the **Individual with Disabilities Act (IDEA),** which was most recently revised in 1997. Under this federal law 13 handicapping conditions are described. One of these conditions is referred to as **emotional disturbance.** School personnel use IDEA to qualify individuals for services. Therefore, familiarity with the law's contents is important. The federal definition of emotional disturbance is provided below.

IDEA defines emotional disturbance as

(1) A condition exhibiting one or more of the following characteristics over a long period of time and to a marked degree, which adversely affects educational performance:
   (a) An inability to learn which cannot be explained by intellectual, sensory, or health factors;
   (b) An inability to build or maintain satisfactory relationships with peers and teachers;
   (c) Inappropriate types of behavior or feelings under normal circumstances;
   (d) A general pervasive mood of unhappiness or depression; or
   (e) A tendency to develop physical symptoms or fears associated with personal or school problems
(2) The term includes children who are schizophrenic or autistic. The term does not include children, who are socially maladjusted, unless it is determined that they are seriously emotionally disturbed

This description of emotional disturbance has been criticized for its lack of clarity and its exclusion of individuals who are socially maladjusted (Council for Children with Behavioral Disorders, 1987, 1989; Forness & Knitzer, 1992; Webber & Sheuermann, 1997). Like all IDEA categories, professionals must demonstrate that the disorder adversely affects students' school performance. At this juncture of identification, the SLP can be effective in the diagnosis. Knowledge of speech and language risk factors that may occur concomitantly with obvious behavioral and emotional characteristics should be considered and assessed. Awareness of the co-occurrence of deficits in both speech-language and emotional and behavioral issues allow the professional to see multiple perspectives that may be contributing to the child's academic success and socio-emotional development. An SLP may assess a speech-language deficit and conclude that the diagnosis is impacting the emotional /behavioral problem. On the other hand, an SLP may recognize the impact of the emotional and behavioral problem on the child's language development.

The Council for Exceptional Children (CEC) proposed another definition upon which professionals frequently rely. CEC's definition for emotional disturbance is less vague and more inclusive than the federal definition; it states that **emotional or behavioral disorders** (EBD) refer to a condition in which behavioral or emotional responses of an individual in school are vastly different from his or her generally accepted age-appropriate, ethnic, or cultural norms. Consequently, educational performance is adversely affected in such areas as self-care, social relationships, personal adjustment, academic progress, classroom behavior, or work adjustment. The council further expresses:

> EBD is more than a transient, expressed response to stressors in the child or youth's environment and would persist even with individualized interventions, such as feedback, the individual, consultation with parents or families, and/or modifications of the educational environment. The eligibility decision must be based on multiple sources of data about the individual's behavioral or emotional functioning. EBD must be exhibited in at least two different settings; at least one of which must be school related.

EBD can coexist with other handicapping condition as defined elsewhere in this law. "This category may include children or youth with schizophrenia, affective disorders, or with other sustained disturbances of conduct, attention, or adjustment" (Council for Exceptional Children, 1991, p. 10).

After reviewing the two definitions, it is evident that the one developed by CEC is more inclusive, claiming ownership for youth presenting with emotional as well as behavioral symptoms. Proponents for the inclusion of the individual who is socially maladjusted have argued that current research has run counter to the exclusionary clause found in the present IDEA definition (Duncan, Forness, & Hartsbough, 1995; Rosenblatt, Robertson, Bates, Wood, Furlong, & Sosna, 1998; Terrasi, Sennett, & Mackin, 1999; Webber & Scheuermann, 1997). **Social maladjustment** is merely a construct that appears to change depending upon the interpretation of any one individual. When the behavior of an individual is contextualized within a specified environment (i.e., school) the focal point centers on appropriate behavior for academic and social success rather than on semantic distinctions. With this distinction in mind, children served under the IDEA definition are youth with both emotional and behavioral disorders. This chapter will refer to individuals with psychiatric disorders as youth with EBD. Prior to describing the four areas of psychiatric disorders, two systems of categorization will be reviewed.

METHODS OF CATEGORIZATION

Categorization of ideas, people, images, or words is an efficient method that allows one to retain and recall information (Seiler & Beal, 2002). Categorization of behavior also allows individuals to label the behavior and describe it. Unfortunately, when describing behavior or a particular handicapping condition many individuals do not fit neatly into any one category. Within the classification of EBD there are many subgroupings. Achenbrach and Edlebrock (1983) made one of these subcategories popular when they published the Child Behavior Checklist. This diagnostic tool consists of 113 behavioral descriptors, which consequently identifies an individual as exhibiting internalizing behaviors or externalizing behaviors. Internalizing and externalizing behaviors are broad terms used to describe a set of behaviors.

Externalizing and Internalizing Behaviors

Externalizing behaviors describe the more overt actions children use. Externalizing behaviors are outward expressions that are obvious to anyone observing the individual. Adjectives used to describe this sort of behavior are: oppositional, impulsive, inattentive, aggressive, and combative. In contrast, internalizing behaviors reflect one's internal state, and someone unknown to the child may not observe these actions as easily. These adjectives would include: withdrawn, unresponsive, anxious, or sad. While there is some merit to all classification symptoms, it would be an oversimplification to place a child in one specific category.

Internalizing behaviors are often viewed as synonymous with emotional disturbances, while externalizing behaviors are often viewed as synonymous with behavioral disorders. Recognizing that the lines between emotional disturbances and behavioral disorders are often blurred will give the SLP better insight into the child's behavior. Children and adolescents can be identified with both internalizing and externalizing behaviors. For example, a student identified with a conduct disorder (oppositional, impulsive) may also have a coexisting depression (sad, anxious). Though the externalizing behaviors are more visible, an underlying depression frequently contributes to the child's behavior. Frequently, children's behaviors will cycle from one category (i.e., externalizing) to another (i.e., internalizing).

Diagnostic and Statistical Classification System of Mental Disorders

Several clinically derived classification systems have been developed. The system most widely used by the medical community is the American Psychiatric Association's Diagnostic and Statistical Manual of Mental Disorders-Text Revision (DSM-IV-TR) (2000). The categories and subcategories of the **DSM-IV-TR** (2000) were developed after years of investigation and field testing. The manual continues to be updated as the field of psychiatry evolves. The most recent text revision includes the latest in technological advances in the field. One particularly helpful feature of the manual is the descriptive text that follows the criteria for each disorder. Another helpful feature of the DSM-IV-TR is the common language it provides among professionals. These characteristics provide a basis on which to describe and compare children when communicating about them. This is especially important for aspiring professionals who have just mastered their own technical language within their chosen profession. This additional mastery of concepts and vocabulary improves the lines of communication between professionals and adds credibility to one's profession.

The current manual identifies 10 major groups of disorders that may be exhibited by infants, children, and adolescents (Hardman, Drew & Egman, 2002). This chapter will deal primarily with four major categories of psychiatric disturbance: disruptive behavior disorders, psychotic disorders, mood disorders, and anxiety disorders. Prior to looking at each of the four categories in more detail, some explanation of how psychiatric disorders and speech-language disorders became a relevant area of study for the SLP is provided.

CONCOMITANCE OF PSYCHIATRIC DISORDERS AND LANGUAGE

Speech-language disorders, learning deficits, and EBD frequently co-occur in children. The concomitance of these disorders has been the subject of much interest and study in the past several decades, resulting in two basic research strategies. The first involves identifying youth with psychiatric problems in samples of individuals with known speech and/or language disorders. Youngsters identified with speech and language diagnoses demonstrated a high prevalence of EBD that ranged from 50 to 70 percent (Camatra et al., 1988; Cantwell & Baker, 1987; Mattison, Cantwell, & Baker, 1982). The second strategy identified children with speech and language disorders in populations previously described with psychiatric disorders (Camarata et al., 1988; Cohen, Davine, Horodesky, Lipsett, & Isaacson, 1993; Cohen, Lipsett, & Dipp, 1991). Similarly, these children have shown an equally high or higher prevalence of speech-language and learning problems. The language-learning connection is not a new one. It is a firmly established finding that children with language disorders are known to develop learning problems (Aram & Nation, 1980; Fessler, Rosenberg, & Rosenberg, 1991). Children with learning problems are themselves at-risk for psychiatric disorders, which may be one reason why children with language involvement have higher rates of psychopathology (Cantwell & Baker, 1987; Cohen & Lipsett, 1991). Further, Cantwell and Baker (1987) point out that children with language disorders are more likely to have difficulty playing symbolic games and are more likely to have difficulties with the subtle nuances of social interaction than children without language disorders or children with pure speech disorders. Clearly, difficulty with peer relationships is a strong correlate of psychiatric disorders in children. Baker and Cantwell's landmark study in the 1980s, connecting psychiatric disorders with speech and language disorders, provided future researchers and clinicians with additional insight into the population they treat.

DISRUPTIVE BEHAVIOR DISORDERS

Based on the DSM-IV-TR (2000) classification system, the category of disruptive behavior disorders consists of oppositional defiant disorder and conduct disorder. Broadly defined and understood, the disruptive behavior disorders are often synonymous with behavior disorders. The observed behaviors associated with the disorder (noncompliant, aggressive, disruptive) are the same behaviors linked to the juvenile offender who is also described as an individual who is socially maladjusted. Are these juveniles socially maladjusted or do they have a behavior disorder? Perhaps it is only a semantic distinction, but it is one often faced by professionals. Regardless of the continuing arguments, the savvy SLP will recognize that individuals who are frequently characterized as having either oppositional defiant disorder or conduct disorder most likely have an underlying language-based learning disability. This finding is consistently revealed in the literature stating that anywhere from 30 to 80 percent of those identified with disruptive behavior disorders also have an identified language-based learning disability (Camarata et al., 1988; Cantwell & Baker, 1987; Cohen, Lipsett, & Dipp, 1991). These areas of difficulty include expressive semantics, syntax and articulation, auditory comprehension, reading, writing, and spelling (Camarata et al., 1988; Cantwell & Baker, 1987; Cohen & Lipsett, 1991). All of these skills are necessary for successful completion of an academic program.

In a study conducted by Cohen and Lipsett (1991), 237 4- to 12-year-olds who sought treatment in various mental health centers also received language assessments. Of the children referred solely for a psychiatric disorder, 38 percent had previously unrecognized language impairment. Further, findings revealed that the mothers viewed these children as more delinquent, and the teachers viewed the children as having more externalizing behaviors than individuals previously identified with either a language disorder or with a language disorder and a psychiatric disorder. It can be concluded that if a language disorder is not diagnosed, then the child's behavior may be interpreted negatively.

In a correlational study, Giddan, Milling, and Campbell (1996) illustrated that language-processing problems frequently co-occurred with various psychiatric categories, particularly those that fall under the category of disruptive behavior disorders. Poor peer relations and the inability to process speech adequately appear to make a large contribution to individuals with disruptive behavior disorders. The inability to make and sustain social relationships is often seen as the crux of the problem for children with disruptive behavior disorders. Recent research that has assessed children's ability to use language effectively has confirmed deficits in pragmatics or social use of language. Rinaldi (in press) replicated these findings supporting the notion of problematic social skills, which are further exacerbated by semantic and syntactic deficits. These findings appear to support the theoretical explanation put forth by Prizant and colleagues in 1990, which indicated that children with delayed and/or disordered language skills may have a difficult time establishing peer relationships, thus putting them even farther behind their peers in the area of socio-emotional development.

DISRUPTIVE BEHAVIOR DISORDERS AND THE JUVENILE JUSTICE SYSTEM

The majority of students with a handicapping condition of EBD served in schools, and the majority of referrals to mental health clinics, are students identified with disruptive behavior disorders (Cohen & Lipsett, 1991). That is really not all that surprising given the fact that these students are quite difficult to manage in the typical classroom, despite experienced teachers with specialized training. The sheer numbers in the classroom (25 to 30 students) make a disruptive, unruly student difficult to ignore at best and more difficult to teach at worst.

A 1994 report by the U.S Department of Education (1994) reported that 20 percent of students with EBD are arrested at least once before they leave school as opposed to 9 percent of students with disabilities and 6 percent of all students. Fifty-eight percent of youngsters with EBD are arrested five years after leaving school, as opposed to 30 percent of all students with disabilities. Of those with EBD who drop out of school, 73 percent are arrested within five years of leaving school.

Cohen, Davine, and Meloche-Kelly (1989) sampled the language skills of 37 5- to 12-year-old students in a center for children with mental health issues. High rates of the children with language disorders were detected only upon routine and systematic examination of their speech and language skills. A review of the records proved to be an unreliable measure in determining language deficits if the examiner relied on a verbal/performance discrepancy on IQ tests. Cohen and colleagues (1989) questioned why so many individuals' speech and language problems were overlooked. It was hypothesized that the children's language difficulties in this particular sample may have been missed due to the more salient conduct problems they demonstrated. The Cohen et al. study (1989) revealed two important considerations: (1) children who act out may not be considered for further testing of other underlying learning issues; and (2) professionals may overlook language-learning difficulties if they are relying on a verbal/performance discrepancy formula.

This bleak picture of high arrest rates and underidentified language learning deficits depicts the incredible odds educators face when dealing with this very high-risk group. Unfortunately, children with EBD are the most likely group of all the 13 identified under IDEA to drop out of school. However, as mental health professionals become more knowledgeable about the possibility of language learning deficits co-occurring with EBD, more attention can be given to collaborative assessment and intervention plans for children that present with emotional and/or behavioral disorders.

Oppositional Defiant Disorder

The essential feature of **oppositional defiant disorder** is the continuing pattern of negativistic, defiant, disobedient, and hostile behavior toward authority figures such as parents and teachers. The oppositional behavior is generally directed more toward figures the child knows well. The disorder is more prevalent in males, especially when they have exhibited difficult temperaments in their early elementary school years. Another indicator of oppositional defiant disorder is difficulty in being calmed once behavior has escalated, as well as extreme reactions, usually aggression for minor incidences. **Attention deficit/hyperactivity disorder** is common in children with oppositional defiant disorder. The number of oppositional symptoms generally increases with age. It is reported (American Psychiatric Association, 2000) that oppositional defiant disorder is frequently a developmental antecedent to conduct disorder.

Conduct Disorder

The behaviors associated with **conduct disorder** are more severe in nature than oppositional defiant disorder. The characteristics noted in conduct disorder show repetitive and persistent patterns of behavior, where the basic rights of others or major societal norms or rules are violated (American Psychiatric Association, 2000). These behaviors fall into four major groupings:

- Aggressive conduct that causes or threatens physical harm to other people or animals
- Nonaggressive conduct that causes property loss or damage
- Deceitfulness or theft
- Serious violations of rules

Individuals with conduct disorder may have little empathy and show little concern for the feelings of others. Intentions of others are often misperceived; they feel threatened and often respond aggressively. These children and adolescents should be tested routinely for speech and language deficits. Self-esteem of these individuals could be low, or may appear inflated. They may exhibit temper outbursts for no apparent reason, frustrate easily on tasks, and appear impulsive in their thinking. Conduct disorder may be associated with lower than average intelligence, with affected individuals showing a greater percentage of difficulties in the areas of reading, verbal problem solving, and language than their same-age peers.

PSYCHOTIC DISORDERS

Schizophrenia

Less common than disruptive behavior disorders is psychosis in children and adolescents. The presenting speech and language features particular to **psychosis** have classically diagnosed the disorder and have aided psychiatrists in its diagnosis. Difficulties in producing a clear and coherent message are often a primary indicator of psychosis, and in clinical terms, this has been referred to as a formal thought disorder. While some have debated whether these individuals have a speech-language or thought disorder, it has been concluded through decades of research that individuals with schizophrenia have a thought disorder rather than a language disorder (Schwartz, 1982).

Features
The essential features of **schizophrenia** are a mixture of positive and negative signs and symptoms. The positive symptoms appear to reflect an excess or distortion of normal functions. These symptoms include distortions in thought content (delusions), perception (**hallucinations**), language and thought

processes (disorganized speech), and self-monitoring of behavior. Two dimensions commonly associated with the positive symptoms are the delusions and hallucinations, known as the psychotic dimension, and disorganized speech and behavior, known as the disorganized dimension (American Psychiatric Association, 2000). The negative symptoms include restrictions in the range and intensity of emotional expression, in the productivity of thought and speech, and in the initiation of goal-directed behavior.

Language Characteristics

Some argue that disorganized thinking is the single most important feature in schizophrenia. In almost all clinical settings inferences about thoughts are based primarily on an individual's speech. The qualitative interpretation of speech has become a principal means of assessing disorganized speech. Researchers have assessed and quantified speech and language characteristics of the patient with schizophrenia.

Caplan (1996) analyzed the discourse of children with schizophrenia. He assessed their discourse using Halliday and Hasan's (1976) linguistic devices, and compared their use of these devices that speakers employ to tie references made to people, objects, events, and ideas together. In Caplan's sample, 31 10-year-old children with schizophrenia were matched with normally developing peers. The findings showed that the children with schizophrenia spoke less and did not provide the listener with enough links to previous utterances. Children with schizophrenia also provided the listener with fewer references to people, objects, or events mentioned in earlier utterances. In addition, the children appeared easily distracted by their immediate surroundings with little regard to the topic of conversation. Those children exhibiting loose associations confused the listener by using unclear and ambiguous references more than the children with no loose associations. These same findings were compared to other studies examining the language of adults with schizophrenia (Harvey, 1983; Rochester & Martin, 1979). Interestingly, the findings concluded that these youngsters did not have the "poverty of speech" found in the adult population with schizophrenia. Further, it was speculated that the onset of schizophrenia in middle childhood might also be associated with impaired maturation of social cognitive skills, including the development of logical thinking and topic maintenance. In conclusion, Caplan (1996) indicated that children with schizophrenia demonstrated deficits at the macrostructural and microstructural levels. The macrostructural deficits involved poor organization of topic maintenance and inadequate reasoning. The microstructural deficits involved impaired use of linguistic devices that link the contents of continuous speech and neighboring speech. Consequently, it was difficult to follow the line of thinking, which included whom subjects were talking about, what they were talking about, and how their topic was related to the topic of conversation.

Related Characteristics in Thought-Related Disorders

Individuals with thought disorders frequently exhibit emotional lability. **Affect** may range from blunted and flat to euphoric and manic. Those who experience a flattened affect are frequently unable to experience pleasure. Anxiety, agitation, and confusion may be observed in these individuals. Exaggerated speech may also be characteristic of these individuals as they lose themselves in their delusions, rituals, and hallucinations.

Schizophrenia, a disorder of thinking, can often be diagnosed through a person's speech and writing. The SLP's contribution to the diagnosis of schizophrenia can be substantial because these are two modalities that are well within the domain of the SLP. France (1992b) discusses four divisions when examining an individual's speech: stream, connection, possession, and content of thought.

- The stream of thought is how fast one thought follows another, which can be slowed down in depression or accelerated in a manic state.
- Disorders of connection involve a characteristic loosening of associations where two or more subjects can be woven together to combine thoughts, or where intruding stimuli become part of the thought process and adhere to the topic already initiated. Concrete thinking may be observed where the schizophrenic person cannot think in abstract terms.
- Disorders of possession include thought insertion, thought withdrawal, and thought broadcasting. Thought insertion is the belief that the thoughts one experiences come from someone else or somewhere else. Thought withdrawal, or the absence of thought, is the experience of one's thoughts being taken out of one's head. Thought broadcasting is an extension of thought withdrawal where thoughts travel outside the head only to have other people access them.
- Abnormalities of content of thought include delusions. **Delusions** are false beliefs, which may be either persecutory or paranoid, and reflect a distorted relationship between individuals and the world around them.

The more severe examples of psychosis are rare in the school setting. A clinician is more likely to see a child in the earlier stages of psychosis, or after the child has experienced some severe symptoms for which she or he is medicated. Continued monitoring of the child's speech and language functioning often provides helpful input for the consulting psychiatrist charged with the medical management of the child.

Individuals with schizophrenia are sometimes physically awkward and may display neurological **"soft signs"** such as left/right confusion or poor coordination. Some minor physical anomalies have also been noted, such as a highly arched palate, narrow or wide-set eyes, or subtle malformations of the ears (American Psychiatric Association, 2000).

As stated previously, the symptoms of psychosis are manifested in all aspects of communication. Speech and language characteristics prior to the onset of schizophrenia are helpful in diagnosing the illness. If this is not possible, awareness of what constitutes a formal thought disorder is useful. Finally, knowledge of the impact of medication on speech and language functioning is also beneficial.

MOOD DISORDERS

Mood disorders are a group of conditions in which a disturbance of affect is prominent. These may include major depressive disorder, dysthymic disorder, and bipolar disorder. Rather than define each of the characteristics of these mood disorders, general characteristics will be provided for each mood disorder, immediately followed by definitive speech-language characteristics.

Depressive Disorder

Depressive disorder is characterized by depression, including the loss of the ability to enjoy life, feelings of sadness and grief, and possible suicidal ideation. As in all of the DSM-IV-TR categories, these characteristics must be present for a sustained period of time, generally 6 months.

Individuals who are depressed communicate less frequently than those who are not. Avoidance of social situations is not uncommon because of the energy required to socialize and make conversation. Overall speech rate may be slowed, responses short, and repetition necessary because of the decrease in the ability to concentrate. Less affect will manifest in a reduced range of pitch and other suprasegmental features. Breznitz and Sherman (1987) found that speech of depressed patients is often punctuated by long pauses. It is hypothesized that this may be due to the interjection of depressed thoughts that interfere with thinking and speech.

Loss of interest or pleasure is almost always present in depression. Family members may notice social withdrawal. Appetite may be reduced whereas others with depression may experience increased appetite or cravings for specific foods. The most common sleep disturbance is insomnia. SLPs may notice the psychomotor changes, which commonly include agitation or a slowing down of speech, thought, and body movements. There may be increased pauses before answering. Other speech characteristics include a decrease in volume, flat inflection, and a decrease in the amount of content (France, 1992a; Pennel & Creed, 1987; Scherer, 1987). France (1992a) also reported that pitch changes may be evident, and resonance will sometimes be abnormally nasal or pharyngeal. In addition, many individuals report impaired ability to think, concentrate, or make decisions. They may appear easily distracted or complain of memory difficulties. The school-age child may show a drop in grades. Cognitive tests, such as IQ tests, may show lower verbal and performance scores.

Nonverbal communication will also provide insight into how an individual feels. Restricted affect, flattened affect, reduced eye contact, and stooped or hunched posture may be apparent in an individual with depression (France, 1992a). Poor nonverbal communication may be more evident in close relationships than in less superficial relationships, where the nonverbal interactions are not interpreted as abnormal (Segrin & Flora, 1998).

Dysthymic Disorder

Dysthymic disorder is typically thought to be less severe than depression. This is diagnosed after the child or adolescent has experienced low-level distress, irritability, self-criticism, or low self-esteem for longer than a year. Symptoms may include poor appetite or increased appetite, disruptive sleep patterns, and a decrease in activities. Other signs include a tendency to give up easily, an inability to cope with routine tasks, and becoming easily frustrated with simple problems.

Speech and language characteristics are similar to those found among individuals with a major depressive disorder. The characteristics described above (i.e., sleep disturbances, appetite changes, and psychomotor symptoms) are less common. Dysthymic disorder is of many years' duration, so the mood disturbance may be seen as part of the person's personality rather than as a depressive disorder. It is also noteworthy to point out those children who are viewed as aggressive by their peers and teachers experience higher levels of peer rejection and have more depressive symptoms than their nonaggressive peers (Dumas, Bechman, & Prinz, 1994). The research specific to speech and language functioning has been in the area of severe depressive illness rather than dysthymia.

Bipolar Disorder

The essential feature of **bipolar disorder** is the presence of one or more manic or hypomanic episodes. These include mood disturbances that are sufficiently severe to cause marked impairment in social function or to require hospitalization (American Psychiatric Association, 2000). These episodes can occur once, or they can reoccur following a depressive episode. Further, the DSM-IV-TR divides bipolar disorder into either Bipolar I or Bipolar II. The reader is referred to the manual for more specific information. The point of diagnosis (manic, hypomanic, or depressive episode) determines the psychiatric classification at the time. For the purposes of this chapter characteristics will be provided for both manic/hypomanic and depressive episodes.

Manic and Hypomanic Episodes

It appears that the major distinction between manic and hypomanic episodes is the heightened state of the elevated mood and the duration of the mood. The criteria for manic episodes call for a "distinct period of abnormally and persistently elevated, expansive, or irritable mood, lasting at least one week" (American Psychiatric Association, 2000, p. 362), whereas the hypomanic phase calls for a "distinct period of persistently elevated, expansive, or irritable mood, lasting throughout at least four days" (American Psychiatric Association, 2000, 368).

Manic Episode

Individuals experiencing a **manic** episode frequently do not recognize the presence of a problem. Elevated mood, decreased need for sleep, and inflated self-esteem are typically present. Manic speech is pressured, louder than normal, rapid, and difficult to interpret. The individual may talk for long periods of time frequently without any regard for the listener. Difficulty with topic maintenance and increased distractibility may also be evident.

Hypomanic Episode

In contrast to a manic episode, a **hypomanic** episode is not severe enough to cause marked impairment in social or occupational functioning, or to require hospitalization (American Psychiatric Association, 2000). The elevated mood in a person with hypomania is described as an unusually good mood, which is a distinct change from normal moods and behavior. Further, rapid changes in speech or activity may be present.

By definition, bipolar consists of both depressed and manic states. Therefore, the speech and language characteristics correspond to the particular phase the individual is in. For instance, during the depressed state the individual would present with characteristics typical of depression, whereas in the heightened manic phases speech characteristics present with more pressured speech and thought bouncing or the rapid shifts in topics.

ANXIETY DISORDERS

Anxiety disorders consist of a subgroup of disorders that reflect abnormal and extreme responses to hypothetical and real stimuli. The triggers for the associated anxious feelings are either externally or internally generated. The focus of the anxiety often helps to differentiate the array of anxiety disorders. Generalized anxiety may be brought on by excessive worry. Post-traumatic stress disorder is triggered by exposure to an extremely traumatic event that may involve death, witnessing a violent crime, or physical or sexual abuse. Generalized anxiety and post-traumatic stress disorder will be discussed later in this chapter.

Generalized Anxiety Disorder

Excessive worries and concerns about real-life circumstances characterize **generalized anxiety disorder.** The anxiety and worry are accompanied by at least three additional symptoms that include restlessness, being easily fatigued, difficulty concentrating, irritability, muscle tension, and disturbed sleep, with only one of these symptoms required in children. Many individuals with generalized anxiety disorder also experience somatic symptoms such as nausea, diarrhea, and sweating. Disorders of autonomic hyperarousal, which include accelerated heart rate, shortness of breath, and dizziness, are less prominent in generalized anxiety disorders than in other anxiety disorders such as post-traumatic stress disorder. However, fidgety behavior and an inability to keep still may be apparent as a result of hyper-vigilance and the feeling that something is going to occur. The person is on constant alert and also may startle easily.

Anxiety disorders appear frequently in the general population and the disorder is often linked with depression. Twenge (2000) studied anxiety in young adults and has seen a substantial increase in the levels of anxiety since first tracking clients in the 1950s. This increase in anxiety will most likely remain high as divorce rates remain elevated, youth continue to experience heightened levels of crime rate, and fear of further terrorist attacks continue. With the increases in anxiety, professionals are beginning to look at symptoms in very young children. While very young children cannot always articulate what is wrong with them, regressive behavior and mood changes may signal anxiety or depression in youngsters.

The rate of anxiety disorders among children ages 1.7 to 15.9 with diagnosed communication disorders was high in Cantwell and Baker's (1987) study of 600 children and adolescents. Parent and child interviews indicated that 30 percent of the subjects had at least one symptom of anxiety, while 10 percent of the subjects qualified for a diagnosis of anxiety disorder. Further, in a 14-year follow-up of speech/language impaired and control children, subjects with language and speech impairments showed significantly higher rates of anxiety disorders into young adulthood when compared to their peers with no impairments (Beitchman et al., 1996).

The causal connection remains unclear, but speech and language issues may often be overlooked when treating individuals with anxiety. An overrepresentation of anxiety in the individuals with speech and language disorders is evident based on the research discussed.

Post-Traumatic Stress Disorder

Post-traumatic stress disorder (PTS) is the development of characteristics following exposure to an extreme traumatic event (American Psychiatric Association, 2000). The response to the event involves intense fear, helplessness, and horror, and in children this response also includes disorganized or agitated behavior. Typically, the individual reexperiences the traumatic event repeatedly, and then may avoid stimuli associated with the trauma. A general numbing of responsiveness is seen. These events may include sexual and physical abuse, torture, terrorist attack, natural or man-made disasters, severe automobile accidents, or being diagnosed with a life-threatening illness. Impaired affect modulation, impulsive behavior, and impaired relationships with others are some of the symptoms that may occur, and may be overlooked as part of another disorder.

PTS is a relatively new area of study in the psychiatric arena but many children who experience traumatic and stressful events such as physical and sexual abuse may manifest anxiety in more overt ways such as noncompliance and defiance of authority. Care must be taken to consider anxiety as the source of the problem rather than a disruptive behavior or attention disorder. Sexual abuse is one of the most common causes of post-traumatic stress in children (Majcher & Pollack, 1996). When the abuse occurs before age 11 the event is three times more likely to result in PTS (Davidson & Smith, 1990). This matter is further complicated because researchers have shown that actual onset of anxiety and panic may not surface until neuronal activity matures in adolescence. This developmental model of anxiety corresponds to neurophysiological factors associated with animal studies (Kimura & Naka-mura, 1985, 1987).

Certain temperament types identified in children under age 2 are thought to have a nervous system that is more easily aroused, which would predispose these children to greater anxiety. This argument also makes sense when considering the large number of youth with pervasive developmental disorders who are also treated for anxiety. These youth have demonstrated hyper- or hypoarousal states to different sensory stimuli, which in turn creates anxiety.

SLPs may be among the first to observe cognitive symptoms of stress that may include poor attention span, difficulty concentrating, difficulty in naming common objects, academic difficulties, lowered IQ, and poor communication skills (Richards & Bates, 1998). Affective symptoms may include panic and irritability, tension, constricted emotions, inability to express feelings, and avoidance of pleasurable activities (Richards & Bates, 1998). Regardless, it is important to consider why the child is performing the way he or she presents. This information may result in an altered form of intervention.

DIFFERENTIAL DIAGNOSIS

A **differential diagnosis** between what is a speech and/or language disorder and what is a psychiatric disorder is not always discernible based upon the information observed. As a critical member of a multidisciplinary team, the SLP's job is to provide useful information that will contribute to the diagnosis and treatment of the individual. As a practitioner it is critical to have some background and awareness of the DSM classification system which is widely used in the diagnosis of psychiatric disorders. In addition to having a global understanding of characteristics particular to the DSM classification system, background in how impressions are formed is useful. Impressions and perceptions influence how data are interpreted, which in turn is filtered through a background of experiences unique to that individual. Awareness of impression and perceptions is important, but additional knowledge of different cultural patterns further illuminates the diagnostic process.

IMPRESSION FORMATION

Impressions are collections of perceptions about others that are maintained and used to interpret information. Broad impressions are formed through perceptions of both physical qualities and behavior. Relevant pieces of information are selected and then organized and interpreted. The interpretation formed is filtered through a unique set of background experiences, which include attitudes, beliefs, and general upbringing. These elements of the environment shape one's value system, which in turn influences how we perceive others. The SLP is put in the position to interpret formal and informal findings of test results. Interpretation of a loose association or what constitutes poor social skills influences individual interpretation. What appears to be gross disorganization of thinking to one person may only seem somewhat disorganized to another, or the disorganization may be dismissed altogether as the person having a bad day.

The implicit personality theory (Seiler & Beall, 2002) explains how personality is interpreted and described. Qualities in an individual are observed, and then these qualities are linked with other frequently associated characteristics. For instance, if a child is jumping in and out of his or her seat, dropping pencils on the floor, and not completing the assigned task, one may consider the child to be rude or noncompliant. Essentially, this is a form of stereotyping.

Caution should be exercised to avoid interpreting information based on preconceived notions without input from other professionals. Understanding the human reaction to make sense of the information we observe, and then to form conclusions, is the job of the appropriate professional. Recognizing that preconceived notions can substantially alter a final diagnosis should lead the professional to keep an open mind so an accurate diagnosis can be generated.

MULTIDISCIPLINARY APPROACH

Frequently, there is an overlap between psychiatric diagnoses. This is seen more often between the disruptive behavior disorders and mood disorders, as well as between the mood disorders of depression and anxiety. Similarly, there is overlap between the psychiatric diagnosis and speech, language, and learning difficulties. That is why a team approach in which group members wait to form their final diagnosis until all the pieces across disciplines is necessary.

ASSESSMENT

Language is central to human communication and development. The empirical research that is available supports a strong association between speech and language impairment and psychiatric disorder in childhood (Baker & Cantwell, 1987; Beitchman et al., 1996; Camarata et al., 1988; Fessler et al., 1991; Giddan et al., 1996; Prizant et al., 1990). Given this information, in any mental health setting or school setting specializing in care of students with emotional and behavioral disorders, a speech and language assessment should be part of the medical evaluation of referred individuals. Likewise, SLPs evaluating youngsters with speech and language disorders must be aware of the issues and prevalence of psychiatric disorders that occur within this population.

Optimum circumstances encourage a multidisciplinary approach to assessment, including a psychologist, a psychiatrist, and an SLP, a clinical social worker, a general and/or special educator, parents/caregivers, and any other appropriate related service personnel, such as the occupational therapist or physical therapist.

Of obvious significance is the large role language and communication play in the team's diagnosis. An SLP has the unique training and expertise to be sensitive to this relationship and can be instrumental in interpreting findings. The SLP does not work in isolation. Diagnosis and treatment is not successful unless all perspectives are considered, each one being different, coming from a unique training perspective.

The Team

Psychiatrist

A psychiatric evaluation usually begins with the mental status examination, a tool most commonly used by **psychiatrists** (Folstein, Folstein, & McHugh, 1975). This examination presents a series of questions revolving around orientation of time, place, and person. In addition, keen observations of other characteristics are noted, such as hygiene, posture, affect, and general appearance. Characteristic behaviors are noted, and the quality of responses is judged. Psychiatrists regularly interpret the content of thought of their clients, questioning them about persistent thoughts, obsessions, hallucinations, or other occurrences that may help contribute to the diagnosis of one disorder over another. The information gleaned from this interview is used in conjunction with other observations and diagnostic information from other team members.

Occupational Therapist

The **occupational therapist** assesses the child both informally and formally. Observation in the child's classroom or another natural setting is important to assess how well sensory information is integrated for productive learning. The occupational therapist may look at motor planning, fine motor skills, visual motor skills, and ability to follow multistep directions. Formal assessment may involve tests such as Developmental Test of Visual Motor Integration-VMI (Beery, 1989).

Social Worker

The **social worker** is a key individual in accessing important family information through face-to-face and phone interviews with family members. The social worker obtains information on developmental history, previous academic and behavioral history, and family dynamics. Additionally, the social worker will meet with the child, dialoguing to gain additional insights and to get the child's perspective on observed and reported difficulties she or he may have.

Nurse

In some settings the **nurse** may also play a role in the team assessment. Current health and general observations are made. The nurse can provide information on medical issues related to the child's academic setting. Additional medical diagnosis such as diabetes or seizure disorders may need to be understood by the team and the nurse can provide this information. If medication is taken, the type and dosage is reported, as well as the child's compliance in taking the medication.

Special Educator

The **special educator,** or diagnostician, in charge of diagnostic testing is important for obtaining present levels of performance in major academic areas such as reading, math, and written language. One common instrument used is the Woodcock-Johnson-Psychoeducational Test (Woodcock & Johnson, 1990). Achievement tests yield standard scores, age scores, or grade scores that help in defining academic strengths and weaknesses, as well as identifying or supporting an existing learning disability.

Classroom Teacher

With the exception of the primary caregivers, the classroom **teacher** spends the most time with the child. Teachers are able to provide vital information on classroom performance, test results, and general observations of the child's behaviors. These may include reactions to situations and peers or recorded comments made by the child.

Psychologist

The **psychologist** provides information on cognitive functioning. Psychologists use a formal measure of intelligence such as the Wechsler Intelligence Scale for Children Revised (WISC-III) (Wechsler, 1998) that provides a global measure of intelligence using various subtests to cumulatively reflect a child's general intellectual ability. In addition to the IQ scores yielded from intelligence tests, other assessments are often completed. These tests may include projective tests, which are interpreted by the psychologist to gain insights into the child's personality.

Speech-Language Pathologist

The SLP figures prominently in the multidisciplinary team. Each team member uses language in his or her evaluation of the child. Oral responses from the child are interpreted by members of the team. Likewise, oral language is used to communicate information from the professional to the child. The levels of syntactic complexity and the length of utterances used by the professionals must be monitored or considered when weighing how well the child responded. SLPs are uniquely qualified to communicate what they observe in the language of youngsters to the health professionals and educators working with them (Cohen et al., 1989; Giddan, Trautman & Hurst, 1989). In addition to the assessment process, treatment plans used with children and families rely almost exclusively on verbal communication. The SLP must help professionals make informed decisions regarding appropriate language-based assessments matching the child's comprehension level to the therapy offered.

The SLP should screen the child's hearing or make a referral to the audiologist for a hearing assessment. Assessments of the child's receptive and expressive language should be made. Tools such as the TOLD-P III (Newcomer & Hammill, 1997) or the CELF-R (Wiig, Wayne, & Semel, 1992) are good starting points, depending upon the child's age. However, in addition to traditional receptive and expressive measures, inclusion of pragmatic functioning, narrative analysis, and assessment of the child's ability to problem-solve (i.e., [Test of Problem Solving] (Zachman, Jorgenson, Huisingh, & Barrett, 1984) is necessary to obtain a complete picture of language functioning. These formal test results are combined with informal findings completed through observation and conversation with individuals involved in the child's daily care. Informal observations provide a measure of social validation to formal test results. Observations take place in settings where communication occurs naturally. If direct observations of the child's home environment are not possible, obtaining information from the child's primary caregivers helps to complete the communication picture. Participation by family members should be encouraged as they are an integral part of diagnosis and intervention.

MULTIDISCIPLINARY TEAM–THE FINAL STAGES

After all formal and informal tests are performed it is necessary to review the information in a multidisciplinary meeting. These steps include:

- Convening with all the accumulated information
- Sharing information with an open mind until all perspectives are heard
- Coming to a consensus on diagnosis
- Developing an appropriate treatment plan

INTERVENTIONS

Early Intervention

Early language intervention has been consistently reported in the literature as a preventative method in the development or exacerbation of socio-emotional problems (Beitchman et al., 1996; Carson, Klee, Perry, Muskina, & Donaghy, 1998). New initiatives are constantly being developed that address early identification. For example, several studies that set out to identify and treat children with both conduct disorders and anxiety disorders indicated positive outcomes when the intervention involved parent training (Kendall, Flannery-Schroeder, Panichelli-Mindel, Southan-Gerow, Henin, & Warman, 1997; Stratton & Hammond, 1997). Unfortunately, not all professionals have access to information alerting them to appropriate referral sources and programs for very young children. Many times youngsters reach school age before help is available; however, with revisions to IDEA, early intervention is becoming more accessible.

Functional Behavior Assessments

When IDEA was most recently reauthorized, **functional behavior assessments** (FBAs) became a recommended form of treatment to address the behavior of children who are suspended or expelled from school for disciplinary reasons. Functional behavioral assessments will be described in the next section in relation to positive behavior interactions. These two interventions are frequently developed together when addressing students with emotional and/or behavioral issues.

Positive Behavior Interactions

Positive behavior support (PBS) is the application of behavior analysis to achieve socially important behavior change. The behaviors targeted with PBS prohibit or impede academic performance and social development (Wilcox, Turnbull, & Turnbull, 2000). PBS is not considered a new intervention plan. It is an application of a behaviorally based approach to improve the teaching and learning environment for all students systemically by increasing prosocial behavior, thereby decreasing problem behavior (Sugai et al., 2000). The basis of an effective PBS begins by defining the team's knowledge of the problem. Horner, Sugai, Todd, and Lewis-Palmer (2000) outline four parts in this definition:

- First, the team identifies positive contributions of the individual.
- Second, the team must come to agreement on all the problem behaviors that prevent that child from learning. These behaviors must be observable and measurable.
- Another important consideration is the context in which the behaviors are observed. The team defines the environment where the problem behavior is occurring.
- Last, a functional behavior assessment is performed to identify the events that reliably predict and maintain problem behavior.

According to Horner et al. (2000) these assessments occur most frequently around problem routines and result in a summary statement that describes what the student does, the conditions that are likely to trigger the problem behavior, and an assumption about what consequences appear to maintain or reinforce the behavior. This assessment is also the result of direct observation of the student to support the assumptions made. Within a program utilizing positive behavioral intervention, a comprehensive functional behavioral assessment is included.

Social Skills and Pragmatic Language Therapy

The lack of necessary social skills often serves as a deterrent in forming and maintaining adequate relationships for individuals with psychiatric disorders. For younger children social skills may involve greeting others, turn-taking skills in both play and conversation, and regulating emotions in a socially appropriate way. The child may exhibit avoidance of others or may not show a healthy skepticism when first meeting strangers. Older children may exhibit similar patterns of behavior with additional difficulties taking another person's perspective, an inability to generate multiple solutions to problems, or an inability to work logically through a problem. Students have social skills deficits for many reasons. One reason may be lack of exposure to appropriate models, or a choice not to comply with social and cultural norms. Other individuals manifest a lack of awareness of the social expectations in a particular setting, due to primary language deficits. While the reason for poor social skills may have a different origin, all of these children can benefit from social skills training. Typically, if the child demonstrates lack of social awareness due to primary language deficits he or she has a pragmatic language deficit.

Many programs are available to address pragmatic language skills such as role playing and using scripts. Ciechalski and Schmidt (1995) were able to demonstrate that using role playing along with performance feedback from guidance counselors positively affected the social interactions of students with disabilities. Using a student's strong literacy skills, Donahue, Szymanski, and Flores (1999) were able to foster a student's social interaction skills with another student by cooperatively working on a joint writing assignment. Regardless of the form of direct instruction used to promote stronger social interaction skills, most professionals agree that the key to generalizing the newly developed prosocial skills is adequate experience in several natural environments. Therapy, involving the clinical social worker, the art therapist, or the special educator, are natural ways to include pragmatic language skills in the child's intervention plan. Co-treatment is also a reciprocal process that allows different disciplines to learn from each other.

Cognitive and developmental levels must be considered when developing programs. The use of pictures and physical props may be necessary when instructing developmentally young children. Social skills stories developed by Carol Gray (1995) are a popular method for introducing some youngsters to appropriate social responses in various contexts and situations. Older children and adolescents more skilled with basic conversation skills often benefit from taking ownership in the choice of their own target areas that parallel their interests, needs, and development.

Language of Feelings

Many youngsters, particularly those with pragmatic language deficits, cannot identify or articulate their feelings or the feelings of others. These skills develop in children as young as age 2. The language of feelings can be taught directly by the SLP either in individual therapy, group therapy, or a larger context (Giddan, Bade, Rickenberg, & Ryley, 1995; Giddan & Ross, 2001). It is important for children to understand the impact of their emotional outbursts on others. Addressing this issue and teaching alternative prosocial behaviors are encouraged (see positive behavior supports).

Preschoolers ages 3 to 5 can be taught the language of emotions in a purposeful manner by identifying facial features, vocal characteristics, and body postures associated with different emotions. The intervening professional should adapt lessons based on the different developmental levels when teaching the subtle nuances and shades of emotions. Co-treating with therapists skilled in expressive therapies (art, music, dance/movement) is also beneficial for generalization of these activities. This becomes more important for the child who has limited language and needs a nonverbal method of expression.

Pharmacological

Psychotropic medication is an important factor in the intervention of individuals with emotional and behavioral problems. Many of the above mentioned interventions are most effective when paired with the appropriate medications. However, a few studies have investigated the effects of medication in relation to the psychiatric diagnosis. One recent study by Hallfors, Fallon, and Watson (1998) showed that children who received a diagnosis of ADHD, schizophrenia, bipolar, or major depression were six times more likely to receive medication than other children in the study; children with conduct disorders were less likely to receive medication. While this study did not address the effectiveness of the medications, it did show that children with conduct disorders were prescribed medication far less frequently than those with other disorders.

The developments in psychiatry have advanced from a psychoanalytical approach to one that is increasingly more grounded in medical-neurobiological findings. Scientists continue to make strides in discovering how medicine can be used to manage behaviors. A very brief overview of some of the common psychotropic medications is provided:

- Tricyclic antidepressants. Tricyclic antidepressants were formerly some of the most widely used drugs for treatment of depression. They have been used to treat enuresis, school phobia, and disruptive behavior disorders as well as some affective disorders (Hallfors et al., 1998). Tricyclic antidepressants include clomipramine (Anafranil), desipramine (Norpramin), imipramine (Tofranil), and nortriptyline (Pamelor).
- Other antidepressants. These drugs consist mostly of drugs referred to as selective serotonin retake inhibitors (SSRIs), such as fluoxetine hydrochloride (Prozac), paroxetine (Paxil), and sertraline (Zoloft). These popular drugs are used for depression and anxiety syndromes (Hallfors, Fallon, & Theodore et al., 1998); other common antidepressants are bupropion (Wellbutrin) and trazodone (Desyrel).
- Lithium. Lithium has been considered the first mood stabilizer. Physicians discovered that various medications used to treat seizure disorders (anticonvulsants) also regulated mood disorders.
- Anticonvulsants. Anticonvulsants are used with a variety of psychiatric disorders such as impulse and bipolar disorders. Some of these include carbamazepine (Tegretol), phenytoin (Dilantin), and valproic acid (Depakote).
- Stimulants. Stimulants have been the primary choice of treatment for attention problems. They have been shown to improve focus and decrease motor activity observed in many children with attention problems. Long-term effects are not as well documented especially with regard to social issues often associated with attention problems (Hallfors et al., 1998). Some common stimulant medications are methylphenidate (Ritalin) pemoline (Cylert), amphetamine (Adderall), and dextroamphetamine (Dexadrine).
- Neuroleptics. These medications are used in major psychiatric disorders characterized by mania and psychosis (Hallfors et al., 1998). Common neuroleptics used are chlorpromazine (Thorazine), thioridazine (Mellaril), haloperiodol (Haldol), triflueperazine (Stelazine), perphenazine (Trilafon), thiothixiene (Navane), riperidone (Risperdal), clozapine (Clozaril), fluphenazine (Prolixin), and loxapine (Loxitane).

SLPs should be aware of the range of medications available to clients with psychiatric disorders as well as some of the side effects and the affect they may have on speech.

Side Effects

Dry mouth is a frequent side effect of many medications in all categories. Janicak, Davis, Preskorn, and Ayd (1997) point out that this particular side effect affects speech production and can contribute to dental cavities. Dysarthria may occur with drugs that sedate. Neuroleptics may cause movement disorders, which may affect the jaw or tongue. Any change in speech language functioning after the introduction of medication is worth documenting and sharing with the consulting psychiatrist. Slurred speech may be an indication of overmedication; however, a side effect of some psychostimulants may result in pressured speech or a rapid rate of talking with overmedication.

Interface Between School and Mental Health

Ideally, there should be meaningful communication between mental health facilities, private treatment professionals, and schools, but unfortunately this is not always the case. Communication between professionals that treat youth with psychiatric disorders is essential. A problem exists when federal guidelines for eligibility for special education are not followed. The problem seems to be one of diagnosis and the subsequent eligibility for services. Children who are diagnosed in facilities outside of school may not be eligible for services unless communication between clinics and schools is consistent (McGinnis & Forness, 1988). The psychiatric diagnosis determined in the *Diagnostic and Statistical Manual* and eligibility for special education under the federal guidelines is not always easily transferable. While many day treatment programs have their own staff psychiatrist who can communicate meaningfully with the day treatment staff, hospital and clinic professionals are not always versed in IDEA eligibility practices. Incorrect terminology between professionals and schools may result in a psychiatric diagnosis without securing needed services for the child.

Eligibility is particularly problematic for those children and adolescents identified with the disruptive behavior disorders (opposition defiant disorder, conduct disorder, and ADHD) because of their identification with social maladjustment. Socially maladjusted youth are excluded from service under the federal definition of SED [EBD] unless they are also determined SED [EBD] according to the five other criteria listed in the definition. This play for services becomes a semantic game. Professionals must document accurately, thoroughly, and carefully to meet the definition under the IDEA. Ironically, the children with disruptive behavior disorders are among those most frequently identified in classrooms for youth with EBD (Mattison, Humphrey, Kales, Handford, Finkenbinder, & Hermit, 1986; Mattison, Morales, & Bauer, 1992). It is imperative that all professionals work toward a common language and understanding, so the child can be served comprehensively, at home, in the community, and at school.

As mental health issues continue to indicate an upward trend, services to treat those with mental health issues will continue to increase as well. SLPs need to feel confident of the vital role they play in the diagnosis and treatment of individuals with psychiatric disorders. Continued work and research continues to promote a greater level of confidence and understanding of the relationship between communication and socio-emotional development.

Case Study 1: Adolescent with Psychiatric Disorders

Rex is a 15-year-old 10th grader recently referred to a day school for students with emotional and behavioral disorders. Rex was referred to the program because of increasing concerns over his "unusual behaviors and responses" in his previous public school setting. Past school history is positive for language-based learning disabilities in the areas of math and written language. Records also indicated previous speech and language therapy in the early elementary grades.

A multidisciplinary team that included the school psychologist, special educator, occupational therapist, SLP, and psychiatrist completed diagnostic testing. These assessments were completed both formally and informally while observing Rex during structured and unstructured times. Rex's parents were also interviewed to obtain a more complete family history and to discuss current concerns.

Results of the psychological assessment indicated a young man in the average range of intellectual functioning as demonstrated on the WISC-III. In fact, his ability to handle verbal abstractions and his fund of general knowledge was in the superior range of functioning. In contrast, performance areas including attention to detail, nonverbal reasoning, and ability to sequence items visually were comparatively low. Educational testing utilizing the Woodcock-Johnson Tests of Achievement-Revised concurred with classroom observations and previous reports of below age level performance in the areas of math and written expression. Measures used by the occupational therapist assessed fine motor skills, sensory motor skill, and visual-perceptual skills. Rex demonstrated delays in letter formation, slow handwriting speed when copying, and poor cursive skills. Visual-perceptual skills were determined to be functional. Anecdotally, the OT noted inconsistent attention to tasks as well as tangential responses to questions. The psychiatrist reported behaviors consistent with a psychotic illness, including thought blocking, anxiety, and mental confusion.

Speech and language assessments completed the multidisciplinary testing. The Clinical Evaluation of Language Fundamentals-Revised (CELF-R) was administered to provide an overview of Rex's receptive and expressive language functioning. Rex demonstrated average skills perceiving semantic relationships between single words as well as the ability to interpret word relationships at the sentence level. However, Rex demonstrated a severe deficit in the ability to interpret, recall, and execute oral commands of increasing length and complexity. Expressively, Rex scored in the average range for all three subtests, indicating an average ability to understand and formulate original sentences using simple but appropriate syntax and morphology. Speech, voice, and fluency were assessed informally. Rex demonstrated adequate articulation skills but his prosody, rate, and inflection were flat and his rate of speech was judged to be slow.

The multidisciplinary team convened to review and discuss each discipline's finding. It was concluded that indeed Rex was indicating a psychotic disorder that was affecting his performance across all academic and social settings. While speech and language results showed evidence of a receptive language disorder it was the team's consensus that the receptive language problem was secondary to an emerging thought disorder. Because Rex showed a strong fund of general information and expressively showed average skills in sentence formulation, he was expected to be able to maintain himself in a structured classroom setting. The team recommended academic and psychiatric interventions including (a) a small, self-contained setting; (b) goals addressing attention and organization; (c) indirect speech language services to provide comprehension strategies for the classroom teacher and suggestions for modifying written language assignments; (d) weekly sessions with the licensed clinical social worker; and (e) antipsychotic and antistimulant medications prescribed by and followed by the staff psychiatrist. Additionally, the SLP suggested that Rex participate in a weekly pragmatic language group to work on topic maintenance and appropriate responses, while improving his ability to take another person's perspective. The team agreed to meet about Rex on a quarterly basis to monitor his progress.

Case Study 2: Psychiatric Disorder

Josh is a 13-year-old seventh grader enrolled in a program for individuals with emotional and behavioral disorders. Josh presents with a long history of involvement in the juvenile justice system, where he has been charged with theft and breaking and entering. Josh presently lives with his maternal grandmother.

His mother is unable to care for him and his father is incarcerated. School records are incomplete, as Josh has relocated five times in his seven years of schooling. Records note consistently poor academic performance. A recent psychological test indicates a full-scale IQ of 67; however, the examiner felt test results were not valid because Josh "did not fully cooperate" during all tasks. A diagnostic assessment was recommended because of Josh's poor academic record, terse verbal output, and increasing aggression toward his grandmother and staff.

The school's special educator, psychiatrist, and SLP conducted assessments over a four-week period. Because of Josh's lack of trust in formal testing situations, much of the testing was completed informally. The special educator and SLP met daily with Josh to review his schedule, letting him know when he was in class and when he came to "speech." During speech diagnostic sessions Josh initially spent a good deal of time manipulating objects in the clinician's office such as Legos and three-dimensional puzzles. As he warmed up to the clinician he would respond to questions regarding likes, dislikes, and how he spent his time. When Josh was willing, the clinician would have him demonstrate some of his skills by reading words from standardized word lists and typing responses on a portable word-processor (Alpha-Smart Pro). It was evident that Josh was functioning three to four years below grade level in some academic tasks. Josh was able to complete the Peabody Picture Vocabulary Test, which assesses one-word receptive vocabulary. He received a standard score of 85, demonstrating a low average performance in his understanding of words. Academically the special educator was able to assess classroom math and reading work. Josh was able to add, subtract, multiply, and divide two-digit numbers. He was able to use the calculator for multiplication and division tasks. Josh demonstrated the ability to read material at the fourth grade instructional level.

The psychiatrist met with Josh several times. He was unsuccessful in getting Josh to respond to him, deferring the psychiatric diagnosis of Josh at the time. The team met to discuss Josh's placement and educational plan. The team concurred that continued diagnostic assessment was needed to aid in a comprehensive picture of Josh's strengths and weaknesses. At the time continued support for a restrictive placement in a facility for emotionally and behaviorally disturbed children was clear. The team agreed to continue to assess skills through dynamic and portfolio assessments to supplement formal testing.

Several months later formal testing was completed indicating a language-based learning disability based on the Woodcock-Johnson Tests of Achievement, the Clinical Evaluation of Language Fundamental-Revised, and the Lindamood Auditory Conceptualization Test. Further, Josh demonstrated difficulty with short-term auditory memory, word retrieval, and phonological production of multisyllabic words. These phonological core deficits contribute to a severe language-based learning disability affecting receptive and expressive language as well as academic skills, particularly reading. The following recommendations were made: (a) continued treatment in the day program for students with emotional and behavioral disorders; (b) enrollment in the Orton Gillingham Method of reading; (c) speech and language therapy targeting phonological awareness and strategies for word retrieval and memory; (d) special education help with math and written language; (e) weekly therapy with a licensed clinical social worker and an updated DSM diagnosis from the staff psychiatrist.

REVIEW QUESTIONS

1. Why do you think the author chose to use the term *individual with emotional and behavioral disorder* as opposed to *individual with emotional disturbance*?
2. What language or label is used in the federal definition (IDEA) for children with psychiatric disorders?

3. Why is the study of psychiatric disorders relevant for the SLP?

4. Which of the four categories of psychiatric disturbance occur most frequently among speech-language disordered youngsters?

5. What are some of the speech and language characteristics associated with anxiety disorders?

6. Why might a language assessment be difficult to interpret when a child also has symptoms of psychosis?

7. What is the likelihood of a school-based SLP working with students with emotional and/or behavioral disorders?

8. Name three interventions used with this population. How are they the same or different as working with children with learning disabilities? ADHD?

REFERENCES

Achenbach, T. M., & Edlebrock, C. (1983). *Manual for the Child Behavior Checklist.* Burlington: University of Vermont Press.

American Psychiatric Association. (2000). *Diagnostic and statistical manual of mental disorders* (4th ed.). Washington, DC: American Psychiatric Association.

Aram, D., & Nation, J. (1980). Preschoolers with language disorders and subsequent language and academic difficulties. *Journal of Communication Disorders, 13,* 159–170.

Baker, L., & Cantwell, D. P. (1987). Factors with the development of psychiatric illness in children with early speech/language problems. *Journal of Autism and Developmental Disorders, 17*(4), 499–510.

Baltaxe, C., & Simmons, J. Q. (1988). Communication deficits in preschool children with psychiatric disorders. *Seminars in Speech and Language, 8,* 81–90.

Beery, K. (1989). *Developmental Test of Visual-Motor Integration-3rd Revision* Cleveland: Modern Curriculum Press.

Beitchman, J. H., Wilson, B., Brownlie, E. B., Walters, H., Inglis, A., & Lancee, W. (1996). Long-term consistency in speech/language profiles: II. Behavioral, emotional, and social outcomes. *Journal American Academy of Child and Adolescent Psychiatry* 35(6), 815–970.

Breznitz, Z., and Sherman, T. (1987). Speech pattern of normal discourse of well and depressed mothers and their young children. *Child Development, 58,* 395–400.

Camarata, S. M., Hughes, C. A., & Ruhl, K. L. (1988). Mild/moderate behaviorally disordered students: A population at risk for language disorders. *Language, Speech, and Hearing Services in Schools, 19,* 191–200.

Cantwell, D. P., & Baker, L. (1987). Prevalence and type of psychiatric disorder and developmental disorders in three speech and language groups. *Journal of Communication Disorders, 20,* 151–160.

Cantwell, D. P., & Baker, L. (1987). The prevalence of anxiety in children with communication disorders. *Journal of Anxiety Disorders 1*(3), 239–245.

Caplan, R. (1996). Discourse deficits in childhood schizophrenia. In J. H. Beitchman, N. J. Cohen, M. M. Konstantareas, & R. Tannock (Eds.), *Language, learning, and behavior disorders* (pp. 156–177). New York: Cambridge University Press.

Carson, D. K., Klee, T., Perry, C. K. Muskina, G., & Donaghy, T. (1998). Comparisons of children with delayed and normal language at 24 months of age on measures of behavioral difficulties, social, and cognitive development. *Infant Mental Health Journal, 19*(1), 59–75.

Ciechalski, J. C., & Schmidt, M. W. (1995). The effects of social skills training on students with exceptionalities. *Elementary School Guidance and Counseling, 29*(3), 217–223.

Cohen, N. J., Davine, M., Horodezky, N., Lipsett, L., & Isaacson, L. (1993). Unsuspected language impairment in psychiatrically disturbed children: Prevalence and language and behavioral characteristics. *Journal of American Academy Child Adolescent Psychiatry, 32*(3), 595–603.

Cohen, N. J., Davine, M., & Meloche-Kelly, M. (1989). Prevalence of unsuspected language disorders in a child psychiatric population. *Journal of the American Academy of Child and Adolescent Psychiatry, 28*(1), 107–111.

Cohen, N. J., Lipsett, L., & Dip, C. S. (1991). Recognized and unrecognized language impairment in psychologically disturbed children: Child symptomatology, maternal depression, & family dysfunction. Preliminary report. *Canadian Journal of Behavioral Sciences, 23*, 376–389.

Council for Children with Behavioral Disorders. (1987). Position paper on identification of students with behavioral disorders. Reston, VA: Council for Children with Behavioral Disorders.

Council for Children with Behavioral Disorders. (1989). Best assessment practices for students with behavioral disorders: Accommodation to cultural diversity and individual differences. *Behavioral Disorders, 14*, 263–278.

Council for Exceptional Children. (1991). Report of the CEC advocacy and governmental relations committee regarding the new proposed United States federal definition of serious emotional disturbance, Reston, VA: Council for Exceptional Children.

Davidson, S., & Smith, R. (1990). Traumatic experiences in psychiatric outpatients. *Journal of Traumatic Stress Studies, 3*, 459–475.

Donahue, M. L., Szymanski, C. M., & Flores, C. W. (1999). When "Emily Dickinson" met "Steven Spielberg": Assessing social information processing in literacy contexts. *Language, Speech, and Hearing in Schools, 30*, 274–284.

Dumas, J. E., Bechman, E. A., & Prinz, R. J. (1994). Aggressive children and effective communication. *Aggressive Behavior, 20*(5), 347–358.

Duncan, B. B., Forness, S. R., & Hartsough, C. (1995). Students identified as seriously emotionally disturbed in school-based day treatment: Cognitive, psychiatric, and special education characteristics. *Behavioral Disorders, 20*(4), 238–252.

Fessler, M. A., Rosenberg, M. S., & Rosenberg, L. A. (1991). Concomitant learning disabilities and learning problems among students with behavioral and emotional disorders. *Behavioral Disorders, 16*(2), 97–106.

Folstein, M. E., Folstein, S. E., & McHugh, P. R. (1975). Mini mental state: A practical method for grading the cognitive state of patients of the clinician. *Journal of Psychiatric Research, 12*, 196–197.

Forness, S. R., & Knitzer, J. (1992). A new proposed definition and terminology to replace "serious emotional disturbance" in Individuals with Disabilities Education Act. *School Psychology Review, 21*(1), 12.

France, J. (1992a). Depression. In R. Gravell & J. France (Eds.), *Speech and communication problems in psychiatry* (pp. 156–171). Clifton Park, NY: Delmar Learning.

France, J. (1992b). Psychoses. In R. Gravell & J. France (Eds.), *Speech and communication problems in psychiatry* (pp. 113–155). Clifton Park, NY: Delmar Learning.

Giddan, J. J., Bade, K. M., Rickenberg, D., & Ryley, A. T. (1995). Teaching the language of feelings to students with severe emotional and behavioral handicaps. *Language, Speech, and Hearing in the Schools, 28,* 127–133.

Giddan, J. J., Milling, L., & Campbell, N. B. (1996). Unrecognized language and speech deficits in preadolescent psychiatric inpatients. *American Journal of Orthopsychiatry, 66*(1), 85–92.

Giddan, J. J., & Ross, G. J. (2001). *Childhood communication disorders in mental health settings.* Austin, TX: Pro-Ed.

Giddan, J. J., Trautman, R. C., & Hurst, J. B. (1989). The role of the speech and language clinician on a multidisciplinary team. *Child Psychiatry and Human Development, 19*(3), 180–185.

Gray, C. (1975). Teaching children with autism to "read" social situations. In K. Quill (Ed.), *Teaching children with autism: Strategies to enhance communication and socialization.* Clifton Park, NY: Delmar Learning.

Hallfors, D., Fallon, T., & Watson, K. (1998). An examination of psychotropic drug treatment for children with serious emotional disturbance. *Journal of Emotional and Behavioral Disorders, 6*(1), 56–72.

Halliday, M. A. K., & Hasan, R. (1976). *Cohesion in English.* London, UK: Longman Group.

Hardman, M. L., Drew, C. J., & Egman, M. W. (2002). *Human exceptionality: Society, school and family* (7th ed.). Boston: Allyn & Bacon.

Harvey, P. D. (1983). Speech competence in manic and schizophrenic psychoses: The association between clinically rated thought disorder and cohesion and reference performance. *Journal of Abnormal Psychology, 92*(3), 368–377.

Horner, R. H., Sugai, G., Todd, A. W., & Lewis-Palmer, T. (2000). Elements of behavior support plans: A technical brief. *Exceptionality, 8*(3), 205–215.

Individuals With Disabilities Education Act of 1997, P.L. 105-17, 105th Cong., 1st Sess., H.R.5 (1997).

Janicak, P. G., Davis, J. M., Preskorn, S. H., & Ayd, F. J., Jr. (1997). *Principles and practice of psychopharmacotherapy* (2nd ed.). Philadelphia: Williams & Wilkins.

Kendall, P. C., Flannery-Schroeder, E., Panichelli-Mindel, S. M., Southan-Gerow, M., Henin, A., & Warman, M. (1997). Treatment of anxiety disorders in youths: A second randomized clinical trial. *Journal of Consulting and Clinical Psychology, 65,* 366–380.

Kimura, F., & Nakamura, S. (1985). Locus coeruleus neurons in the neonatal rat: Electrical activity and responses to sensory stimulation. *Developing Brain Research, 23,* 301–305.

Kimura, F., & Nakamura, S. (1987). Post-natal development of δ-adrenlceptor mediated auto inhibition in the locus coeruleus. *Developing Brain Research, 35,* 21–26.

Majcher, D., & Pollack, M. H. (1996). Childhood anxiety disorders. In L. Hechtman (Ed.), *Do they grow out of it? Long-term outcomes of childhood disorders* (pp. 139–169). Washington, DC: American Psychiatric Press.

Mattison, R. E., Cantwell, D. P., & Baker, L. (1982). A practical method for screening psychiatric disorder in children with speech and language disorders. *Journal of Abnormal Child Psychology, 10*(1), 25–32.

Mattison, R. E., Humphrey, F. J., Kales, S. N., Handford, H. A., Finkenbinder, R. L., & Hernit, R. C. (1986). Psychiatric background and diagnoses of children evaluated for special class placement. *Journal of the American Academy of Child Psychiatry, 25*(4), 514–520.

Mattison, R. E., Morales, J., & Bauer, M. A. (1992). Distinguishing characteristics of elementary schoolboys recommended for SED placement. *Behavioral Disorders, 17*(2), 107–114.

McGinnis, E., & Forness, S. (1988). Psychiatric diagnosis: A further test of special education eligibility, hypothesis. *Monographs in Behavioral Disorder, 11*, 3–10.

Newcomer, P. L., & Hammill, D. D. (1997). *Test of Language Development-Primary* (3rd ed.). Austin, TX: Pro Ed.

Pennel., I., & Creed, F. (1987, August). *Depressive illness.* Medicine International.

Prizant, B. M., Audet, L. R., Burke, G. M., Hummel, L. J., Maher, S. R., & Theadore, G. (1990). Communication disorders and emotional/behavioral disorders in children and adolescents. *Journal of Speech and Hearing Disorders, 55*, 179–192.

Richards, T., & Bates, C. (1998). Helping children's post-traumatic stress. *Education Digest, 63*(8), 62–67.

Rochester, S., & Martin, J. R. (1979). *Crazy talk: A study of the discourse of schizophrenic speakers.* New York: Plenum Press.

Rosenblatt, J., Robertson, L., Bates, M., Wood, M., Furlong, M. J., & Sosna, T. (1998). Troubled or troubling? Characteristics of youth referred to a system of care without system-level referral constraints. *Journal of Emotional and Behavioral Disorders 6*(1), 42–54.

Scherer, K. R. (1987). Vocal assessments of affective disorders. In J. D. Maser (Ed.), *Depression and expressive behavior* (pp. 59–82). London, UK: Lawrence Erlbaum Associates.

Schwartz, S. (1982). Is there a schizophrenic language? *Behavioral and Brain Sciences, 5*, 579–626.

Seiler, W. J., & Beall, M. L. (2002). *Communication making connections* (5th ed.). Boston: Allyn & Bacon.

Segrin, C., & Flora, J. (1998). Depression and verbal behavior in conversations with friends and strangers. *Journal of Language and Social Psychology, 17*(4), 492–503.

Stratton, C. W., & Hammond, M. (1997). Treating children with early-onset conduct problems and a comparison of child and parent training interventions. *Journal of Consulting and Clinical Psychology, 65*(1), 93–109.

Sugai, G., Horner, R. H., Dunlap, G., Hieneman, M., Lewis, T. J., Nelson, C. M., Scott, T., Liaupsin, C., Sailor, W., Turnbull, A. P., Turnbull, H. R., III, Wickman, D., Ruef, M., & Wilcox, B. (2000). Applying positive behavioral supports and functional behavioral assessment in schools. *Journal of Positive Behavior Intervention, 2*(3).

Terrasi, S., Sennett, K. H., & Mackin, T. O. (1999). Comparing learning styles for students with conduct and emotional problems. *Psychology in the Schools, 36*(2), 159–166.

Twenge, J. M. (2000). The age of anxiety? Birth cohort change in anxiety and neuroticism. *Journal of Personality and Social Psychology, 79*(6), 1007–1011.

Webber, J., & Scheuermann, B. (1997). A challenging future: Current barriers and recommended action for our field. *Behavioral Disorders, 22*(3), 167–178.

Weschler, D. (1998). *Weschler Intelligence Scale for Children-3rd edition*. San Antonio, TX: The Psychological Corporation.

Wiig, E. H., Wayne, S., & Semel, E. (1992). *Clinical evaluation of language fundamentals—preschool*. San Antonio, TX: Harcourt Brace Jovanovich.

Wilcox, B. L., Turnbull, R., & Turnbull, A.P. (2000). Behavioral issues and IDEA: Positive behavioral interventions and supports and the functional behavioral assessment in the disciplinary context. *Exceptionality, 8*(3), 173–187.

Woodcock, R. W., & Johnson, R. W. (1990). *Woodcock-Johnson Test of Achievement*. Allen, TX: DLM Teaching Resources.

Zachman, L., Jorgenson, C., Huisingh, R., & Barrett, M. (1984). *Test of Problem Solving*. East Moline, IL: Lingui Systems, Inc.

Appendix A

Assessment of Cognitive Communication Skills

Initial Questions

1. What is the real-life experience for which this person is preparing or in which she or he is currently participating?
2. What are the communication demands of this experience or situation?
3. How can I determine the capabilities and needs of this person in this situation?

After answering the first two questions, consider the cognitive-communicative strengths and needs from the following perspective to answer the third question.

Perception

Is there evidence of perceptual problems that will interfere with performance in communication?

If NO, look at other matrix behaviors.

If YES, is formal assessment necessary?

If NO, consider informally:
1. Ability to focus visually or auditorially on pictures, objects, voices.
2. Ability to visually track across a page or among several pictures or objects.
3. Ability to discriminate visually or auditorially among pictures, sounds, objects.

If YES, consider:
1. Medical evaluation to rule out vision or hearing problems.
2. Constructional Praxis Tests, such as Test of Visual Motor Skills (ages 2–13) or TVMS: upper level (ages 12–40) (Psychological and Educational Publications)
3. Central auditory processing battery.

Courtesy of Blosser, J. L., & DePompei, R. (2003). *Pediatric Traumatic Brain Injury 2E*. Clifton Park, NY: Delmar Learning, pp. 120–31.

4. Developmental Test of Visual Motor Integration (Follett Publishing Co.)

Are data sufficient to define strengths, needs, and direct treatment?

If NO, consider

If YES, develop goals and initiate treatment.

Attention

Are there problems with impaired attention skills that will affect performance in communication?

If NO, look at other matrix behaviors.

If YES, is formal assessment necessary?

If NO, consider informally:
1. Level of arousal (to people, time of day, stimulus presented)
2. Vigilance: Can attention to task completion be maintained?
3. Distractibility: Unable to maintain attention to task in noisy, busy environment?
4. Perseveration: Unable to shift from one task to another or one topic to another?

If YES, consider:
1. Attention Deficit Disorders Evaluation Scale (Hawthorne Educational Services)
2. Fisher's Auditory Problems Checklist (Life Products)
3. Wisconsin Card Sorting Test (PAR)

Are data sufficient to define strengths, needs, and direct treatment?

If NO, consider

If YES, develop goals and initiate treatment.

Memory

Is performance indicative of memory problems that will affect performance in communication?

If NO, look at other matrix behaviors.

If YES, is formal assessment necessary?

If NO, consider informally:
1. Short-term memory skills:
   a. Able to follow increasingly complex directions?

If YES, consider:
1. Oral Commands CELF (Psychological Corporation)
2. Oral Commission DTLA-2 (PRO-ED)

b. Able to respond to verbal or written directions one at a time, two at a time, etc.?

2. Working memory
   a. Can direction be held long enough to complete task?
   b. Can piece of information (phone number, page of math assignment) be recalled long enough to complete task?
   c. What is memory span for unrelated words (numbers, random words, visual symbols)?

3. Long-term memory
   a. Episodic:
      (1) Can retell events of the day, week?
      (2) Can recount experiences of interest (outings, parties) from past?
      (3) Can recount experiences from present—new game, classroom activity, work experience?
   b. Semantic:
      (1) What vocabulary is retained in conversation?
      (2) Where are gaps in previously learned information?
      (3) How is previously learned skill (addition, typing) completed now?
      (4) How are rules for games learned preinjury recalled?
      (5) What is present academic achievement level?

4. Retrieval
   a. What is skill in recalling information given or activity performed immediately versus, a half hour later, end of day, next day?
   b. Is ability to retrieve information aided by visual or auditory cueing?
   c. What is recalled best—facts, main idea, little details, episodic events?
   d. Is information retrieved by recognition, free recall, or cueing?
   e. Is recall increased with:

3. Visual Auditory Subtest: Woodcock-Johnson Psychological Test Battery III (DLM Teaching Resources)
4. Token Test for Children (DLM Teaching Resources)
5. Digit span TOLD (PRO-ED)
6. Numbers Reversed subtest: Woodcock-Johnson Psychological Test Battery (DLM Teaching Resources)
7. Denman Neuropsychology Memory Test (Denman, 1984, Charleston, NC)
8. PPVT (R) (American Guidance Service)
9. Language Tests-TOLD (PRO-ED); CELF (The Psychological Corporation)
10. Academic achievement based on curriculum already studied
11. SAT or ACT (compare to previous scores)
12. Group achievement tests (compare to previous scores)
13. Selective Reminding Test: Woodcock-Johnson Psych-Educational Battery III (DLM Teaching Resources)
14. Test of Word Finding (DLM Teaching Resources)
15. Test of Adolescent/Adult Word Finding (DLM Teaching Resources)
16. Test of Word Finding in Discourse (DLM Teaching Resources)

- difference in task (recall as many fruits as you can versus recall the ones that are fruits from the word list presented)?
- giving a reward as incentive to recall?
- giving a memory strategy (chunking, imagery) as help?

f. Does academic pressure, such as answering questions or recitation in class, decrease efficiency of word finding?

g. Does allowing less time to formulate a response decrease efficiency of word recall?

h. Does a stressful social situation with peers, family, or teachers decrease word finding efficiency?

Are data sufficient to define strengths, needs, and direct treatment?

If NO, consider

If YES, develop goals and initiate treatment.

Speed of Information Processing

Is there evidence that slowed processing of information affects performance in communication?

If NO, look at other matrix behaviors

If YES, is formal assessment necessary?

If NO, consider informally:

1. Are responses based on visual input different from auditory?
2. If pauses are inserted when being given information, is response more accurate?
3. If response is not cued or question not repeated, how long does it take for response?
4. Is question forgotten if too much time elapses?
5. Are directions requested for same task frequently?

If YES, consider:

1. Ross Information Processing Test (PRO-ED)
2. Formally time responses while giving information rapidly and with pauses

Are data sufficient to define strengths, needs, and direct treatment?

If NO, consider

If YES, develop goals and initiate treatment.

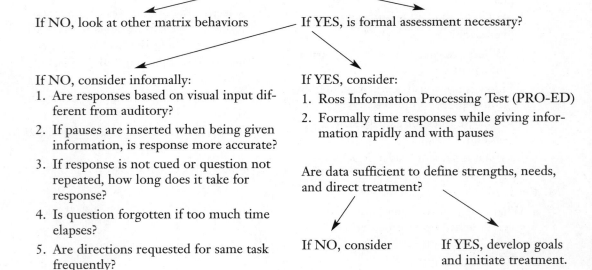

Executive Functioning

Does behavior demonstrate possible problems with executive functioning that may affect performance in communication?

If NO, look at other matrix behaviors.   If YES, is formal assessment necessary?

If NO, consider informally:

1. What is cognitive understanding of personal strengths and needs?
2. Prior to formalized test how does child predict he or she will do?
3. How does child evaluate how he or she performed after subtest or test?
4. Can child set goals to achieve completion of a task (work or play) without external direction?
5. Is plan devices to attempt goals?
6. Is plan self-initiated and appropriate to age?
7. Is problem-solving skill used if a problem with the plan arises?
8. Do inappropriate behaviors interfere with completion of plan and does child try to inhibit these behaviors?
9. Is self-talk employed to monitor behaviors during an activity?
10. Are there demonstrated abilities to evaluate self on completed test or therapy tasks?
11. Organization
    a. Is there ability to describe steps in an activity such as baking a cake?
    b. Is there ability to describe tools needed to complete activity such as mowing the lawn?
    c. Is there ability to sequence steps for activity such as studying for a test?
    d. What ability to categorize (by class, function) is present?
    e. What ability to associate within and across categories is noted?

If YES, consider:

1. Ask for written or verbal analysis of perceived strengths and needs.
2. Concept Formation subtest: Woodcock-Johnson Psycho-educational Test Battery III (DLM Teaching Resources)
3. Likeness/Differences subtest: DTLA-2 (PRO-ED)
4. Associations subtest: Word Test (Lingui-Systems)
5. Functional Assessment of Verbal Reasoning and Executive Strategies (FAVRES) (Clinical Publishing)

Are data sufficient to define strengths, needs, and direct treatment?

If NO, consider

If YES, develop goals and initiate treatment.

Receptive Language

Does understanding verbal or written communications suggest performance in communication may be affected because of receptive language problems?

If NO, look at other matrix behaviors.

If YES, is formal assessment necessary?

If NO, consider informally

1. Is vocabulary at age level?
2. Does vocabulary development keep up after injury?
3. Are there gaps in curriculum-specific vocabulary?
4. Is there a difference in ability to follow written versus verbal directions?
5. Is there a difference in following directions if gestural or tactile information is provided?
6. Does rate, amount, or complexity of information presented verbally or in writing affect receptive abilities?
7. Is there a difference in ability to comprehend based on communication demands of a person or environment?
8. Is comprehension of facts different than comprehension of inferences when presented either verbally or in writing?

If YES, consider:

1. PPVT (American Guidance Service)
2. Woodcock-Johnson Psycho Educational Test Battery III (DLM)
3. Token Test for Children (DLM Teaching Resources)
4. Directions subtests, CELF (The Psychological Corporation)
5. Spelling and vocabulary tests from previous and present grade levels
6. PIAT (American Guidance Service)
7. Test of Auditory Comprehension of Language: TACL-R (DLM Teaching Resources)
8. Refer to reading teacher for testing

Are data sufficient to define strengths, needs, and direct treatment?

If NO, consider

If YES, develop goals and initiate treatment.

Expressive Language

Do verbal or written communications suggest performance in communication may be affected because of expressive language problems?

If NO, look at other matrix behaviors.

If YES, is formal assessment necessary?

If NO, consider informally:

1. Are there oral motor weaknesses (dysarthria, apraxia) noted?
2. Is there a problem swallowing various textured foods?
3. What is ability to use words in naming tasks related to familiar or unfamiliar contexts?

If YES, consider:

1. Comprehensive Apraxia Test (Praxis House Publishers) Dysarthria Test
2. Frenchay Dysarthria Assessment (College-Hill Press)
3. Formal dysphagia assessment

4. Is there a difference in verbal versus written output? (Using a detailed picture, if story is told, then written, what changes in ideas, word choice, details, and grammar occur?)

5. What differences are noted in verbal output when topic of conversation is structured versus unstructured?

6. When asked a question, is response tangential or on-topic?

7. Is confabulation present and can it be redirected?

8. What is amount of verbalization? Is being withdrawn or hyperverbal in a conversation a concern?

9. Can information from several sentences be condensed into main idea (telegram)?

4. Test of Word Finding (DLM Teaching Resources)

5. Word Association: CELF-R (The Psychological Corporation)

6. Rapid Automated Naming Test (Denckla & Rudel, 1974)

7. TOLD (PRO-ED)

8. TOWL (PRO-ED)

9. The Word Test (Lingui-Systems)

10. The Adolescent Word Test (Lingui-Systems)

11. Discourse analyses of varying complexity and length

Are data sufficient to define strengths, needs, and direct treatment?

If NO, consider   If YES, develop goals and initiate treatment.

Pragmatic Language

Do pragmatic language skills indicate potential difficulty in communication?

If NO, look at other matrix behaviors.   If YES, is formal assessment necessary?

If NO, consider informally

1. Is disinhibition observed in conversation?

2. Is there a problem understanding use of social space (proxemics)?

3. Are nonverbals used appropriately?

4. Are nonverbals understood and responded to adequately?

5. In unstructured conversation:
   • what is ability to introduce topic?
   • what is ability to maintain topic?
   • what are turn-taking skills?
   • what are turn-giving skills?
   • what are repair/revision strategies?
   • what are specificity/accuracy skills?

If YES, consider:

1. Pragmatic protocol (Prutting & Kirschner)

2. Ross Test of Higher Cognitive Functions (Academic Therapy Publications)

3. Reviewing expressive segments of language tests

4. The Adolescent Test of Problem Solving (TOPS) (Lingui-System)

5. Complete analysis of language sample

6. Does increased stress in social situations with family and peers (observe in natural settings of different types and circumstances) affect interactions?

Are data sufficient to define strengths, needs, and direct treatment?

If NO, consider

If YES, develop goals and initiate treatment.

Discourse Analysis

Does use of expressive and pragmatic language suggest possible deficits in discourse abilities?

If NO, look at other matrix behaviors.

If YES, is formal assessment necessary?

If NO, consider informally:
1. Does the child talk a lot, but fail to include the most important information?
2. Does the child seem to lose train of thought while talking?
3. When the child gives instructions (e.g., how to play a game) can sequence of steps be followed?
4. Does child have difficulty paraphrasing information from his or her textbook?
5. Is he or she able to sequence ideas to make a coherent response during class discussion?

If YES, consider:
1. Listening Test (Lingui-System)
2. Gray Oral Reading Test (GORT)
3. Test of Problem Solving (TOPS) (Lingui-System)
4. The Strong Narrative Assessment Procedure (SNAP) (Thinking Publications)
5. Guide to Narrative Language Procedures for Assessment (Thinking Publications)
6. Discourse measures:
   • Select important/unimportant details
   • Answer explicit and implicit questions
   • Provide gist interpretations main idea, lesson, proverbs
   • Determine outcomes of functional/social situations
   • Problem-solving tasks
   • Figurative language and multiple meaning tasks

Are data sufficient to define strengths, needs, and direct treatment?

If NO, consider other portions of the matrix.

If YES, develop goals and initiate treatment.

Appendix B
Internet Resources

Chapter 1: Traumatic Brain Injury

Brain Injury: Medical, Legal, and Informational Resource for Traumatic Brain Injury (TBI)
http://www.braininjury.com
National Resource Center for Traumatic Brain Injury
http://www.neuro.pmr.vcu.edu
The Center for Outcome Measurement in Brain Injury
http://www.tbims.org/combi
Traumatic Brain Injury Model Systems: Traumatic Brain Injury National Data Center
http://www.tbindc.org
Traumatic Brian Injury Resource Guide: Centre for Neuro Skills
http://www.neuroskills.com
Traumatic Brain Injury Survival Guide
http://www.tbiguide.com

Chapter 2: Cerebral Palsy

National Institute of Neurological Disorders and Stroke: Keyword Cerebral Palsy
http://www.ninds.nih.gov
The National Information Center for Children and Youth with Disabilities (NICHCY)
http://www.nichcy.org/pubs/factshe/fs2txt.htm
United Cerebral Palsy Association
http://www.ucpa.org

Chapter 3: Attention-Deficit/Hyperactivity Disorder

Attention Deficit Disorder Association
http://www.add.org

Internet Mental Health: keywords Attention Deficit Disorder; Tourette's Disorder
http://www.mentalhealth.com
Internet Resource for Special Children: Keyword Tourette's Syndrome
http://www.irsc.org
Pediatric Neurological Associates: Tics and Tourette's
http://www.pediatricneurology.com/tics.htm
Tourette Syndrome Association, Inc.
http://www.tsa-usa.org
Tourette Syndrome "Plus"
http://www.tourettesyndrome.net
WebMD: keywords ADHD; Tourette Syndrome
http://www.webmd.com

Chapter 4: Language Learning Disabilities

KidSource OnLine: Keyword Language Learning Disorders
http://www.kidsource.com
LDOnline: The Leading Website on Learning Disabilities for Parents, Teachers, and Other
  Professionals
http://www.ldonline.org
Pediatric On Call: Child Health Website for Everyone: Keyword Language Learning Disorders
http://www.pediatriconcall.com
The American Speech and Hearing Association: Professional Site Keyword Language Learning
  Disabilities
http://professional.asha.org

Chapter 5: Autism Spectrum Disorders

Autism/PDD Resources Network
http://www.autism-pdd.net
Autism Society of America
http://www.autism-society.org
Center for the Study of Autism
http://www.autism.org
Cure Autism Now Foundation
http://www.canfoundation.org
Division TEACCH (Treatment and Education of autistic and related Communication handicapped
  Children)
http://www.teacch.com

Families for Early Autism Treatment (FEAT)
http://www.feat.org
Family Village—A Global Community of Disability Related Resources: Keyword Autism
http://www.familyvillage.wisc.edu
Internet Resource for Special Children: Keyword Autism
http://www.irsc.org
National Alliance for Autism Research (NAAR)
http://www.naar.org
OASIS: Online Asperger Syndrome Information and Support
http://www.udel.edu/bkirby/asperger
Office of Special Education and Rehabilitative Services: Keyword Autism
http://www.ed.gov/offices/OSERS
The National Autistic Society: UK
http://www.nas.org.uk

Chapter 6: Mental Retardation

American Association of Mental Retardation
http://aamr.org
President's Committee on Mental Retardation
http://www.acf.dhhs.gov/programs/pcmr
The ARC: The National Association of and for People with Mental Retardation and Related
    Developmental Disabilities and their Families
http://www.thearc.org

Chapter 7: Cleft Lip and Palate

Cleft Palate Foundation
http://www.cleftline.org
Kids Health for Kids
http://www.kidshealth.org (Keywords: cleft lip and palate)
UC Davis Health System Health and Wellness Information: Keyword Cleft Lip and Palate
http://wellness.ucdavis.edu
Wide Smiles: Cleft Lip and Palate Resource
http://www.widesmiles.org

Chapter 8: Substance Abuse

Arium: A Non-profit Organization for the Prevention of Fetal Alcohol Syndrome
http://www.arium.org

National Organization on Fetal Alcohol Syndrome

http://www.nofas.org

The ARC: Keyword Fetal Alcohol Syndrome

http://www.thearc.org

The National Library of Medicine: Keywords Fetal Alcohol Syndrome; Pregnancy and Substance Abuse

http://www.nlm.nih.gov

Chapter 9: Psychiatric Disorders in the Speech-Language Impaired Youngster

American Psychiatric Association

http://www.psych.org

Depression and Related Affective Disorders Association

http://www.drada.org

National Alliance of the Mentally Ill

http://www.nami.org

National Institute of Mental Health

http://www.nimh.nih.gov

National Mental Health Association

http://www.nmha.org

Glossary

Abruptio placenta: separation of the placenta from the uterine wall

Adaptive functioning: skills in real-life situations

ADD: attention deficit disorder without hyperactivity

ADHD. *See* attention deficit/hyperactivity disorder

Adiadochokinesia: the inability to perform rapid, alternating muscle movements

Affect: an expressed emotional response

Akinesia: a dyskinesia that results in a reduction in movement

Alveolar bone grafting: a surgical procedure that grafts bone into the cleft site at the alveolar ridge

Ankle foot orthosis: a brace used to maintain the proper positioning of the ankle and calf

Apraxia: a disorder of sequenced movement of body parts in the absence of muscle weakness or paralysis

Arcuate fasciculus: a long subcortical tract that connects the posterior and anterior speech and language areas in the cerebrum

Articulation therapy: treatment that focuses on speech production, that is, learning to make the sounds of the language

Asperger's syndrome: a neurobiological, developmental disorder that primarily affects social skills, particularly in the areas of social reasoning and social adaptation, but is not associated with any delay or deviance in language acquisition

Asphyxia: lack of oxygen to the brain

Aspiration: the entry of food, liquid, or foreign objects into the airway that can lead to chronic lung damage

Association: a cluster of anomalies often present together but that have not been identified as either a syndrome or a sequence

Ataxia: disturbed balance; general incoordination of motor acts

Attention deficit/hyperactivity disorder: a neurobiological condition characterized by developmentally inappropriate level of attention, concentration, activity, distractibility, and impulsivity

Auditory processing disorder: one or more of the central auditory processes responsible for generating the auditory evoked potentials and the behaviors of sound localization and lateralization, auditory discrimination, auditory pattern recognition, temporal processing, auditory performance with competing acoustic signals, and auditory performance with degraded acoustic signals

Augmentative and alternative communication: communication methods that supplement or substitute for natural speech

Autism (autistic disorder): a complex developmental disorder that appears in the first 3

years of life (though it may be diagnosed much later) which affects the brain's normal development of social and communication skills. Autism is considered the "prototype" of the PDD disorder and most clearly defines the core impairments of social interactions, impaired verbal and nonverbal communication, and restricted and repetitive patterns of behavior

Autosomal dominant: traits that are manifest when the trait is present in either copy of a gene

Axon: a projection that conducts a nerve impulse away from the neuron and synapses to another neuron, gland, or muscle

Basal ganglia: a group of subcortical nuclei that influence the initiation and maintenance of movement

Bipolar disorder: a DSM-IV-TR category classified under Mood Disorders. This disorder is characterized by one or more manic or hypomanic episodes. These episodes can occur once or they may reoccur following a depressive episode

Bifid uvula: a cleft in the uvula; frequently associated with a submucous cleft palate

Bolus: a chewed piece of food ready to be swallowed

Bradycardia: slow heart rate

Broca's area: a speech and language center in the brain that is important for the expression of language

Cerebellar system: a system that works in conjunction with the pyramidal and extrapyramidal systems to provide coordination for motor speech

Cerebral palsy: a nonprogressive motor disorder caused by damage to the motor systems of the brain

Cheiloplasty: cleft lip repair

Childhood disintegrative disorder: regressive developmental disorder marked by a pro-

longed period of normal development; age of onset and pattern of development are the critical factors differentiating CDD from autism

Chronic obstructive pulmonary disease: an irreversible lung disorder

Cleft lip: a congenital malformation involving incomplete closure of the upper lip

Cleft palate: a congenital malformation involving incomplete closure of the soft and/or hard palate

Closed head injury: an injury where there is no penetration or opening from the outside through the dura mater

Cognitive-behavioral modification: general category of intervention techniques that attempt to modify behavior by altering the thought patterns of individuals

Coma: a period of unresponsiveness or unconsciousness resulting from injury to the brain stem

Communication and Symbolic Behavior Scale (CSBS): behavior scale developed by Wetherby and Prizant in 1993 that is used to assess the communicative, symbolic, and social-affective abilities of "developmentally young" children

Compensatory articulation: atypical articulation as a response to structural or functional inadequacies, often of the velopharyngeal mechanism

Conduct disorder: a DSM-IV-TR category, whereby an individual demonstrates repetitive and persistent patterns of behavior, where basic rights of others or major societal norms or rules are violated

Conductive hearing loss: a hearing loss caused by a problem in the outer or middle ear that prohibits the conduction of sound into the inner ear or auditory nerve

Congenital: occurring before birth

Congenital malformations: defects seen in the physical development of the fetus

Concussion: a mild head injury, which may or may not include a brief loss of consciousness, and may be followed by a short period of change in mental status without any focal neurological signs

Content enhancement strategies: the use of semantic information and discussion for organizing information in class

Conversational discourse: an interaction between two individuals in which speaker/listener roles and topics change frequently

Coprolalia: speaking of obscenities

Cortical blindness: a disorder caused by damage to the brain that prohibits the conversion of visual stimuli into a visual image

Cranial nerves: nerves that originate in the brainstem and provide sensory and motor information to the oral, pharyngeal, and laryngeal musculature

Cricopharyngeal sphincter: the opening at the top of the esophagus

Cul-de-sac resonance: abnormal resonance caused by acoustic energy being trapped in a pouch with an entrance but no outlet; cul-de-sac resonance may occur when sound entering the nasal cavity is trapped due to an anterior nasal blockage; speech generally sounds "muffled"

Delusion: a false belief based on misinterpreting reality of varying intensity, and seen in schizophrenia, the manic stage of bipolar disorder, and substance abuse

Dendrites: projections from the neurons that receive neural stimuli

Developmental apraxia of speech: a motor speech disorder characterized by atypical sounds, voicing, and repetition errors that can result in delayed development of speech and language and developmental milestones of language

Developmental apraxia of speech: difficulty in voluntarilty programming, combining, organizing, and sequencing movements necessary for speech production

Developmental pediatrician: a doctor who works with children with developmental disabilities

Differential diagnosis: systematic comparison of symptoms to distinguish between diagnoses

Diffuse axonal injury: injury that occurs diffusely throughout the brain rather than in one localized area

Diplegia: paralysis affecting the same limbs on both sides of the body

Diplopia: double vision

Discrete-trial teaching: traditional method of language instruction incorporating drills, often with large numbers of trials until a child reaches a high level of performance

Down syndrome: a genetically based syndrome involving the 21st chromosome that affects an individual's overall development, as well as speech and language development and function

DSM-IV-TR: *Diagnostic and Statistical Manual,* fourth edition, text revision—a text published by the American Psychiatric Association providing descriptions of diagnostic categories used by clinicians and investigators to classify, diagnose, and treat individuals with various mental disorders

Dysarthria: a group of motor disorders characterized by disturbed muscle control resulting from damage to the central or peripheral nervous systems or to the speech musculature

Dysgraphia: a disorder characterized by severely impaired writing skills

Dyskinesias: involuntary movement disorders

Dyslexia: a disorder characterized by severely impaired reading skills

Dysthymic disorder: a DSM-IV-TR category classified under Mood Disorders. This disorder is characterized by a feeling of pervasive sadness following low-level distress, irritability, or low self-esteem for longer than a year

Echolalia: parrot-like repetition of what is heard; often a characteristic of autism

Ecological communication model: language intervention model that applies to families in naturalistic settings; focuses on the child and parent during play and addresses activity level, joint focus of attention, balance of turns, imitation, initiated communication, and topic selections

Edema: swelling of the brain due to fluid leakage

Emotional and behavioral disorder. *See* emotional disturbance.

Emotional disturbance: an emotional disorder that affects an individual's ability to learn; characterized by inappropriate behaviors or feelings under normal circumstances

Executive function: a cluster of cognitive processes necessary for organized, goal-directed behavior

Expressive language therapy: treatment that focuses on language formulation and production, that is, language output

Externalizing behaviors: a set of behaviors displayed by outward expressions including impulsive, aggressive, and fleeting attention

Extrapyramidal system: a part of the nervous system that is responsible for regulating extraneous movements, including posture and facial expressions

Fetal alcohol effect: a diagnosis given when not all, but some of the deficits of fetal alcohol syndrome are present

Fetal alcohol syndrome: a profound birth defect with specific patterns of disability manifested in physical growth and development secondary to maternal use of alcohol during pregnancy

Fistula: an abnormal hole or passage between two cavities

Fragile X syndrome: genetic condition characterized by mental retardation, which is caused by changes in the long arm of the X chromosomes

Functional behavioral assessment: a technique that analyzes the situations that come before and after a behavior with the goal of assessing the fucntion that the behaviors are serving for the child

Gastrostomy tube: a feeding tube placed directly into the stomach

Generalized anxiety disorder: a DSM-IV-TR category classified under Anxiety Disorders whereby an individual experiences anxiety and worry often accompanied by restlessness, fatigue, irritability, muscle tension, and difficulty concentrating

Glottal stop: a compensatory articulation produced by a forceful release of air trapped beneath the vocal folds

Hallucination: a false sensory perception characterized by a distortion of real stimuli. Can include hearing voices or sounds not present (auditory hallucinations) or seeing people or objects (visual hallucinations); occurs in schizophrenia and the manic phase of bipolar disorder

Head injury: traumatic damage to the head that may fracture the bones of the skull or face, and may or may not include injury to the brain

Hemiplegia: paralysis of one side of the body

Herniation syndrome: syndrome that occurs if a localized mass or area of swelling pushes on and deforms the shape of the brain

Hyperkinesia: a dyskinesia that results in decreased movement

Hypernasality: excessive nasal resonance during speech caused by sound entering the nasal cavity inappropriately; the perception of hypernasality is most obvious during vowel production

Hypertelorism: excessive distance between the eyes

Hypertension: high blood pressure

Hypertonia: increased muscle tone

Hypokinesia: a dyskinesia that results in decreased movement

Hypomanic: a persistently elevated, or an irritable mood for a continuous period of at least four days

Hyponasality: reduction in nasal resonance due to blockage or occlusion in the nasopharynx or nasal cavity; the perception of hyponasality is most obvious during nasal consonant production

Hypopharynx: the portion of the throat below the base of the tongue

Hypospadias: malpositioning in the opening of the urethra of the penis

Hypotonia: decreased muscle tone

Hypoventilation: inadequate ventilation

Hypoxic-ischemic encephalopathy: a brain dysfunction from insufficient oxygen and blood flow during the birth process

IDEA: Individuals with Disabilities Act of Public Law 101-46; the new name for Public Law 94-142 (the Education for All Handicapped Children Act) as per the 1990 amendments to the Education of the Handicapped Act; IDEA also added two new categories of disability—autism and brain injury

Impaired abstraction: an inability to generalize thinking to other situations

Incidental teaching: intervention technique incorporating naturally occurring interactions designed to facilitate language use; different than discrete-trial teaching because it allows the child to initiate the interaction and choose the location and content of the teaching

Inclusion: placement of children with disabilities in general education classrooms

Internalizing behaviors: a set of behaviors displayed by inward expressions including withdrawn, anxious, and sad

Intrauterine growth retardation: a condition that occurs when the fetus is deprived of oxygen and other nutrients resulting in low fetal weight and decreased size

Intraventricular hemorrhage: a bleeding into ventricles within the brain that occurs when blood vessels in the brain burst

Joint attention: communicative skill that occurs before development of speech and allows a child to share objects and events with another person

Language learning disability: a disorder characterized by delayed phonological acquisition, difficulty with perception and production of complex phonemic configurations, and difficulty in phonological awareness

Learning disability: a disorder characterized by normal cognitive functioning with isolated deficits in learning

Low birth weight: a baby who weighs less than 2500 grams (approximately 5 pounds, 5 ounces) at birth. Low birth weight can result from prematurity (and may be average for the baby's gestational age) or from intrauterine growth retardation (and be small for gestational age)

Lower motor neurons: neurons that send motor axons to the peripheral nerves

Maxillary advancement: a surgical procedure that advances the midface area to establish an appropriate upper jaw and lower jaw relationship

Mechanical ventilation: the process by which negative or positive pressure is provided to assist or substitute for the inspiratory muscle function needed for breathing

Mental retardation: below average intellectual functioning that includes adaptive limitations

Metathesis: transposition of phonemes in words

Microcephaly: an abnormally small head size, resulting in poor brain growth. Microcephaly is nearly always due to a small brain size associated with prenatal factors such as intrauterine infection, PKU, FAS, chromosomal abnormalities, brain injury, or disease

Middorsum palatal stop: an abnormal articulation produced by a forceful release of air trapped behind a closure formed with the back of the tongue up against the middle of the hard palate; often a compensatory articulation for anterior oral crowding

Mixed hearing loss: a hearing loss that occurs when a person with a sensorineural hearing loss develops a conductive hearing loss

Morphology: the study of word structures

Morphosyntax: the structure of a language including word roots, prefixes, suffixes, word order, and sentence composition

Narrative discourse: orderly, continuous account of an event or series of events

Nasal emission: the inappropriate escape of air into the nasal cavity during attempted production of high-pressure consonants

Nasogastric tube: a feeding tube placed through the nose

Neologisms: the creation of words that are meaningless to the listener

Neurons: the basic nerve cells of the nervous system that are responsible for all neural behaviors, including speech, language, and hearing

Nonverbal communication: behaviors, attributes, or objects (except words) that communicate messages that have social meaning

Nurse: a medical professional who cares for and treats injured and ill individuals

Nystagmus: an eye disorder that causes jerking movements of the eye in either a vertical or a horizontal direction

Occupational therapist: a therapist who provides assessment and intervention for fine motor impairments

Open head injury: an injury where the skull is penetrated and the damage is localized to the site of penetration

Oppositional defiant disorder: a DSM-IV-TR category, whereby an individual demonstrates a continuing pattern of negativistic, defiant, and hostile behavior directed toward authority figures

Optic atrophy: damage to the optic nerve that prohibits the brain from receiving visual stimuli and transferring it into a visual image

Oral motor: involving the normal and abnormal patterns of the lips, tongue, jaw, and cheeks for eating, drinking, facial expression, and speech

Orthognatic surgery: surgery involving the bone structures of the upper and lower jaws

Orthopod: a doctor who specializes in medical and surgical treatment of the bones, joints, and ligaments

Otitis media: a bacterial infection and inflammation of the middle ear; otitis media with effusion also involves a buildup of fluid in the middle ear

Palatal lift: a prosthetic appliance used to raise the velum; used when the velum is structurally, though not functionally, adequate to achieve velopharyngeal closure

Palatal obturator: a prosthetic appliance used to cover a palatal cleft or palatal fistula

Palatoplasty: surgical repair of the palate

Palilalia: repetition of one's last word or phrase

Pervasive developmental disorder not otherwise specified: a pervasive developmental disorder that extends from the prototype of autism, with a decrease in both the severity and number of specific domains affected (which includes deficits in social reciprocity, communication, and repetitive behaviors or interests)

Pervasive developmental disorders: general group of disorders characterized by severe impairment in reciprocal social interaction and communication, with the possible presence of stereotyped behavior, interest, and activities

Pharyngeal affricates: a compensatory articulation produced by forcing air through a narrow opening created between the base of the tongue and the back pharyngeal wall

Pharyngeal flap: a surgical procedure performed to aid the individual in achieving velopharyngeal closure; a flap of tissue is excised from the back pharyngeal wall and joined with the velum to close some of the velopharyngeal space

Pharyngeal fricative: a compensatory articulation produced by forcing air through a narrow opening created between the base of the tongue and the back pharyngeal wall

Pharyngeal stop: a compensatory articulation produced by a forceful release of air trapped beneath a closure with the base of the tongue against the back pharyngeal wall

Pharyngeal wall augmentation: a surgical procedure involving an implant or injection in the velopharyngeal area to aid in velopharyngeal closure

Phonological processes: the simplification rules that children use as they learn speech sounds, such as leaving out final sounds in words

Phonology: the study of speech sounds, sound patterns, and rules used to create words with those sounds

Physical therapist: a therapist who provides assessment and intervention for gross motor impairments

Platoplasty: palate repair

Postconcussion syndrome: short period of changed mental status without any focal neurological signs

Post-traumatic amnesia: a period of memory disturbance occurring after trauma

Post-traumatic stress disorder: a DSM-IV-TR category classified under Anxiety Disorder whereby an individual develops extreme fear, helplessness, and horror in response to a traumatic event

Pragmatics: the study of the rules that govern the use of language in social situations

Prenatal drug exposure: maternal use of legal or illegal drugs during pregnancy without the consent of a physician

Primary injury: injury that occurs at the time of trauma due to the direct movement of the brain inside the skull

Proprioception: awareness of the position of the body in space

Prosody: variations in rate, pitch, loudness, stress, intonation, and rhythm of continuous speech

Prosthodontist: a professional who develops appliances to replace or improve oral and facial structure or function

Protodeclarative function: utilization of gaze and/or gesture to obtain an object or event; typically the only type of gaze/gesture used by children with autism

Psychologist: a person who provides counseling and makes recommendations for issues relating to behavior

Psychosis: a symptom associated with a number of psychiatric disorders characterized by the inability to perceive reality accurately

Psychotropic: affecting a person's psychic function, behavior, or experience

Psychiatrist: a physician who specializes in psychiatry

Pyramidal system: a part of the nervous system that is responsible for voluntary movement of the speech muscles

Quadriplegia: paralysis affecting all four limbs of the body

Receptive language therapy: treatment that focuses on language comprehension and understanding, that is, language input

Reciprocal gaze: looking at communication partner when speaking and listening; must be present to discern a conversational partner's facial expressions

Resonance: voice quality resulting from vibration of sound in the pharyngeal, oral, and sometimes nasal cavities during speech

Retinopathy of prematurity: a condition that commonly occurs in children born prematurely and results from oxygen-related damage to the blood vessels of the retina caused by oxygen administration

Rett's syndrome: an inherited disorder affecting only females; characterized by initial normal development followed by deceleration of head growth, loss of previously acquired hand skills, loss of social engagement, and severely impaired expressive and receptive language development

Schizophrenia: a group of psychotic disorders characterized by disturbances in thought, perception, affect, behavior, and communication lasting longer than 6 months

Seizure: an episode of disorganized activity in the brain that results in abnormal involuntary movements

Self-injurious behaviors: chronic and repetitious behaviors that a person self-inflicts to cause physical harm

Semantics: the study of meaning in language

Sensorineural hearing loss: a hearing loss that occurs when the inner ear or auditory nerve is damaged

Sequence: a series or pattern of secondary anomalies that result from one initial anomaly or mechanical factor

Simonart's band: a bridge of soft tissue extending across an otherwise open cleft; due to partial, incomplete fusion of the upper lip

Sleep apnea: intermittent interruptions of breathing during sleep

Social maladjustment: term used to describe the problem behaviors of individuals, particularly youth, who have difficulty with the law; juvenile delinquency is an associated term

Social worker: a person who assists families in coping with social, emotional, physical, or financial needs

Soft signs: health information, especially related to neurological conditions, that is mainly subjective

Special educator: a person who provides specialized education services for people with emotional, physical, or social disabilities

Speech bulb obturator: a prosthetic appliance consisting of a retainer portion and an attached acrylic bulb that fills a large portion of the velopharyngeal space

Speech intelligibility: whether or to what extent a person's speech is comprehensible to a listener

Speech-language pathologist: a therapist who provides assessment and intervention for speech, language, oral motor, and communication skills

Sphincter pharyngoplasty: a surgical procedure that creates a sphincter in the center of the velopharyngeal area

Stoma: a hole

Strabismus: an eye muscle imbalance resulting in inward or outward turning of one eye

Stuttering/dysfluency: communication disorder in which the smooth flow of speech is interrupted by blocks, repetitions, or prolongations

Submucous cleft palate: a defect in the underlying structures of the secondary palate (bone and muscles) with the oral surface structures still intact

Substance abuse: a consistent abusive pattern of drug use

Substance dependence: the continued use of drugs and/or alcohol even when significant problems related to the abuse are evident

Syndrome: a pattern of anomalies or malformations that generally occur together and have a common known or suspected cause

Syntax: the arrangement of words to form meaningful sentences

Tachycardia: a condition in which the heart rate is excessively rapid (though the rhythm of the heart's contractions is normal). For an infant, tachycardia is a heart rate over 180 to 200 beats per minute. It occurs when infants are upset or excited, but can also be an indication of infection, heart disease, or breathing problems. An increased heart rate may also be a side effect of certain drugs or fever

TEACCH (Treatment and Education of Autistic and Communication Handicapped Children): a North Carolina state program of services for autistic people that is dedicated to improving communication skills and autonomy to the maximum of the child's potential, and using education as the primary means to achieve the goal

Teratogen: an external substance or factor that may interfere with embryological development, resulting in a congenital malformation

Teacher: a professional who is trained in educating individuals

Tics: involuntary, rapid, and repetitive movements that occur slowly and irregularly

Tracheotomy: surgical placement of a plastic or metal tube through the outer surface of the neck and into the trachea to create an airway

Traumatic brain injury: an acquired brain injury caused by an external force, resulting in total or partial functional disability, or psychosocial impairment, or both, that adversely affects a child's educational performance

Triplegia: paralysis affecting three limbs of the body

Unconventional verbal behaviors (UVBs): behaviors frequently manifested by children with autism; may include echolalia, perseverative speech, and language with private meaning

Upper motor neurons: neurons that send axons from the cerebral cortex to the nuclei

Variable expression: variability in the presentation of individuals with a specific genetic disorder; different structures and functions may be affected, and to varying degrees

Vasoconstriction: constricted blood vessels

Velopharyngeal dysfunction: inability to achieve velopharyngeal closure, regardless of cause

Velopharyngeal insufficiency: inability to achieve velopharyngeal closure due to a short velum relative to the posterior pharyngeal wall

Veloplasty: palate repair

Ventricles: inner fluid spaces of the brain

Videofluoroscopy: a videotaped X-ray procedure used to examine deep structures of the body during movement

Wernicke's area: a speech and language center in the temporal lobe responsible for comprehension

Whole language: treatment approach in which reading, understanding, writing, and expressive language are taught as a whole, often using experiential activities and children's literature to help teach language concepts

X-linked recessive disorder: an X-linked disorder inherited from genes located on the X chromosome; an X linked recessive disorder results when the defective gene has no normal counterpart gene present; such disorders generally only affect males since males have only one X chromosome and females have two X chromosomes (with one generally possessing a nonaffected gene)

Index